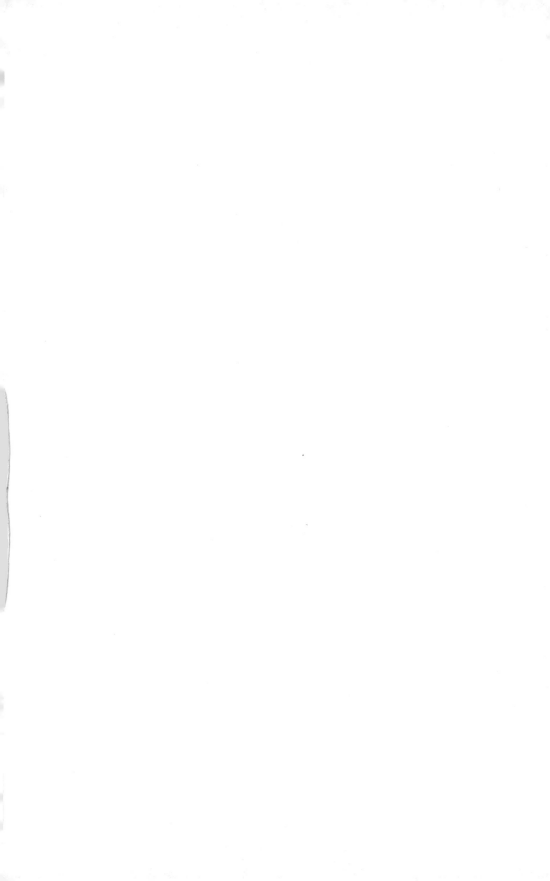

Cultivating Mindfulness to Raise Children Who Thrive

Cultivating Mindfulness to Raise Children Who Thrive introduces an expanded view of human development and health, which begins before conception and moves through pregnancy, early childhood and adulthood.

This book is a call for all prenatal and perinatal professionals and policy makers to appreciate indigenous ways of knowing, being and doing and integrate them with scientific evidence in the care of expectant parents and their babies. It explains how this could also tackle pressing social issues facing the modern world and favour social innovations through a revaluation of preconception, pregnancy, birth and childcare practices. Sansone presents the reader with scientific discoveries of epigenetics, interpersonal neuroscience, quantum physics, attachment, anthropology, prenatal and perinatal psychology and mindfulness, which interestingly resonate with the intuitions of primal wisdom.

The book will be of interest to clinicians, policy makers, researchers, parents and those interested in the prenatal and perinatal roots of human development and well-being.

Antonella Sansone is a mother, clinical psychologist, researcher, mindfulness teacher/facilitator and author. Her work with expectant and new parents and infants in the UK and Italy, empirical studies of African indigenous cultures and inspiring motherhood have led to the writing of this book and the design of a PhD drawing on it. She has been granted the *International Excellence Award* from Central Queensland University in Australia.

Cultivating Mindfulness to Raise Children Who Thrive

Why Human Connection from Before Birth Matters

Antonella Sansone

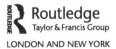
Routledge
Taylor & Francis Group

LONDON AND NEW YORK

First published 2021
by Routledge
2 Park Square, Milton Park, Abingdon, Oxon OX14 4RN

and by Routledge
52 Vanderbilt Avenue, New York, NY 10017

Routledge is an imprint of the Taylor & Francis Group, an informa business

British Library Cataloguing-in-Publication Data
A catalogue record for this book is available from the British Library

Library of Congress Cataloging-in-Publication Data
A catalog record for this book has been requested

ISBN: 978-1-138-59823-2 (hbk)
ISBN: 978-1-138-59827-0 (pbk)
ISBN: 978-0-429-48646-3 (ebk)

Typeset in Baskerville
by Apex CoVantage, LLC

To the mothers, fathers and children of the world, and those who walk with them in their sacred journey through pregnancy, birth and beyond.

—

Contents

x *Contents*

Foreword

As a practising obstetrician for over three decades, I have often observed how and why experiences and mental health of women during pregnancy and in the postnatal period are of utmost importance for the well-being of both the mother and her child. Depression, stress or anxiety in pregnancy have been associated with an increase in obstetric complications, such as stillbirth, preterm delivery, low birth weight and admission to special care baby units, besides susceptibility to more adverse neurodevelopmental outcomes, including behavioural, emotional and cognitive problems: well into adulthood.

Sansone's excellent book, through its 11 engrossing chapters, takes the reader through a wonderful journey of mindfulness, by caring about the mother's mind, emotions and mental health. The book also shows how paying attention to these attributes in a non-judgemental way reduces tension and fear by promoting emotional positivity and stability.

While a systematic review and meta-analysis of 14 articles on the subject in 2017 demonstrated improved foeto-maternal outcomes with the application of mindfulness, Sansone's careful analysis found that by incorporating traditional birthing wisdom across cultures, and in neuronal chemistry of attachment and pregnancy neuro-psychology, mindfulness-based interventions reduce ruminative thinking and trait anxiety, as well as increase empathy and self-compassion.

Her personal narratives of interactions with indigenous cultures, of weaving music into child-rearing and of her immersive experience with Nature and everything natural lets her admirably walk the tightrope between soul and science. Her writings reflect the emotional connectivity that finds its intelligence in deep-rooted cultural traditions, and how these influences work on the foetal brain as it develops in its neural chemistry and complexity, absorbing innate maternal connectedness and bonding. Sansone's approach and analysis is therefore quite detailed, well-researched and an exemplary piece of work.

Her stellar book reinforces what has been known across continents and cultures for centuries: that relaxation, breathing and self-hypnosis are intelligent choices of coping with pain during labor and birth.

What Sansone adds in her piece of latest work is that maternal psychoneu-roimmunology not only reinforces consciousness control of the immune system function, but also that "embracing the present" allows the mother to concentrate on herself. This enables her to be more receptive to the outer and inner sensations of the instant, thereby strengthening the relationship between her and her baby. The enhanced perception during mindfulness allows her to have total attention and presence during childbirth and feed-ing, creating a secure link of trust with her baby.

The concept of sustained protection, a trustworthy ally, is a recurrent message in the chapters of the book. The author reiterates how mindful-ness is an inner force, which can be reactivated on demand: a shelter that increases psychological flexibility, which is a fundamental aspect of health. Psychological flexibility is adaptable to a variety of situational needs, which by promoting consistent behaviours like awareness and openness, sig-nificantly benefits psychological health during pregnancy and postnatal periods.

Should caregivers in maternal and child health worldwide be made famil-iar with and trained in Sansone's mindfulness approaches as outlined in her sterling book, pregnant women, their partners and their infants would experience important, multiple and sustained benefits, including improved psychological well-being and economic solvency for generations.

At a time of increasing strife among nations beset by the behemoth of an all-consuming pandemic, it is more important than ever for communi-ties, governments and healthcare systems to heed to the lucid messages of maternal consciousness, acceptance and compassion so adroitly articulated by Sansone in her book.

A book that should be on the shelves of any individual concerned with the future of a tumultuous world, and who wishes to leave it a better place than they found it.

Mr Dib Datta MD FRCOG
Consultant Obstetrician and Gynaecologist
Past Member, Board of Trustees and College Council,
Royal College of Obstetricians and Gynaecologists, London

Foreword

You have a precious book in your hands. It is one of the very few works in which parenting and perinatal are addressed with an anthropological perspective, integrating attachment theory, infant research and neuroscience and finally taking into account the function not only of the mother, but also that of the father in child development and well-being.

Antonella Sansone is a pioneer who, as a true researcher, has been able to use her own personal and family experiences (born in Italy, subsequently lived in the UK, Africa and Australia) to outline a complex transcultural, biopsychosocial and systemic vision of parenting, integrating primal wisdom with the modern scientific Western Worldview.

In a period in which the COVID-19 pandemic changed the way of life around the world and put the Western way of life (influenced by economic and commercial factors) in serious crisis, Sansone referred to the enhancement of past experiences and to the wisdom that can be found in ancient habits and cultures, but still present in many populations of Africa and Asia.

The author also highlights sociological and philosophical problems and promotes a vision of parenting which, by integrating different cultures, leads to changing our Western stereotypes. In particular, the early (also prenatal) relationship between mother and baby is influenced, enhanced not only by the mental health of the mother, but also of the father, the healthcare practitioners and the entire community. In fact, research has shown that the relationship between parents, especially in romantic love, tends to be configured as an attachment relationship in which, during the perinatal period, both protect the partner and their mental states influence each other. Mothers' and their infants' well-being have also been supported since pregnancy and beforehand by the entire village for millennia.

Pregnancy and the perinatal period can be times of joy and anticipation but also of challenge and stress for the mother, father, infant and family. A pregnant mother's own unresolved childhood trauma and birth trauma can pose a risk to her life cycle and that of the child, having lasting and serious consequences. In these moments of personal and relational danger, when maternal affective disorders are frequent, the function of the father as an attachment figure is fundamental. This is particularly true in

Western culture where the extended family (grandparents, uncles, cousins) has been gradually replaced by the nuclear family and both parents work. In other parts of the world, particularly in Africa and Asia, the situation is very different and ancient patterns of offspring care are more common. The same fathers, however, can frequently manifest perinatal affective disorders, even if in different ways from maternal ones. In these cases, the father may not be able to play his protective role towards the mother and even interfere with the development of the newborn and the mother-child relationship.

In this perspective, Sansone proposes an innovative mindfulness relationship-based model rooted in the most ancient practice, enhancing mother-foetus communication and connection to support parental mental health and the mother-father-baby triad relationship in pregnancy and beyond birth.

This book is invaluable reading not only for psychologists and health professionals (gynaecologists, paediatricians, obstetricians, midwives, neonatologists, nurses) who deal with perinatal, but also for new parents who want to grow their babies healthy and safe and thus contribute to a healthier society.

Prof Franco Baldoni, MD, PhD
Head of the Attachment Assessment Lab,
Department of Psychology, University of Bologna, Italy

Preface and acknowledgement

This is not the book I planned to write. My original manuscript was a memoir of my first pregnancy and relationship with my unborn baby with some links to scientific evidence. The expansion of my embodied knowledge acquired through motherhood; my experience with the Himba, an African indigenous culture; the mindfulness retreats; mindfulness teaching training and practice; and the inspiration of many scholars' work have given the original manuscript a very long gestation.

Meanwhile I was invited with other professionals in the field to attend at the House of Commons "The 1001 Critical Days – from Conception to Year Two – a Cross-Party Manifesto" and its All Party Parliamentary Group both founded by Member of Parliament Andrea Leadsom. This manifesto highlights the importance of the period from conception to age two in shaping brain development and health and supporting this period to enhance the outcomes for children and next generations and prevent many societal and economic problems. I highly acknowledge Andrea Leadsom's inspiring work condensed in her quote, "The early years, ensuring good support for every pregnancy and every baby, is something I am passionate about. Experiences in the period from conception to the age of two will have a profound impact on the lifelong emotional wellbeing of each of us. I do encourage you and congratulate you on the work you are doing".

Parallel to these political experiences, I had the unique privilege to share the life of the Himba of Northern Namibia – a lightning revelation consolidating my knowing that mothering among indigenous cultures supported by the entire community produced much healthier human souls than mothering practices in the modern West. Like any creative endeavour, a new manuscript had a mind of its own and listened to the call: sensitising all those who play a significant role in parental and infant health and well-being – not just the parents themselves, but the prenatal and perinatal healthcare professionals, the policy makers and every member of the community so that every prospective and new parent and every child are welcomed and embraced by the village. It was a new call for our community to support and nurture the mother-foetus relationship and maternal and paternal mental state.

Science confirms what indigenous people worldwide have known for millennia: the deep realm of consciousness and mindfulness practices before conception, during life in the womb, birth and beyond play a critical role in human development and health and well-being outcomes. Our sense of self, trust in the world, our ability to be mindful, kind and compassionate towards others, the way our immune systems respond to pathogens, including stress, and our spiritual development, are all rooted in that critical time, though neuroplasticity makes us open to change at any age through repeated experience.

How can we all contribute to nurture mindful awareness and heal ruptures caused by traumas during these sensitive periods of human development? First of all, we need healthcare practitioners and science, the entire world, to acknowledge the unborn baby as a sentient being and the mother-baby relationship prior to birth, and adopt a trauma-informed compassionate care approach towards mothers, fathers and their babies in the womb. The best outcomes are when knowledge becomes coherently embodied in our *Being*.

This book is intended to provide an exploration of many disciplines and the connections among them and attempts to weave them with my own ideas. It invites the reader to develop an in-depth interdisciplinary integrative mindset which overcomes the reductionism of a hyper-specialistic perspective, integrates science with primal wisdom and lets wisdom be the leader. I hope this book will offer answers to many challenges – political, economic, environmental, mental health – which humans face today. It addresses questions about human development, human basic needs and wisdom virtues and ultimately, human nature. Only reflection upon the human condition and self-development can lead to societal, environmental and political changes. Exploring answers through insights from different disciplines and perspectives has been a very challenging work, a work that, weaving with mothering, the experience with indigenous cultures and mindfulness practice, has created a preventive model and programme for expectant parents that can be tested but also leaves space to commonsense knowing. This wisdom way of knowing that has guided humans for millennia cannot and does not need experimentation.

Many people have contributed to the making of this book, some perhaps without knowing it. I am deeply grateful to my daughters Gisele and Sahara, who have been my *Muses* in the writing of this book and any other writings. Without them I wouldn't have experienced the depth, beauties, and art of motherhood with all its challenges. My gratitude goes to my husband David Southwood, who was born and grew up in the wilderness of Africa and let me access the cradle of primal wisdom and mothering through the most remote indigenous areas. His contagious knowledge and passion for African culture, safari and conservation, and his photographic talent allowed me altogether to learn the marvels and wisdom of this ancient continent through his artwork. But most importantly, I thank him for having shared with me the creation of our daughters.

I thank my parents Raffaele and Rosa, whose internal presence, nurture and Italian traditional family values have been transmitted to my mothering, thus exerting an epigenetic influence on my daughters. I value the influence of my older brothers in enriching my childhood.

I would particularly like to thank all the expectant and new parents and babies at the birth unit of St John and St Elizabeth Hospital in London and all those over the years who have taught me so much. That experience would have not been possible without consultant obstetrician Yehudi Gordon's interest in the psychological aspects of obstetrics and invitation to undertake my project at his birth unit. There are many thanks to be given to the Himba women and children, who offered me and my family insights into our essence and a transformational experience. As I ventured with my husband and our young girls in their lands, capturing timeless images, I realised we were entering a world where the essence of Africa – the essence of being human – was still intact.

I thank many scholars and thinkers, artists and mindfulness teachers whose work I benefitted from. Many are not mentioned in the text yet have been my guidance. I would like to thank Dr Allan Schore for having recognised the need for this book and encouraged me to submit it to Routledge. I acknowledge Prof Franco Baldoni's important work on paternal mental health and its influence on maternal mental health and child development. I was inspired by his conference presentations and his studies he generously shared with me. I appreciate the inspiring work of Professor of Psychology Darcia Narvaez, which highly values indigenous wisdom and its integration with modern culture as the route to restoring humanity's well-being. I was honoured to meet eminent neuroscientist Jaak Panksepp, a most passionate advocate for an affect-centered view of brain development. He made a valuable contribution to our understanding of how much we share with animal emotional feelings, how this acknowledgement helps us understand human emotions and the physiology of love, separation and grief. After an interesting conversation about my new book, Panksepp showed his delight in writing a foreword. Sadly, he died a few months later leaving a heavy grief in the hearts of those who met him and in the scientific world.

I also owe so much to my regular yoga and mindfulness practice and the teachings of Eastern approaches in the therapeutic and healing relationship between therapist and client. They have provided me with insights about how to creatively integrate them into Western theories and approaches in my work with expectant and new parents and infants. I would have never understood the essence of mindfulness without the intense practice on the retreats at Sharpham House in Devon, England, during the Youth Mindfulness one-year Teaching Course.

I am deeply appreciative of Prof Susan Kinnear, dean of Research of Central Queensland University in Australia for having offered me an

International Excellence Award, which encouraged me to undertake a PhD. This PhD aims to put some headways made in this book into a rigorous study, in particular to investigate associations between maternal mindfulness, mental health, and mother-foetus/infant relationship, and between these and interoception and adult attachment style, in support of the pilot Pre- and Perinatal Mindfulness Relationship-Based (PMRB) programme I developed. Research is focused on creating an impact on individuals, communities and healthcare services across the world by providing solutions to meet complex social, economic and environmental challenges and identifying new opportunities for advancement. But research has to be led by wisdom and heart qualities in order to have the highest impact. Clinical practice teaches us that it is the life force which drives us human beings to create a meaningful life and healthy communities, regardless of the challenges we encounter. I hope that both the emotional connectivity seeking its wisdom in deep-rooted cultural traditions of this book and my PhD will inform future preventive creative strategies to support maternal well-being, a healthier society, our very home Earth, economy, and a sustainable life.

In my professional work, I would also like to thank Dr Vivien Sabel, psychotherapist, author and creator of the Blossom Method, for her steady presence, support and encouragement, and all my colleagues at the Association of Prenatal and Perinatal Psychology and Health (APPPAH), International Society of Prenatal and Perinatal Psychology and Medicine (ISPPM), in particular MD and psychotherapist Ludwig Janus, for his valuable contribution to Prenatal Psychology, the Mother and Child Foundation, in particular Prof Michael Crawford and Simon House, for their essential work on the importance of preconception nutrition and emotional well-being, and Olga Gouni, founder of the College of Prenatal Sciences, for her devoted work in the prenatal field. They all have helped me sustain a commitment to this book through their continued dialogue on social media, conferences and meetings. I especially thank consultant obstetrician Dr Dib Datta, for having understood the importance of this work, his continued inspiration, invaluable warm support and encouragement and his receptiveness to maternal and infant mental health.

I would like to thank Dr Rosina McAlpine for generously supplying important feedback on my original broad manuscript, which helped me reorganise the scope and specific contents and narrow the focus, leading to a new book. I thank my editor Sophie Leighton for her understanding and patient waiting for my delayed work due to my move to Australia and commitment to my PhD. Many thanks to Routledge editor Joanne Forshaw who has believed in this cutting-edge project in perinatal care, understood its challenges and those of moving to Australia with my family and undertaking a PhD. I also appreciate the work of Routledge editorial assistant Daradi Patar in preparing the book for production, project manager Aruna Rajendran, and proof-reader Cynthia Harasty. The book cover picture wouldn't sum up the pre-birth mindful mother-child bond in the lap of Nature so beautifully without the much-appreciated collaboration of pregnant Karly Pfeffer.

Behind the scenes, I would like to thank all my friends on social media and in real life for their encouragement, mentors and companions who brought me where I am today.

I am deeply grateful to Mother Nature and the opportunity I have been offered to see and sense its glamorous beauty in all its essence in Australia, home to the Aboriginals, some of the greatest holders of primal wisdom and humanity heritage. Here Nature has offered me material on which to base observations and reflections and has taken care of me in challenging times.

Towards a new paradigm of human development and health

This book introduces an expanded integrative view of human development and health, which begins before conception and moves through pregnancy, early childhood and adulthood with an unbroken continuum in care. It is this continuum, as traditional wisdom as well as modern science have begun to show, that contributes to a healthy pregnancy, birth and healthy life for the child, mother and society. This view embraces wisdom and mindfulness practice, attachment theory and interpersonal neuroscience. The practice of mindfulness is the most ancient among all cultures, in which physical, mental, emotional, spiritual, social and natural environmental elements form one whole – a respected continuum of life and interconnected experience. I explain in this book how maternal mental health issues, birth and developmental trauma, a product of our modern society and obstetric practices, can alter this continuum and have an impact on parents' wholeness and consequently on their relationship with the baby prior to birth and on his or her development, and I suggest some methods of prevention and healing.

The reader is offered an opportunity to understand prenatal life and birth as an embodied narrative between mother and baby and to explore the prenatal roots of human connection through an unprecedented journey into the lives of our indigenous cousins. I consider ways in which we can learn from traditional practices to develop attunement, empathy and compassion, as the foundations of a secure attachment, and fundamental for parents, children and communities to thrive, and to integrate them with modern Western advances. I present the reader with scientific discoveries in epigenetics, interpersonal neuroscience, attachment, anthropology and mindfulness, resonating with the intuitions of primal wisdom. Interestingly, by learning about the existing research in the growing field of mindfulness-based clinical and non-clinical intervention, we discover that it overlaps with research in attachment, as both secure attachment and mindful-awareness practice promote well-being, attunement, empathy and resilience (Siegel, 2007), and both are spontaneously fostered in indigenous cultures.

We shall look at parenting and child health in the context of our lives and society. I explore primal wisdom as the best available window into the social lives of our ancestors, sustaining uncomplicated birth, motherhood and secure attachment, and I use it as a model of sustainability that is much needed in our modern society. We learn how society and community, its rituals and beliefs, influence the experience of pregnancy, birth and human development. We can be inspired by the sociocultural lives of our ancestors and cousins in societies with small bands of hunter-gatherers, or the pastoralist tribe I visited – the norm for 99 per cent of human history – and the way they value and organise child-rearing. Although universal until about 10,000 years ago, such societies have continued to coexist to the present day (Fry, 2014). They allow us to see how the human nervous system functions in a relatively stress-free environment, at least free of the kind of stresses our society imposes, and where human resources lead to great resilience.

Indigenous societies also offer a baseline model to see the epigenetic effects of early caregiving, responsive parenting and childcare practices, as well as how knowledge is transmitted through generations and real human interactions, becoming genetically inherited, unlike our culture, where information is passed on virtually through social media and books. Today we know that early caregiving has long-term epigenetic and developmental effects, some of which emerge only later, as in adolescence, as late-forming psychopathologies (Schore, 2003a).

This book challenges our understanding of prenatal and perinatal processes through cross-cultural comparisons and as something necessary to implement in care providers' as well as parents' practice and to integrate with modern science. It presents us with inspiring stories of motherhood and communal childcare among the Himba of Northern Namibia, with whom I spent some time with my husband and young daughters. Stories of integrated and shared motherhood and childcare offer insights into the quest of how connected in our society we are to motherhood. Do young girls in our society have an opportunity to practise childcare and nurture maternal mental representations? How does this have an impact on women's perception of themselves as mothers and on bonding with their babies?

At a time in history when rates of perinatal mental illness and infant developmental problems are soaring, this book illuminates what pregnancy, birth and parenting experiences can be like, when provided with a mindful facilitating environment, a source of fulfilment and well-being, which significantly affects the welfare of our society. It explains why we must all work together, with synergic compassion and empathy, to ensure that every parent gets appropriate and timely care to optimise their health and competence and prevent the adverse effects of postnatal psychological distress. Why? Because the importance of maternal mental health before and at conception, during pregnancy and in the perinatal period for the well-being of individuals and societies has been recognised in the literature (Mental Health Taskforce (MHTF), 2016; Bauer et al., 2014). Poor maternal mental health during pregnancy, in particular depression, anxiety and stress, is associated with poor foetal and infantile neurodevelopmental outcomes (Glover et al., 2010; Stein et al., 2014).

Parents' trauma experienced long before conception can be transmitted through subsequent generations (Yehuda et al., 2016). The lifelong consequences of adverse developmental outcomes have a huge impact on society and economy. Perinatal and mental health problems, such as depression, anxiety and psychosis, carry a total cost to society of about £8.1 billion for each one-year cohort of births in the UK (MHTF, 2016). Therefore, supporting maternal and paternal mental health to foster optimal child development since long before birth by identifying effective preventive strategies should be a research, social and economic priority.

My intention in writing this book is to provide practitioners, parents-to-be and everyone else with a deep understanding of the importance of the earliest period of human development: from conception through the early postnatal period. I take the reader through a detailed journey, linking current research from diverse disciplines with the experiences of mother and baby from conception through the postpartum period, including references to personal experience and the follow-up of my child. Prenatal and perinatal psychology, the study of the origins of human development, is presented within the context of our lives and society and the full breadth of its interdisciplinary nature. I invite the reader to look at the prenatal period, birth, parenting and mother-infant mental health within a multilayered context. My experience with Caucasian and indigenous African mothers and my own pregnancy and motherhood give further credence to the theory that the mother-baby relationship is interwoven along a continuum that begins before conception and that examining one aspect exclusively misses its complexity. Our exploration of the earliest period of human development must be guided by our awareness that the mother and the developing foetus form a dynamic system, open to the environmental influences – physical, emotional, social and cultural. These connections have profound implications for a systemic paradigm shift in the way our society and policy makers invest in this crucial period of human development. I am calling for a mindfulness relationship-based, body-centred approach and compassionate care for mothers and babies during the conception, prenatal and perinatal period that are also informed by an understanding of trauma. Such resonating compassionate care should involve all layers of the community and be the common ground for all healthcare providers.

One of the primary goals in writing this book is to present to the reader the findings of modern science that reaffirm the intuitions of age-old wisdom so as to implement them into actual practice to help mothers, families and our humanity. Knowledge is still very fragmented and hyper-specialised, creating huge gaps in social services and maternity care often unable to meet basic human needs such as compassion, empathy, listening and connection. These capacities are usually never emphasised, taught or even mentioned during healthcare professional trainings. Yet, love, compassion, kindness and cooperation have been represented in our collective social consciousness for most of the history of humanity. Awareness has to shift towards a new collective intelligence inspired by age-old wisdom and human essential ingredients of sustainability. I suggest that a revolutionary change can occur by revising the way we think about and experience pregnancy, birth, parenting and child development, based on the components and insights offered by wisdom traditions, mindfulness, prenatal and perinatal sciences, interpersonal neuroscience, epigenetics and attachment theory. As Albert Einstein pointed out, "The mindset that causes the problem cannot cure it".

Since the middle of the twentieth century, a number of phenomena have been converging to suggest that something is going wrong. Humans are not who they used to be. Childhood experiences do not always support evolved basic needs, causing developmental trauma and creating species-atypical outcomes (Narvaez, 2014). So do prenatal experiences. Literature on maternal mental health and child behaviour indicates that both antenatal and postnatal psychological distress and consequent poor mental health have significant consequences on maternal well-being, mother-foetus relationship (Alhusen, 2008), bonding formation (Ammaniti & Gallese, 2014), parent sensitivity and responsiveness (Zeanah & Zeanah, 2009), mother-infant emotional availability (Barfoot et al., 2017) and child development (Glover et al., 2010). In addition, maternal chronic stress, including antenatal depression, is likely to be a predictor of postpartum depression, postpartum increases in couple conflicts and the quality of mother-infant attachment (Austin et al., 2005, 2007). Antenatal psychological distress is known to affect obstetric/neonatal outcomes, which often have significant consequences on perinatal bonding, attachment and child development (Dayan et al., 2006).

Links between maternal poor nutrition before and during pregnancy, in particular deficiency of omega-3, and foetal and child brain development and behavioural problems, and perinatal mental health have been found (Crawford & Sinclair, 1971; Hibbeln et al., 2007). However, the effects of nutrition on early brain development and mental health have received very little attention and thus many health practitioners as well as parents-to-be are not aware of its importance. Even modern processed food and eating habits have distanced us from the mindful eating as nature intended, revealing a broken relationship between humankind and Mother Earth. An eco-mindful approach to parenting embraces reconciliation with the caregiving quality of Mother Nature.

The overall goal of this book is to suggest ways to shift ourselves towards greater embodied presence, relational attunement, communal imagination and ecological cooperation. These human qualities have characterised our indigenous cousins for 99 per cent of their existence and still do today. Our materialistic stress-driven and soul-sucking culture separates the mind from the body, the individual from the community and natural environment, and hinders collective imagination. We are at a turning point where human beings are yearning for a shift towards an empathic and cooperative prenatal and perinatal care system that can meet human needs.

My several years of research and observational study of the "dance of attunement" between mother/father and their infant, years before my visit to the Himba, had led me to astounding insights into non-verbal mother-infant communication. My subsequent experience of pregnancy and motherhood gave me a vivid sense of the link between life-enhancing maternal emotions and the reflective function (e.g. fostered by the practice of mindfulness, yoga, connection with nature, favourite music listening, healthy nutrition), and child well-being. All these nurturing experiences consolidated my discovery that attuned bonding can be nurtured during pregnancy and prepare for the postnatal mother-baby relationship, thus preventing both maternal and infant mental health issues. Therefore, it is essential that prospective parents and the whole community become aware of the preborn baby as a conscious sentient being who needs emotional care as much as he does healthy nutrients. He is sensitive and responsive to maternal emotions, thoughts, consciousness, stress, nutrition and the physical and social environment.

This book calls for all prenatal and perinatal healthcare providers' commitment to support this early relationship long before birth because it is a concern to all of us, and for its impact on the well-being of our society and Earth. It is aimed at aiding professionals as well as parents to understand more in relation to implicit non-verbal communication (mindful movements, posture, gesture, facial expression, voice inflection and the sequence, rhythm and pitch of the spoken words), implicit processes – what is behind the word – and the value of connecting and communicating with babies. These communication cues are still highly valued and utilised by indigenous people, while our stress-driven society has distracted us from relying on this implicit (non-verbal) communication system. This communication is supported by a parent-infant-centred approach to care based on wisdom abilities such as compassion, empathy and listening. The empathic, participatory and resonating relationship is necessary to understand the other's experience and is established by non-verbal language (Stern, 2005a). The focus of most healthcare training courses is on technique, but it should be on relationship. The non-verbal channel of communication – not rational thinking and verbal communication – is much more important in human affairs than most people like to think (Buchanan, 2009). It is incredibly naïve to take conscious verbal communications as the primary way that people respond to each other.

I recognise the value of preverbal body responsiveness and attunement as paramount to the well-being of infants, but also to parents' mental health. It is rooted in early life and also becomes a cultural feature, as I learnt from my experience with the Himba and traditional cultures.

What is ground-breaking in this approach is that a mother's feeling of being "seen", "felt" and "valued" through an empathic relationship influences her capacity to connect with and value her baby's needs and experience. This occurs spontaneously among indigenous communities, who still live as human beings have done for most of our existence. Simple human things, like a care provider asking a mother-to-be or new mother how she feels, can make a huge difference to her perception of the birth and baby experience, thus her well-being. I recall a first-time mother whom I used to visit during my research work at the birth unit saying that my visits, listening to her birth story with interest and valuing it, made her appreciate her baby and motherhood. This feeling of "being valued" is crucial in the bonding process (Sansone, 2018a).

Therefore, care providers need to be sensitively attuned to receive prospective and new parents' communications. Their right brain, involved in primary-process communication (intuitions, images and emotions), should be receptive to the music behind the words. In a world that is becoming increasingly multicultural and inhabited by pregnant refugees and parents struggling with linguistic barriers and isolation, practitioners' non-verbal interpersonal skills are vital. These high-quality exchanges require mindful awareness training. *Mindful presence* is a relational stance that is fundamental to evoking an experience and neurophysiological sense of *safety* in the client, which affects pregnancy, birth and parenting. Dr Porges reminds us that feeling safe is an instinctive sense communicated not in words but through facial expression, tone of voice, gesture and gaze (2011). How can parents feel safe in the relationship with their baby and value their parenting experience if health practitioners do not empathically value it in first instance? Or, if a mother is birthing in an environment she perceives as threatening?

Babies have an innate capacity and need for connecting and communicating with their caregivers (Trevarthen, 2009). Although we have evolved to be capable of intersubjective engagement from birth, striking evidence from my experience with the Himba and Caucasian mothers, and from my own motherhood, indicates that the roots of this capacity may be passed down through generations and be set out during *in utero* experiences. Motivated for social interactions, infants are born with capacities to communicate feeling and intention. When parents are receptive, thus in a mindful state, these capacities develop quickly through intersubjective reciprocal proto-communications. These parents tune into the infant's emotions through voice, touch and movement (Stern, 1985), which are the baby's communicative cues.

The attuned interactions channel and enhance physical and visceral energy (Trevarthen & Delafield-Butt, 2013), and thus have a neurophysiological effect and impact on infant well-being. Early experience sets up the growing brain for the capacities (or inabilities) for both self-regulation and social attunement, thus for empathy (Siegel, 2004). Early on, babies' capacity to communicate, connect and show compassion and love form neural pathways that support the development of positive relationships throughout life. This explains the welcoming and friendly attitude of the Himba children, even towards us as strangers, which is very different from that of children growing up in urban technological societies. A core message of this book is that this process of social "connectedness" begins in the womb, through a myriad of physiological cues exchanged between a mother and her preborn, including maternal hormones and nutrients, mediated by her culture and social support.

Our future capacity to tune into relationships, for empathy and compassion, is sown in early life experiences. Therefore, it is extremely important that the whole community, including healthcare providers, mindfully support couple and parent-infant relationships since pregnancy, just as indigenous and traditional communities have done for millennia and still do by default. For the mother, the caregiving behavioural system can be influenced by what happens during pregnancy and birth (Trevarthen, 2001).

While parents and babies have evolved together to "communicate" with each other since time began, under the demands of our fast-paced technological society, parents tend to lose their ability to be present (through their body and senses), thus to "tune into" their baby's cues, needs and feelings. They may be losing their capacity to tune into their own human resources and wisdom. Excessive stress, reflected in jerky gestures and movements and muscular tension, affects the way of holding babies, as well as the tone, rhythm and speed of talking to them, hindering parents' attention, presence and capacity to connect (Sansone, 2018a). If parents can tune into the bodily cues and energy of their preborn and newborn babies and follow their communicative lead, I believe we are offering them the best start in life and reducing the potential for mental illness.

Prenatal and perinatal attunement, understanding and connection are the foundations on which a profound lifelong bond between parents and children can be established, as well as the foundations for social, emotional and moral well-being. Therefore, we need to protect this bonding by enhancing the maternal (and paternal) mental state and well-being through community support fostered by wisdom and mindfulness practices, including the promotion of prenatal and perinatal nurturing practices, just as happens in traditional communities. We cannot promote maternal mental health without focusing on the human foundations we have evolved for millennia and providing an environment for them to flourish.

Most of the unhappy stories I have heard from mums-to-be and new mums reflect failure of compassion on the part of medical and other healthcare personnel. The changing culture of medicine is becoming increasingly responsive to the imperative of business and technology, and less sensitive to the subjective reality of mother and baby. Lack of compassion may have medical consequences on pregnancy and birth outcome, simply because mothers evolved to receive empathic support (Hrdy, 2011). Receiving caring empathic interactions directly affects individual psychobiology and predisposes us to be empathic to ourselves (Adler, 2002). This occurs by conveying emotional-physiological experiences to each other.

The practice of mindful awareness promotes compassionate goals and non-judgemental non-defensive behaviour. This is because the sense of embodied presence and focus on "this" situation allows for an understanding of the "process", in this case prenatal and perinatal, and connection with the state of mind. The practice of wisdom can teach us to open our heart and change the dispositional mindsets established in our life course. By taking up purposeful self-authorship and learning self-calming techniques, we can change our brains, reframe our behavioural patterns, expand our social selves and foster moral behaviour. An important message of this book is that by promoting common-self mindfulness, we promote attuned relationships and secure attachments, thus moral capacities, health and well-being.

Darcia Narvaez (2014) argues that human imagination has significantly to do with the culture human beings create and how children are raised. The practice of mindfulness offers a way to restore human virtues to their full potential. It opens the way to eco-mindfulness, which views human beings as essential part of a cooperative, not competitive, natural world. A sustainable life implies the flourishing of all natural entities, including our *mammalian nature*, sustaining natural birth, breastfeeding and affectionate physical contact – which largely governs the mother-baby relationship. When healthcare practitioners have trained in mindfulness, they become able to bypass intellectualism or verbal barriers by tuning in at the bodily level, which is more expressive and truthful than verbal language.

Deep "listening", curiosity about another human being, is vital as it encourages self-confidence and emotional resonance in the parents, facilitating parents' synchronic responsiveness with their baby, appreciation and enjoyment of the whole experience. The feeling of being valued, rather than judged, corresponds to a physiological condition that may trigger healing. The lack of understanding, especially around birth trauma, of premature babies and baby loss, and its impact on mental health is striking, adding to the major human loss a parent can experience. Raising awareness for all healthcare practitioners of the importance of how these human qualities affect perinatal mental health and bonding/attachment is crucial.

Our modern lifestyle and the influx of electronic devices are making millennial parents miss out on parenting traditional practices such as singing *lullabies* to their children, which have been so important in co-regulating mother and baby psychophysiological systems and mental states and soothing both for millions of years (Persico, 2002). Parents are so overstimulated by media that may have no creative resources left for the baby at the end of a busy day. Lullabies emphasise the importance of sound modulation used by all animals to calm and reassure their young. We need to understand our traditional pregnancy and childcare practices better to enhance mother-child bonds. Our indigenous cousins used to sing a song (and still do) to their "mentally and spiritually conceived" children from before conception, throughout pregnancy and beyond to create a familiar element of continuity to which the child can attach.

A primary focus of all "others" relevant to mothers should be to provide a stress-free environment allowing these resonating activities to unfold naturally. By mirroring and validating the child, the parent helps him become more aware of his own needs and validate himself. But parents also need to be validated in this process. Connection is lost when the child's needs and feelings are rejected and thus invalidated. When given time, mirroring activities during parent-baby attuned interactions can bring about a deep and fascinating state of being. I offer a lyrical narrative of my experience of pregnancy and motherhood. I ponder that while verbal language has given human beings a huge advantage in the battle with their predators and competitors and helped in mastering their environment, it may have suppressed or weakened deeper implicit processes, like those of the communication sensory system, fundamental to understanding the baby's cues. This may have affected a child's emotional, social and moral development. Understanding a baby's preverbal language, through our traditional wisdom and its mindfulness-based practices, offers every mother and father new means of enriching their relationship with their child and gives the child lifelong benefits.

Drawing on contemporary science, observations of other cultures and reflections on my pregnancy and developing baby, this book urges us to understand human beings, in particular mother/father and baby, as dynamic open systems susceptible to environmental influences. Intersubjectivity, reciprocity and love co-regulate all our physiological and psychological systems, having an impact on our physical, mental or social health and well-being. Responsive parenting practices, favoured by a mindfully aware state, optimise neurophysiological systems, including emotions and self-regulation systems (Siegel, 2007). This regulation of our own basic neurophysiological state promotes not only good health, but behaviours such as sociality and empathy, as it allows us to connect with others (Porges, 2011). Joyful encounters (e.g. with healthcare professionals) foster physiological systems underlying positive emotions and self-transcendence. This allows for community bonding and what Narvaez calls a "moral mood", both of which facilitate prosocial behaviour and empathic communal mood (2014). These community bonding and mood promote nurturing practices and self-other development.

I highlight in this book that the way forward is through the conscious development of qualities born of abilities associated with the "heart", such as care and compassion, and replacing judgemental reactivity or fear with loving-kindness. Research has greatly expanded people's understanding of the heart beyond its function as an organ that pumps our blood to include its ability to send important information throughout the body and have a profound influence on our brain. Heart rhythms reflect emotional states and implicit processes and offer a unique window into the communication between the heart, the brain and emotions (McCraty et al., 2009). Positive feelings of love, care, appreciation and other uplifting emotional qualities long associated with the "heart" and wisdom have been found to induce a highly beneficial physical and emotional state called physiological coherence or "heart coherence" (McCraty et al., 1995). This is extremely relevant to physiological co-regulation of emotion between mother and baby, attuned interactions and well-being.

While sharing the life of the Himba, I could witness the links between communal resonance, the capacity to connect with us despite the linguistic and cultural differences and the physical, emotional and relational attunement that indigenous babies develop by default. I found out that the Himba, like all indigenous people, use group rituals, dances and songs, for example to prepare for conception and welcome the baby, as tools to regulate and maintain social ties. Trauma specialist van der Kolk uses dancing and singing within an integrative programme to help traumatised people connect with their bodily sensations and to self-regulate (2014). I use them in my programme to help mothers, and not just those who have mental difficulties, connect with their unborn babies and infants.

When basic human needs are met throughout early life and adulthood, individuals and community develop the resources to thrive. This seems to be the case in hunter-gatherer communities and the pastoralist Himba I visited, where under normal circumstances human needs are met as a matter of routine, especially the needs of infants and young children (Konner, 2005). When care needs are met, the evolved plasticity leads to species-typical outcomes. When these needs are not met, species-atypical outcomes are more likely (Narvaez, 2014). We receive from our ancestors myriad inheritances. Human development comprises a complex set of legacies that interact with maturational timing and with sensitive periods. Recent findings in cell biology, neuroscience and epigenetics suggest that we are influenced by our ancestors' experiences, our mother's experience when we were in the womb, her nutrition and our birth, bonding and attachment with our caregivers. These early and ancestral experiences can influence our genetic code and create implicit memories that, in turn, influence our perceptions, experiences, our capacity to connect and our present-day choices.

Our indigenous cousins intuitively know that they can influence the conceptional and uterine environment with their consciousness of the child. I describe rituals they practise to connect with the soul of the child and boost fertility. I present evidence showing how both the mother and the unborn baby respond to stress and how the baby's development prepares for the environment in which he expects to live outside the womb. I quote research suggesting that this may happen even if excessive maternal stress occurs in the six months prior to conception (Khashan et al., 2009). Furthermore, I present research finding that, "When the predictive adaptive response occurs during prenatal development but does not match the postnatal environment, disease states may occur over the course of the life of the offspring" (Sandman et al., 2012, p. 13). I discuss the development of the prenate's sensorimotor systems and autonomic nervous system, describing my baby's responses to music and to my emotional responses to music, and her developing sense of rhythm as her movements became more fluent with the regular exposure to music in the advanced gestational stage. I describe how the baby's gene expression may be altered by the preconceptional and prenatal/perinatal environment, and how the mind may be embodied from early embryonic stages.

Epigenetics, research on developmental plasticity and indigenous cultures provide increasing awareness of how adult choices and practices influence the well-being of subsequent generations. What a person becomes is the result not only of genes, which play an important but small role, but of how genes are expressed under cultural and environmental influences during sensitive periods. Although much of who a person becomes is malleable, early life establishes many baselines for the life ahead. This is why prenatal and postnatal support (e.g. needed nutrients, hormones, wisdom/mindfulness practices, emotional and social support) can lead to a body and brain that function more optimally, and to a sustainable way of being and way of life.

I take the reader into maternal and preborn/infant experience, not only to enhance awareness of the baby as a sentient being, but also to give a sense of the richness of this experience. The personal narrative, combined with scientific studies, provides a new perspective to look at maternal emotions, consciousness and creativity, and their physiological influences on the unborn baby's development. It also reveals the human story of pregnancy, birth and mothering. The personal and the scientific do intertwine, underlining the fact that science, especially of human development, is a human pursuit and cannot be truly appreciated if it appears as a cold and emotionless abstraction. An important message of this book is that scientific research in prenatal and perinatal development as well as maternal care needs to acknowledge maternal emotions, thoughts, beliefs, age-old intuitive wisdom, expectations and consciousness and their impact on child development.

The topic of *subjectivity* is one that modern neuroscience has avoided. It is generally agreed that there are no direct objective ways to measure the subjectivity of other human beings. Only their words, body language and actions give us clues about their inner experiences. Neuroscientist Jaak Panksepp (1998) suggests that the very nature of the human mind cannot be understood until neuroscience acknowledges the potential contribution of internal representations, some of which are affectively experienced states.

This is a new kind of book that blends expertise with narrated personal experience, bringing the objective of scientific studies into dialogue with the "I" – maternal emotions, soul, compassion and wisdom. It is about bringing a soul into abstract research. In a new trend, scientists are acknowledging the limits of science and the valuable contribution of personal experience in their books. This book reflects an increasing awareness of the necessity for science to embrace subjective experience and intersubjective engagement as the essence of human development and the study of it. The lyrical tone provides a sense of the depth of the unborn baby's life as well as the maternal pregnancy experience.

The scientific data on prenatal development, which has unlocked many secrets of the unborn baby's life, is modest compared to the complexity and wonder of a modern mother-baby relationship. Certain aspects of maternal emotions and their impact on prenatal experiences and child well-being are simply not amenable to scientific investigation. A mother's subjective experience can tell us more than a piece of research, and therefore it deserves to be heard. Intersubjectivity, or the sharing of another's experience, has been a topic of great interest and activity, particularly in its value for development and clinical practice. Only recently has there been a scientific and academic interest in intersubjectivity before birth (Ammaniti & Gallese, 2014). This is another reason making this book timely and necessary.

Today neuroscience is focusing on the fundamental role played by emotion, relationship and experience in child's brain development. Loving, consistent, positive relationships help build healthy brains and protect a baby's brain from the negative effects of stress and trauma (Fleming et al., 1999; Schore, 2001a). Thanks to the brain's neuroplasticity, this process begins during pregnancy, and the seeds can be sown before conception, through the parents' ways of being, and it continues through childhood to early adulthood. The more we understand prenatal and perinatal processes, the more we understand ourselves and our relationships with each other, and the stronger our empathic and compassionate responses will become. The entire culture will also benefit from that knowledge.

Recent technological innovations have allowed scientists to examine the biochemical basis of emotions. Recent neuroscience provides an understanding of how inextricably united the *body and mind* are and the role played by the emotions in health and disease. It is what the Eastern meditators and Buddhism have been teaching for 3,000 years, and now it has become the object of scientific studies. There is increasing evidence that a pregnant woman's placenta can absorb more than just nutrients and oxygen. If the stress hormone cortisol is transmitted to the placenta, altering brain development (Van den Bergh et al., 2005), positive life-enhancing emotions and communications, flooded with feel-good hormones such as endorphins and oxytocin, may foster optimal development. My own subjective account of emotions, mental states and the baby's engagement is free of the limitations of science, though science may provide material for reflection. The narration of my perceptions, projections and consciousness, and my baby's responses – our rich intimate dialogue – cannot be replaced by science but can inspire science.

Recent scientific discoveries have suggested that changes in gene activity can be induced by environmental factors such as the mother's mental states, emotions and their cellular substrate (Lipton, 2015). In his book *The Biology of Belief*, cell biologist Bruce Lipton discusses how a pregnant mother's nurturing thoughts and emotions allow preborn babies to optimise their genetic and physiological development. These findings contradict the common belief that people's genetic make-up is fixed and revolutionises the centuries-old nature-nurture debate consequent to the Cartesian mind-body split. An important message of this book is that parental imagination and consciousness, even around the time of conception, can unlock their creative potential and contribute to create a "*field state*" that may influence their developing baby's genetic predispositions (Emerson, 1996; Lake, 1979; Laing, 1976; Meaney, 2010). Gene activity is designed to be regulated by signals from their immediate environment, some of which, in turn, are profoundly influenced by our social interactions, according to Daniel Goleman (1995) in *Social Intelligence*.

It is interesting that aboriginal and tribal cultures have been aware of the influence of the conceptional environment for millennia. I offer interesting insights from my study of the Himba mothers and children of Northern Namibia and other studies on hunter-gatherers, which also offer a baseline model of secure attachment.

This book explores another uncharted area. Today we still know more about the consequences of toxic substances, physical and psychological impacts than we do about non-harmful or positive influences, for example healthy nutrition, maternal positive emotions such as joy, elation and anticipation, music or maternal singing, or mindfulness. And we still know more about foetal behavioural responses to stress or harmful substances as observed by 4D real-time ultrasound scan. By the sixth month, the preborn can hear and move in rhythm to his mother's voice (DeCasper et al., 1994). Imagine what a difference it makes whether the mother is happily singing or yelling in anger. It is no surprise that sonograms taken while parents yell at each other show the baby's entire body flinching in agitation. Imagine the damage caused by months of feeding this negative energy to a foetus. Likewise, maternal singing of lullabies has been found to have positive effects on the foetus and infant (Persico et al., 2017). Infants who had been exposed to maternal singing during pregnancy showed significantly greater postnatal bonding three months after birth and lower incidence of crying and colic episodes in the first month. Perceived maternal stress was also significantly lower. At the same time, a reduction was observed in the neonatal nightly awakening. In conclusion, mothers singing lullabies during pregnancy could improve maternal-infant bonding and have a soothing effect, thus positively affect neonatal behaviour and maternal stress.

Research in prenatal and perinatal psychology has been incomplete, with its emphasis on vulnerable populations of pregnant women, physical and psychological conditions but not enough on positive influences such as mindfulness or wisdom practices. In my view, the fact that research and policy making have focused mostly on adverse effects, thus on cure rather than health advancement or salutogenesis, may reflect our distancing from our original worldview (still deep in our DNA).

The message is clear: we need to encourage parent-baby ancient nurturing practices as early as possible by providing a mindful facilitating environment that fosters health and well-being. I recall my pregnancy, birth and motherhood experience and the links between my child's personality predispositions, her creative imagination, her gentle, empathic and sociable nature, and the prenatal nurturing fostered by my state of bliss, creative activities, mindfulness meditation, yoga, dancing, listening to piano music, writing and connection with nature. These practices can all foster embodied presence, receptive attentiveness, attunement and reflection, right-brain functions, preparing for motherhood and essential for parenting. Recall that the right hemisphere functions regulate mother-infant attachment for better or worse, by either facilitating resilience to stress or creating a predisposition to affect dysregulation and psychological disturbance (Schore, 1994, 2001a, 2001b).

These practices are aimed at enhancing women's self-discovery, self-belief and self-care, enabling them to take charge of their pregnancies and births and to make a decision independent of Western medical control unless it is really necessary, and of media manipulation and unreliable self-published information online, which is often ambiguous and confusing. More women can be inspired, and so can men, including those working in prenatal and maternal care services, so that cultural change is more likely to occur. This explains why this book is seeking to establish a dialogue between professionals and parents; as long as we maintain the readership gap, no real change is possible.

This book is a blend of scientific knowledge, wisdom, professional and personal experience, but also of art and memoir on what makes us human. I recall that this narrated fusion during my baby's gestation translated into an ongoing embodied narrative between my baby and me, which was the "matrix" for mental development, just as rituals, ceremonies, imagination and wisdom practices during pregnancy have been for thousands of years. Writing a book, composing and reciting a rhyme, listening to music, singing, meditating and other kinds of creative endeavour are pleasurable and meaningful activities that have physiological effects on the mother and consequently on the developing baby. The protective influence of music is documented through individuals' memories of musical pieces they were exposed to during gestation. The indigenous mothers intuitively used to sing the child the same song as before conception and throughout pregnancy to maintain the vital continuum.

In the twenty-first century, dominated by science and technology, we can all learn to integrate neuroscience, psychology, art, poetry and philosophy, as well as our own observations and insights as human beings. To understand the roots of our humanness and make care meet human basic needs, we need this integrative view of life; we need to be at once scientific and lyrical. The paradigm of complexity proposed by Edgar Morin about an awakening consciousness of the necessity of a new model for knowing reality is valid for both scientific and hermeneutic, as well as subjective emotional phenomena (Morin, 1992). Therefore, the split between science and humanities has come to an end. Intuitive wisdom, introspective empathic realisation is no less valid than scientific findings: it is richer. The meaning of a situation is influenced by the context. This is valid for prenatal, birth and postnatal experiences, which manifest through moods, body experience or implicit processes. Therefore, prenatal and perinatal psychology, if conceived in its interdisciplinary integrative nature, may offer a model for knowing complex human reality.

While providing a version of what scientific and professional knowledge has unravelled about the foetus's life and child development, I tell the reader about what this has meant for me as I trod the path of pregnancy and motherhood. Sometimes this knowledge shed light on my journey, but mostly my intuitive age-old wisdom, insights and developing relationship with my baby were the driving forces. It has been so for women for millennia. These forces also provided meanings and philosophical explanations for the whole breadth of the experience, which stands as a bold challenge to the reductionism that continues to dominate the scientific enterprise. The depth of this universal shared essence of femininity was what essentially made me connect with the Himba mothers and opened them to share their culture. Without this connection there would have been no mutual learning. It was this cocktail of intellectual, personal and wisdom endeavours that led me to the development of the Pre- and Perinatal Mindfulness Relationship-Based (PMRB) programme and the design of a PhD.

Science cannot entirely explain and give meaning to mother-baby communications and the intersubjective field. The mother-foetus relationship is primal, not rational; therefore, it involves the deep primal brain systems – the resonating brain stem and limbic (emotion) systems – which, interestingly, are the first to develop in an embryo. In evolutionary terms, the earliest brain and body parts to develop are the most important. It follows that our earliest experiences are embedded from very early intrauterine life and monitor subsequent elaborated cognitive development, contrary to what cognitive scientists used to believe (Delafield-Butt & Gangopadhyay, 2013). This ground-breaking work also seals the gap between mental and physical agency into an integrated embodied mind from prenatal life. This new neuro-philosophical perspective brings neurological issues to bear on the old questions concerning the nature of human mind. If we understand some prenatal and perinatal brain processes at a deep neurological level, we will better understand the fundamentally affective nature of the human mind (Panksepp, 1998).

Chronic anxiety, depression and stress constitute environmental hazards, just like direct hazards to the womb such as pollutants, alcohol, drugs, smoke and radiation (DiPietro et al., 2003). If the world impedes this co-regulating psychophysiological connection between mother and baby, our future health as individuals and families and the cohesion and peace of society are at risk. However, I would remind the reader that mild occasional anxiety and concerns are part of life and offer the prenate a healthy range of stimuli that actually nurture brain development. Mild to moderate levels of psychological distress may promote foetal maturation in healthy populations (DiPietro et al., 2006). What accounts for the different way in which an indigenous mother deals with stress is her resilience and emphatic social support, although that kind of stress is very different from the anxiety and depression of a Western mother.

New findings offer a portrait of the preborn baby that is very different from the passive mindless creature of the traditional paediatric texts. Our indigenous cousins have known this as mothers and communicated with their unborn babies, even before conception, for 99 per cent of our human history. They have retained the sensory communication system and reflective functioning that allow them to nurture this communication. Awareness that the unborn baby is a sentient being – able to feel, learn, memorise and relate to his environment, as studies have shown (Righetti, 1996; Piontelli, 2010) – and fully capable of (non-verbal) communication can motivate prospective parents to establish an embodied dialogue through "communication games" I teach them. Would anyone communicate with a passive unresponsive organism? However, this awareness must involve the whole community and every practitioner with a concern for expectant and new parents. We are all responsible for a child's well-being through the care we provide to the generators of his life and health. The basic tenet that it is possible to communicate with the unborn baby and influence his development is fascinating, revolutionary and full of hope. A notion emerging throughout this book is that the interactions between mother and foetus are *not* unidirectional; that is, the mother may elicit a response from the foetus but not the other way round. I describe my baby's movements as an initiation for engagement after a period of habituation to music, my voice or touch. I recall the Himba mother Badri telling me that when her baby moved in her belly, she knew he wanted to "tell" her something.

This maternal intuitive wisdom is consistent with research showing how a foetus takes motivated and imaginative action, suggesting the individual already has self-organising habits and personality in response to womb experience (Piontelli, 2002, 2010). Human beings have goals expressed in movements, even before birth, and the prenatal imprinting shapes every individual's rudimentary relational engagement and identity. A human foetus, during maturational processes leading to and preparing for birth and life outside the womb, seems to have already a core psychological identity, influenced by the stimuli from the internal environment (maternal psychosociobiology) and the external environment and culture, which contribute to forming his implicit (visceral) memory and nervous system regulation. The genetic imprinting (DNA) passed down by parents during fertilisation, which marks the genetic identity of every individual, would have been over the gestation period already influenced by life inside the mother's body, thus shaping the individual's psychobehavioural predispositions.

Throughout the book, I adopt terms such as "attunement" and "resonance", both deriving from music. Communication is about musicality (Trevarthen, 1999), rhythmic exchange of dynamic (non-verbal) vitality in human interactions and synchronising two people's behaviours. In indigenous cultures, singing and dancing, particularly around the time of conception and gestation, are tools for sharing knowledge and keeping positive social interactions and moods, and they teach us the function of rhythm in maintaining social ties and community life. They also regulate emotional states. I describe how the sensorimotor interactions between mother and unborn baby (e.g. the baby's movement in response to the mother's touch or voice, or to her own emotional response to music) are characterised by a form, intensity, tempo, and by the baby's capacity to integrate such information to create an experience with its own emotional tone (pleasant or unpleasant). These features also belong to music. Musical parameters are in fact intensity, timbre or tone, and duration. Therefore mother-baby interactions are no different from an embodied musical experience.

A study comparing the crying of infants of mothers speaking different languages found that the complex tonal languages pregnant women speak and their melodic patterns are memorised by their unborn babies and show in the crying of their newborn infants (Wermke et al., 2016). The daily practice of ceremonies, dances, singing and listening to music before conception, during pregnancy and beyond (music produced with their own bodies) could explain the intergenerational transmission of the sense of rhythm and the Himbas' agility with rhythmic human interactions, even with people they have never met before.

During my work with both Western and indigenous mothers, I witnessed the astounding power of the mother's speechless wonder at her baby who has just been born and have learnt the richness and truthfulness of non-verbal language. When mothers are stressed, affected by depression or other mental problems in our complex societies, or when mother and baby have experienced a birth trauma, these features of musical synchronisation are jeopardised. Despite loving their babies, suffering mothers can hardly get into the baby's needs, synchronise with the baby's positive emotions, while they are often synchronous with the negative ones, with likely long-term effects on cognition and social emotion (Feldman, 2007; Murray et al., 2010). Musicality is at the basis of sympathy or "feeling with" in both mother and baby, as in all human relationships.

Today there is an increasing neuroscientific interest in attunement, mirroring, resonance and empathy in social interactions and communication.

The mammalian nature we have inherited also requires intersubjectivity with others, reciprocity, and co-regulation of all our physiological and psychological systems (Narvaez, 2014). When any of these basic human needs is not met, this leads to worse outcomes for physical, mental or social health and well-being. Preverbal mother-baby interactions allow us to see the matrix in which the foundation of our capacity to listen, attune and communicate, and intersubjectivity resides. This makes this book extremely timely and interesting for all of us – professionals and researchers, as well as anyone with an interest in how human development unfolds from the earliest stages of prenatal life. I see this book as an opportunity to rekindle the legacy of our original worldview and human abilities that are part of the DNA of all of us before we alienated ourselves from Nature and community.

This book also highlights the deep, spiritual and philosophical meanings of being human, growing a baby and the vital importance for him to receive loving and caring attention. The memory of love and protection becomes the "internal working model" of relationships in a child's mind, which guides social responses throughout life (Bowlby, 1951), but also a primal visceral or bodily memory. What also emerges from this book is that internal working models are not only psychological but also represent the functioning of the nervous system. Siegel describes the mind as embodied and relational. The brain evolved as a "social organ of the body", developing an ability to regulate internal states and attune to the social environment (Siegel, 2004, p. 275). The embodied memory of a loving mother and father will not prevent the challenges of life but will be a rock in times of stress and crisis, which will be perceived as the route to learning and personal growth.

In a society in which many people fear having children due to uncertainties or struggle to have one as a consequence of a stressful lifestyle, which is often incompatible with conception and healthy pregnancy, this book can bring some encouraging hope. Our original worldview and wisdom practices will remind us who we really are so we can begin to reflect on some of the different ways of being in the world. The integration of mind and body reflected in a healthy pregnancy involves, in my view, *a spiritual attainment*. The Australian academic David Tacey (2003) writes that patients/clients tend to express to their therapists/clinicians their sense that a lack of spiritual meaning has something to do with their illness. He addresses the major social issue of spirituality, which requires immediate attention if we are to respond creatively to spiralling outbreaks of depression, suicide, addiction and psychological suffering. Today we can speak of a client-led or grassroots recovery of the spiritual dimension in healing and health. Interestingly, indigenous and traditional societies notice a heightening of spirituality during pregnancy, which could suggest it has a protective function.

According to the new paradigm proposed here, attunement, the very foundation of parenting and secure attachment, is not an intellectual process. Reflective functioning, an ability fostered by the practice of wisdom and mindfulness as early as pregnancy and even before conception, can facilitate attunement and mind-reading, but attunement is mediated by the body and our mammalian caring nature that unfolds in symbiosis with Mother Earth. Mentalising can actually hinder attunement if it is not coupled with sensitivity, which involves the primal sensory communication system. To be able to tune into her baby's needs and cues, thus to be responsive, a mother needs to attune with her own bodily feelings at the present moment, which implies a self-body awareness, and a sense of embodied presence. In fact, in parents who have experienced trauma, the capacity to connect with their bodily feelings as well as with others and self-regulate is impaired, as they had to shut down the painful sensations caused by the trauma for survival (van der Kolk, 2014). Attunement fosters physiological or arousal regulation. Missteps in synchrony are absolutely normal and important for development, as long as they are followed by repair. This flow of life, or feeling of being alive, nourished by responsiveness and attunement, both from the mother and the community, is one of the outstanding aspects of the Himba culture that I witnessed, despite the tough conditions of life.

From beginning to end, this book conveys the important message that a caring empathic society is based on the cultural (communal) consciousness that health derives from the integration of mind, body and spirit, which is fundamental for a baby to develop as a full human being. A healthy society is a reflection of caring attentive parents who are able to sow the seeds of healthily developed children and adults during prenatal life as well as the first years of life outside the womb. This book describes the continuum of development from uterine life and the importance of maintaining the continuum throughout the perinatal transition for health.

In a world increasingly dominated by technology and science, which is easily infiltrating cyberbullying and criminality via the Internet, investing in prenatal and perinatal care inspired by primal wisdom/mindfulness could be the route to preventing many problems. A mother's *being* and *doing* for and with her developing preborn, newborn and infant – along with her mindful eating, attentive love, listening, communicating and all her creative resources – is actually scientific in that it has a huge impact in shaping the baby's brain, her predispositions and capacity for empathy and healthy relationships. We can say that the mother is the holder of science. Therefore, the mother's (and father's) inter-being with her baby matters enormously to society, as the future of a cohesive well-functioning society rests on healthily developed children.

The father also plays an important part directly in a child's life, but even more significantly in creating a supportive environment and relationship around the pregnant and new mother, so as to let her inner resources nourish the baby. A depressed father is less involved in the care of the infant and during pregnancy less motivated in supporting pregnancy and the mother-preborn relationship (Ramchandani et al., 2008a, 2008b). Birth-related paternal depression has been found to be closely associated with maternal depressive symptoms and children's risks for emotional and behavioural problems (Schumacher et al., 2008). However, the father's important role in a child's development is not scientifically and culturally acknowledged enough. I highlight that professionals working with expectant and new parents, birth institutions and government must become aware of the importance of the father. A poor couple relationship, often related to chronic stress, anxiety, depression or trauma and lacking communication and mutual understanding, may sow the seeds of a child and future adult's mental problems. These could be prevented by enhancing parents' awareness of what is happening in intrauterine life and infancy and listening empathically to their stories.

Investment in the preconception, prenatal and perinatal stages is the most cost-effective approach to optimise the health and development of children and adults. It has been demonstrated that preventive prenatal and perinatal problems can be both more achievable and cost-effective than cure (Bauer et al., 2014). The World Health Organization and UNICEF's Nurturing Care Framework for Early Childhood Development (2018) include the mental health of women who are pregnant or who are mothers as a key to the health, growth and development of very young children. It follows that prenatal and perinatal consciousness and healthcare are not just a family concern, but a social as well as economic affair.

It is time we shared information about what works in addressing maternal mental health disorders and child developmental problems. We need innovative programmes in care and care models (both clinical and non-clinical) with strong outcomes for addressing maternal mental health that lend themselves to broader adoption. The wisdom of our indigenous cousins can inspire others with the best practices, which we can integrate with the best of modern technology and capacities.

The practice of eco-mindful awareness, infused with love of Mother Nature, and wisdom abilities could not only enhance the well-being of every mother and father and their relationships with their baby, but also prevent psychological issues that cannot necessarily be assessed during pregnancy. Because the practice of mindfulness is considered a positive activity and a way of life rather than a form of treatment, pregnant and postpartum women may feel less stigmatised than they would if using antidepressants or attending psychotherapy (Misri et al., 2013). They also avoid the side effects of antidepressants which pose a risk to foetal development. Furthermore, through a compassion-based approach to pregnancy and beyond, the healthcare provider can inspire the prospective mother, through mirroring, to nurture a compassionate relationship with her baby. Attuned interactions, healthy relationships, are not just a necessity for survival but a catalyst for growth in family and community.

I argue, drawing on my experience with the Himba as well as my personal experience of birth, that we need to focus on the idea of a culturally recognised and accepted postpartum *rest period* enabling mother and baby to bond undisturbed. This is not possible unless birth professionals have learnt to slow down, connect with the present moment and to be receptive to the parent-infant's needs. We need to acknowledge that natural birth provides a necessary transition from prenatal to postnatal life for both mother and baby and is a psychophysiological facilitator of bonding (Odent, 2015). It is also important for the mother's sense of body-mind integrity. We need to acknowledge that overexertion after labour caused by the pressure to go back to work or rough postpartum practices could lead to depression, infections or increased uterine bleeding, thus jeopardising mother-baby interactions.

Mindful awareness of the importance of the postpartum period as a vital continuum of prenatal life to encourage extended breastfeeding and attuned bonding can stop women feeling the need to return as quickly as possible to "normal" after birth, as many American and some European women do. I suggest that the first step is to value mammalian intersubjective nature and inspire women to believe that they can give birth naturally and use their own inner resources to protect their children – as women have been doing since the beginning of human history. The trend towards elective caesarean births and modern obstetric practices, which are increasingly depriving mother and baby of the vital skin-to-skin contact straight after birth, are having dramatic consequences on mothers, fathers and children. Scientists foresee adverse epigenetic effects. Some things have changed in our society, but the female body and mother-baby psychobiological fit necessary for bonding are not among them. They cannot adapt to these changes without serious health consequences. This book sends powerful messages to counter such prevalent internalised attitudes, which makes it very much needed.

Mothers hold within their own body-self the entirety of the past, present and future. All existence rests within them. They are the keepers of potential. An important message this book aims to convey to a mother-to-be is to rediscover the embodied intimate space and communication with her unborn and child – because it is deep in the DNA and soul, primal and universal, and can be enjoyable, fulfilling and rewarding if experienced with wisdom and creative vitality, and more importantly, because it is crucial for the development of the child's full potential, creativity and humanness. And this is vital for healthy relationships and a healthy society. However, because we evolved to cooperative parenting, to empathic support, this rediscovery of wisdom has to be promoted by communal mindful support, involving governments and policy makers. This message is indeed universal, in that it refers to every society and culture, and thus undoubtedly makes this book open to an international audience. As Dan Siegel states, "Mindfulness awareness is a universal goal across human cultures" (2007, p. xiii).

This book proposes an inspiring and lifelong outcome of intimate bonding and spiritual fulfilment in parenting, which is being dramatically undermined in our Western modern technological societies. It contributes to a new understanding of familiar material. It also offers an excellent opportunity to show how my integrative approach to healthcare and personal mindfulness and motherhood experience contribute new information previously overlooked, and lead to the Pre- and Perinatal Mindfulness Relationship-Based (PMRB) programme. These topical interrelated subjects, addressed from an interdisciplinary perspective, could attract a multi-professional audience. This is a book for mental health, prenatal/ perinatal and other healthcare professionals, those suffering and those seeking clinical, social and political solutions to the cycle of trauma and violence in our society, and parents who seek a book that is beyond instructions but provides answers from the inside out. I am confident that professionals, scientists and parents alike will enjoy the fascinating insights. Those without an integrative intellect could be educated into a new way of conceiving of human science, life and health. And so may anyone who has wondered how the mind develops and how we learn to be human and enjoy it.

The scientific evidence is never a cold description but something fused into a warm, sometimes emotive and poetic style, making it appealing, readable and accessible not just to the expert but also to the layperson. Science, especially of human development, should not only teach us how to master life by means of calculation, but fill our lives with existential meaning. Although science can measure the high level of maternal cortisol (stress hormone) in the placenta and infer that the baby's capacity to deal with stress may be impaired, it does not cover the entire breadth of the dynamic features of a mother-baby relationship. However, investigating multiple associations, such as between maternal mental health, mindfulness and the maternal-preborn relationship during pregnancy, and the mother-infant relationship in my PhD, can depict the complexity of the earliest relationship developing from long before birth. It can highlight antenatal predictors of attuned or disturbed mother-infant relationship and promote antenatal preventive strategies. Besides, inviting women to report their experience of the PMRB programme and the mental health outcomes, birth and bonding can add the subjective dimension that enriches the quantitative data and offers a more comprehensive understanding.

The deeply empathic, insightful and compassionate perspective promises to further humanise the prenatal and perinatal period, parenting and childhood. It is a welcome breath of fresh air and offers possibilities for a new humanity in healing the world. This book contributes to the contemporary revolution in mental health based on the recognition that so many mental problems are the product of developmental trauma, the outcome of unresolved traumatic events in early life (including prenatal) when basic human needs are not met. Because we live in a society that tends to deny human developmental needs – does not even understand them – there will be more and more people affected by adverse factors. This book is a guide to healing and permanently changing how healthcare professionals, psychologists and psychiatrists think about and perceive pregnancy and maternal-infant health. In particular, it will benefit healthcare professionals involved in antenatal/postnatal care and staff working in maternity units who do not have a psychology background. The clarity of vision and breadth of wisdom is much needed. It provides insights and guidance for parents (those who are suffering and those who seek self-development), healthcare practitioners, policy makers, researchers, clinicians and everyone interested in the prenatal and perinatal roots of human development and well-being.

1 Wisdom

The path to unleashing human nature and well-being

The first time my husband drove me across the South African countryside, I was deeply impressed by the closeness of community life, by people's direct face-to-face contact and the large variety of facial and body cues while interacting with each other and by their warmth and resilience towards difficult times. They manifested an embodied feeling of being alive that is being increasingly curtailed by our modern societies. Traumatic stress, mental suffering – including anxiety, depression and all psychological disturbances – and physical illnesses are some manifestations of this biosocial process. Seeing an African mother carrying her baby on her back while washing clothes in the river and smilingly and joyfully waving at us was an ordinary scene. The traditional African mother is far closer to her child and much more aware of what is going on before birth; after birth, she will still be carrying the baby everywhere with her on her back, thus meeting the baby's need for continuous close contact. The benefits for the baby as well as the mother of a period of close physical affectionate contact are supported by research from all over the world.

In his book *Touching*, Ashley Montagu includes some anthropological observations of Balinese children, the Arapesh in New Guinea, the Netsilik Eskimos, the bushmen of the Kalahari and the Ganda children of East Africa (1986). These studies on the babies born in these cultures who are cradled, sung to, stroked, caressed and carried by their mothers and other family members show that their socio-emotional and cognitive development appears well advanced. Jean Liedloff spent two years living with the Yequana Indians in South America (1986). She observed that they worked hard but always with enjoyment and good humour, while intuitively knowing the right thing to do. They lived in close contact with nature, as part of the jungle's system. They enjoyed whatever they did, and work was part of their life. Pregnancy and childbirth were natural and enjoyable, and parents really shared their babies' babyhood and children's childhood.

In India, there are traditions of caring for the embryonic soul of the developing child. We can see another example of openness towards unborn and infant human life in the Mbuti, an African tribe (Turnbull, 1983). Conceiving a baby is considered by the Mbuti a sacred creative act generating life. The baby is conceived in the woman's mind and spiritual practices in Nature, such as dancing, talking and singing to the soul of the baby, surround the period of conception. The same practices accompany pregnancy and the postpartum period to provide the unborn baby with a sense of familiarity and continuum and reassure him or her.

The Himba, the indigenous people of Northern Namibia I spent a few weeks with (Sansone, 2018b), offered a wonderful window to understand some adversities in our modern society. Seeing my young daughters freely playing and connecting with the tribal children – despite the linguistic and cultural barriers – and our human essence revitalised by their unbroken social engagement, was evidence of how mental distress and pathology are mainly a consequence of our modern materialistic, isolating and soulsucking culture. In an African indigenous village, there is a strong social connection, acceptance and warm welcoming in the community, even if you are a stranger. And if you have children, that is a primary reason for sharing, since childhood is very much cherished. The community is always with you and you are never isolated. There is always space for the individual's needs and expression.

Our society cuts us off from our uniqueness by idealising individualism and devaluing social contact and ignoring our emotional needs. This society tends to generate unhappiness and dysfunction. Therefore, mental illness is not an isolated phenomenon but a culturally constructed paradigm. This has to do with the nature of the economic system, where what matters is not your *being* but how you are valued by others, usually on the basis of materialistic productivity. The people who are not productive are devalued and shut down, which causes disconnection from ourselves – our emotions, body and soul. This system does not favour young people raising children, who are subject to huge pressures – working, rushing around, moving very fast and not having the necessary time to "connect" and respond to their children's basic emotional and social needs.

But there is intelligence or wisdom in nature and creation and if we ignore it, we create suffering in ourselves and other people. This intelligence manifests in cosmic connection, social coherence and harmonious alignment of relationships that allows for the efficient flow of energy and communication – in our compassion, love, wisdom. This is what we are meant to be. The recognition of this is what we call spirituality. There is a spiritual nature inside us that needs to be acknowledged and cultivated to prevent adverse consequences on our well-being.

Ignorance and disregard for the essential relatedness of all life has created serious ecological problems on our planet, which have undermined our health. The dirty air and toxic chemicals contained in processed food and other pollutants have poisoned our body-mind. Excessive stress adds to the corrosive effects. Many babies come into this world with developmental problems resulting from micro-traumas (toxic substances and high stress) experienced in their mother's body. We are governed by a culture that erroneously views each of us as an isolated entity, separated from others and from our environment, not part of the whole with which we are connected. By practising wisdom, we can develop a self as well as a collective consciousness of each of us as part of an interconnected social and ecosystem as the route to restoring human essence and well-being.

Love, compassion, kindness and cooperation have been represented in our collective social consciousness for millions of years. We need to prioritise this transformative wisdom or heart-related qualities so as to co-create the best future for our humanity. There needs to be a shift in awareness towards a new collective intelligence based on care, cooperation and acceptance.

> I believe that thinking only of our own comfort and peace to the neglect of other troubles in the world is immoral. The time has come for us to consider seriously how to change our way of life, not through prayer or religious teaching, but through education. Since moral education is sometimes only superficial, we need to devise a systematic approach to exploring inner values and ways to create a more peaceful world.
>
> Dalai Lama (April 16, 2016)

The sense of knowing-how

Wisdom has long been considered a matter of philosophy, just as psychology was until the nineteenth century. Likewise, mindfulness may be still considered a mystical experience. Recently, wisdom and related mindfulness, and their power in inducing bodily experiences and awareness, have become a topic studied by social and neuroscientists (Goldberg, 2005; Stenberg & Jordan, 2005; Kabat-Zinn, 1990; Gilbert, 2010; Goleman & Davidson, 2017). A new understanding of "heart"-related qualities that goes beyond just the philosophical is advancing into a realisation of the heart as a dynamic, connecting and creative intelligence. Coherently connecting the physical, emotional, intuitive and spiritual aspects of the heart can lead to a new way of perceiving, thinking, acting and relating – which we call heart-based or wisdom.

Wisdom includes a great deal of know-how regarding how to live (Kupperman, 2005). In contrast with the "clumsy cousin" of intellectual formulas, "what is needed is a deeply internalised kind of knowing-how that normally does not require pauses and time to think . . . responsive to the moods, needs, and responses of the person with whom one interacts", with "some experiential sense of how various kinds of interaction play out in the long run" (Kupperman, 2005, p. 266). The intellectual brain may think but the heart and related wisdom know.

Throughout this book, I will be discussing how aspects of wisdom, such as empathic affectivity, relational engagement, intersubjectivity, compassion and communal mindfulness, have an impact on early human development and are passed down to successive generations. I will look at how parenting, relationships and behaviours are guided by mindsets, and how these affect development and well-being. The mindsets that dominate many societies today are based on safety, control and ruthless and detached imagination; they are ego-centred and intellectual. By influencing our culture, such attitudes and practice have led to a health and ecological crisis. We live in a society that encourages competition, achievement and success over attachment, compassion and love. Parents' experiences of pregnancy, birth and childcare practices have been dramatically affected by this culture, with adverse consequences on their well-being, and on the foetus and the child's development. But what matters most in pregnancy and caregiving is the art of the journey, the know-how, an intuitive wisdom leading to the creation of a trusting relationship with the baby day by day.

From early life in the womb, even if the baby does not know the world outside, she can sense whether she is loved, rejected or neglected and learns trust and empathy, or distrust, indifference or hatred. These early perceptions form an embodied memory or neurological blueprint, which will not only affect the child's and adult's physical, emotional and mental well-being but also the way in which she relates to the social and natural world (Emerson, 1996). The science of epigenetics teaches us that the genetic imprinting (DNA) passed on by the parents during reproduction is already influenced by the baby's experiences in the mother's body, through which her external environment and culture is transmitted. We now know that traumatic experiences change DNA over generations, unless the trauma is healed or overcome (Yehuda, 2016). Therefore, behavioural patterns, values and wisdom are also learnt through our parents' being and way of treating us, and these are transmitted to our children across generations. The practice of mindfulness and fostered capacities for wisdom can change or mitigate the transmission of the effects of trauma to next generations.

> Environmental and genetic influences are *absolutely inextricable*. The genotype (the design according to which you are built) is open to a wide range of manipulations, as it expresses itself in a particular environmental context, which in turn shapes the phenotype ("you" yourself).
> (Solms & Turnbull, 2002, p. 238)

Even in the womb, human predispositions are being influenced by stimuli from the internal environment – maternal psychobiology, emotions and behaviours, wisdom, morality, love – in turn influenced by her external environment and culture in which she lives. From the viewpoint of neurophysiology, all "life events" are ultimately mediated (registered and translated) by bodily events (Solms & Turnbull, 2002, p. 233). Therefore, because the baby dwells in the mother's body, she can affect her unborn baby's development and orientations with her wisdom practice, encouraging a child's self-knowledge and communal wisdom, and a more nurturing and sociable nature. Children who are, for example innately more nurturing and sociable, as opposed to aggressive and reactive, will literally *create* different environments for themselves and others.

The nine months spent in the womb and the period following birth are the most formative part of a human being's life. What the baby encounters influences her perception of the nature of life. The challenges of the new world outside the womb are huge, but the baby's prenatal experiences prepare her for a continuum provided by the mother's closeness from the moment of birth. "The violent tearing apart of the mother-child continuum, so strongly established during the phases that took place in the womb, may understandably result in depression for the mother as well as agony for the infant" (Liedloff, 1986). This can be observed today in perinatal mental illness and child development problems. We need to acknowledge that experiences in the womb and around birth play a crucial role in a child's development as well as in parents' mental health and well-being.

It follows that there is nothing more important and profound than the bond between the mother and her developing child. This bond begins in the womb and flourishes, and as we grow older, through our relationships and well-being. It will shape our capacity to trust others, for intimacy, to nurture others – humans as well as every creature of the cosmos – and our capacity to foster family, community and the world. Our capacity to deal with challenging life events and recover from traumatic experiences depends to a large extent on the wisdom resources instilled in early life through our relationship with caregivers. Therefore, the intricate relationship between a mother and her developing child must be of concern to everyone – parents, siblings, grandparents, neighbours, practitioners and policy makers – so as to optimise children's development and full potential. Every practitioner with a concern for the pregnant couple and developing child has to embody a compassionate relationship-focused approach.

I envisage that a revolutionary change could be achieved by revising the ways we think about parenting, child development and health based on the components and insights offered by wisdom traditions and prenatal and perinatal sciences, which reveal an unborn baby/infant who is a conscious sentient being. This is, to me, the only way to profoundly have an impact on our next generations and save our humanity. As Albert Einstein pointed out, "We cannot solve our problems with the same thinking we used when we created them".

Primal wisdom

From the Eskimos of Northern Canada to the Bushmen of the Kalahari Desert and other African regions, the survival of hunter-gatherer societies all around the world may have depended on wisdom capacities. These indigenous societies, whose sociocultural lives represented the norm for 99 per cent of human history, developed strikingly similar practices and world views (Ingold, 1999). Their perinatal, childcare and social practices appear to foster survival and well-being at both the individual and the community levels. These communities are known for their social harmony, social cohesion, peace and attunement to each member of the group and other entities of the cosmos. In a world affected by a major individual, social and ecological crisis threatening our fundamental human virtues, we can be inspired by our ancestors' and cousins' wise lifestyles and the way in which they value and organise child-rearing, so as to integrate their wisdom with our modern sensibility (Fry, 2006; Ingold, 1999). Although universal until about 10,000 years ago, such societies have continued to coexist to the present day (Fry, 2014).

These societies also teach us about the epigenetic inheritance of responsive parenting, prenatal/perinatal and childcare practices and their effects on attachment and child development. They can offer us a baseline model, resonating with scientific studies, to see how empathy, connection and morality – prosocial abilities – are not fostered by theoretical teaching or coercion but from the beginning of life through lived experience, through responsive caregiving, care and a society that provides support for basic needs – of mothers, babies and every individual (Narvaez et al., 2013). Like perceived persistent stress, maternal embodied wisdom is transmitted to the unborn baby in subtle ways, consciously and subconsciously. This model resonates with research literature attesting to the fact that mothers with more social support are more responsive to their babies' needs and as more able to handle the daily stress and rely on their inner wisdom. Their children grow up emotionally more responsive and resilient (Olds et al., 2007). Moreover, infants nurtured by multiple significant caretakers, who share childcare, grow up more secure, empathic and independent (Coontz, 1992).

Some might argue that we cannot return to our ancestors' lifestyle, and besides – who wants to live outside with predators? The purpose of using evolutionary baselines is not to romanticise the past but to be inspired by them in order to preserve our essential human nature and shift our mindsets and culture in a way that fosters greater well-being, not only in human beings but also for the natural world. Our respect for our Mother Earth relies on our capacity for empathy and understanding of the essential interdependence of all life, which is nurtured in early life. One of the most revealing discoveries during my visit to the Himba was that wisdom practice permeates all their daily activities and affects children's development and well-being. It was remarkable to observe that both secure attachment and wisdom components are entangled and develop by default among these cultures. It is striking that by learning about the existing research in the growing field of wisdom and mindfulness, we also discover that it overlaps with research in attachment, as both secure attachment and mindful awareness practice promote well-being, attunement, empathy and resilience (Siegel, 2007).

Today we still know more about the effects of toxic substances, physical and psychological insults such as stress than we do about non-harmful or positive influences, for example healthy nutrition or maternal life-enhancing emotions such as joy, awe, curiosity, appreciation of life, elation and anticipation, or simply falling in love with the baby. These are all fostered by wisdom or mindfulness practice, breathing awareness, yoga and other movement therapies, melodic music listening, connection with Nature and social engagement. And we still know more about foetal behavioural responses to stress or harmful substances as observed by 4D real-time ultrasound scan than about feel-good emotions induced by nurturing practices.

By the sixth month, the preborn can hear and move in rhythm to his or her mother's voice and recognises it after birth (DeCasper et al., 1994), showing that he or she is responsive to positive influences. Imagine the different influence this has if the mother is happily singing or yelling in anger. It is no surprise that sonograms taken while parents yell at each other show the baby's entire body flinching in agitation. Imagine the damage caused by months of feeding this negative energy to a preborn baby. Throughout this book, I explore how nurturing practices foster parents' as well as a community's well-being to influence development constructively prior to birth and beyond. When we cannot remove negative chronic stressors, we can empower mothers with human resources and coping strategies.

An accurate longitudinal follow-up of my baby from intrauterine life to her first four postnatal years tracks the links between her emotional and behavioural development and the prenatal nurturing fostered by my mind-body state of bliss, my creative imagination and activities – mindfulness meditation practice, yoga, piano music listening, writing. All these influences formed an "empathic core" through which my baby's early sensory-motor and affective experiences emerged to shape her predispositions (blueprint). These practices, in particular mindfulness, can all foster global attentiveness, receptiveness, attunement and reflection, functions involving the right brain (Siegel, 2007). Activation of the right-brain hemisphere during pregnancy could help to prepare for motherhood, given that the right hemisphere functions regulate mother-infant attachment (Schore, 1994, 2012). It follows that education, as early as during pregnancy, is not a theoretical teaching, but a neurobiological process shaped by early parent-infant meaningful lived interactions. But it is also a cooperative process in which culture and society, including prenatal and perinatal healthcare practitioners, exert important influences.

The continuous changing of an expansive self

The primal wisdom perspective considers the self as expansive, fluid, communal and multidimensional. In fact, the individual cannot be separated from her community and all entities. All things (mountain, animal, river, human being) are interconnected as well as aspects of the common self.

Later on, I describe my unborn baby's attunement with my conscious state of peace while, next to my husband and both surrounded by trees, I was listening to the birds' songs. We are surrounded by a fascinating natural world, made of a highly complex and still mysterious web, vibrating with billions of interacting species that communicate and display the diversity of life and complexity of their being. Sensing these relationships and listening to the song of life translates into energy (physiological state) and forms of vitality. Wisdom has to do with this quality of energy or aliveness, which shapes our perceptions, attitudes and actions. It nurtures a mother-baby relationship during pregnancy, which becomes a neurological blueprint.

In primal wisdom, the development of the self is "understood relationally as a *movement* along a *way of life*, conceived not as the enactment of a corpus of rules and principles (or a 'culture') received from predecessors, but as the negotiation of a path through the world" (Ingold, 2011, p. 146). Darcia Narvaez suggests that in our modern society, we need a path of moving towards common-self wisdom (2014). Understanding love, and extending it to children, isn't just a concern of parents, but a far more important aspect of human beings. For human beings, having children does more than reproducing their parents' genes. When it is experienced as a movement along a path of life, having children also lets us acquire knowledge, enhances our capacity to change and adjust to new environments, to be resilient, to create our own environments and give answers to important philosophical questions. It changes and expands our self. Within a common-self wisdom view, the quality of parenting strongly influences the heart, soul and consciousness of the next generation, their experience of meaning and connection, their deepest feelings about themselves and others, their life skills and the full expression of their potential in the world. This process starts at the moment of conception, although the ground can be prepared by parents' consciousness long before conception. The following is a passage from my journal of pregnancy:

> Like probably many women, I had sometimes thought of a life without children: self-independent, self-focused, carefree, all my love for my partner. But what would be left of me, of us, once passed away? Why not use our genes, our body wisdom, sensibility and creativity to give life to another human being? Is there any other experience comparable to parenting, able to provide us with such an emotional and challenging complexity, the deepest loving bonding, the joy of sharing simple things with your baby, such as smiling, cooing, babbling, or watching her first steps and insatiable curiosity about very small things of reality? Although I hadn't experienced mothering yet, I felt that the loss of part of my 'independent self' could be replaced by a more complex, profound and enriched one. I was anticipating what maternal love is about.

This openness to change permeates every aspect of primal wisdom. In primal wisdom, death is a temporary transition before being transformed into another life form. Therefore, there is no fear of death. Suicide does not make sense for the hunter-gatherers, as there is nothing to escape from (Everett, 2009). All is life. Time is eternal, vertical and *now*, with cycles of birth, life and transformative death to new life. Nothing is constant and there is *life force* or a "power moving beneath the outward appearance of things". (R. H. Whitehead 1988, pp. 9–10, as quoted in Martin, 1999, p. 63). It is what many scientists investigating energy fields refer to the invisible as Spirit from a quantum mechanics perspective (Lipton, 2015). Consistently with this ancient wisdom, cell biologist Bruce Lipton and other epigeneticists offer new insights into the interface between biological organisms, the environment, and the influence of emotions, perceptions, thoughts and subconscious on the expression of our genes and the body's healing potential. It is not the environment itself but our perception of a negative environment that affects the cells by changing their chemistry and may cause disease. Our thoughts and perceptions, implicit processes, are the primary factors in biological processes.

According to primal wisdom, the nature of being is eternal, as life energy shifts in and out of forms or from form to form. There is a deep sense of moving with the flow and of Nature and in union with it. Our suffering and psychological ill-health arise from identifying with a permanent self, possessing it, and seeing our life and world through the lens of this concept, refusing to move with change and impermanence (Watson, 2008). Nowadays, pregnancy, birth and parenting can pose a dramatic challenge to our capacity to change with the flow of experience (resilience). When this challenge is perceived as an opportunity for growth rather than a threat, we significantly contribute to a healthy pregnancy and healthy development of the baby.

Accepting the changing reality of things, even of our moods and mind states, of our physiology, like the dramatic changes induced by pregnancy and birthing, makes us see their meanings and enjoy things more. It is key to well-being and mental health. One major motive for suicide is the illusion/delusion that the depressive state will never change (hopelessness). Understanding the feeling of interconnection as a key to well-being is very important. This tenet of primal wisdom is supported by neuroscience, showing that the brain is a social organ changing its processes or structure in response to lived experience (experience-dependent neuroplasticity) (e.g. Siegel, 2010). The more connected we are with entities, and the more expanded our self, the richer and more resilient we become. We have more resources to rely on in challenging moments. Thus, we can change our brain, mind and body through our consciousness, which is also an important tenet of mindfulness. But this requires continued practice.

Our consciousness of interconnectedness allows us to see ourselves in each other and so to connect with you, rather than judging and confronting.

The latter disconnects. Within the self/collective wisdom view, our well-being depends on others, on our collective nature. So, a mother is able to meet her child's basic needs and promote his well-being if her basic needs are fulfilled and well-being fostered. Our individual happiness is an illusion, related to a materialistic society focused on the accumulation of goods. Epigenetics teaches us that, from gestation, we acquire our predispositions because of our environments. We are the product of the seeds sown by our environment (including the mother's emotions, consciousness and attitudes during pregnancy). When we relinquish the idea of self as a separate entity, instead of being connected, the suffering is diluted. Even at birth, the self is the product of nine months' relationship between a developing body and environment. Like nutrients, stimulation allows for development. And if we consider the influence of our grandparents, we realise that we are the product of far more than nine months' gestation! The self is in a complex relationship from conception onwards. There would be no self without relationship. We interact with an environment because we are only cells. Then we begin to interact with a growing placenta, changing hormones and this already contributes to shape our predispositions (Emerson, 1996). Mother's sense of relational presence in the womb has a protective function. I foster this sense in mothers through mother-embryo/foetus dialogue and *communication games* using visualisations, breathing exercises and awareness of the baby's movement.

A pregnant mother, just like everyone and everything, belongs to something bigger that the self that she is holding. She is part of the life force of the ecosystem. She is an expression of the wisdom of Nature, manifesting through her mammalian nature. So is labour, a natural force that a woman embodies, yet whose power is beyond her self-control. This is a hard reality for many Western modern women to accept, as they have been conditioned to over control every aspect of their lives, with the expectation that everything will follow as they intend. The materialistic and medically oriented mindset that controls the birth industry in our modern world does not help here. Prenatal/perinatal healthcare practitioners, often under the stress of long working hours and impersonal environments, tend to apply cold abstract theory instead of compassion, listening, understanding and presence of mind and body. We must remember that we are mammals and mammals require particular circumstances to thrive. Feeling isolated or under stress, without autonomy or positive social support does not allow us to thrive. Great care should be taken about preparing for pregnancy, childbirth and postnatal care – by the whole community.

Labour is about letting go of life forces, letting go of expectations and fears and being present to let the process unfold smoothly. Pregnancy and birth thus require a resistance-free acceptance of a changing body-self. But how is this possible when women are continuously subjected to the media, which propose a bodily model of perfection, thus a fixed self? Or when our hospitalised birthing practices induce stress in labouring mothers and child and interfere with the unfolding of our mammalian instinct? Although cae-sarean births may be increasingly considered normal in our society, they may be experienced as an intrusion into a woman's body and life, even a trauma, which is far more difficult to process than is generally claimed (Sansone, 2014).

Attitude towards the natural world: relevance to the prenatal relationship

> Look deep into nature, and then
> you will understand everything better.
>
> A. Einstein

Within a holistic perspective of life, the human being is in relationship with all entities. There is no fear of animals or of others – they are all kin, a part of the common self (Ingold, 1999). There is a deep trust in Nature, includ-ing body wisdom and the caring mammalian nature with its benefits. There is no violation of others, whether human or non-human, or lack of courtesy, generosity or respect. The values of extended kinship are strongly devel-oped from early life by a deep understanding of the natural world and of the individual embedded in the environment. Consciousness is attributed to every creature (thus to the unborn baby too!) as well as to the creative forces that brought it about. The presence of energy is acknowledged in all entities, including animals, plants, mountains, clouds, oceans – all of Nature – and each contributing to the common self. It is an ecology of diverse interdependent living selves beyond the human, which allows for ecological harmony, sustainability and human well-being (Kohn, 2013).

In primal wisdom, there is a strong sense of the importance of being in tune with invisible energies as a responsibility to all members of the collec-tive self. Therefore, wisdom is a state of being, which includes the natural world and leads to a way of life. This state of harmony and collective and ecological coherence reflects into a regulated physiological state (van der Kolk, 2014). Our culture emphasises and promotes individualism, but at a deeper level we never exist as an individual organism, even during gestation when we develop in a continuous dialogic narrative with our mother's body, brain and mind. In his book *The Body Keeps the Score*, trauma specialist Bessel van der Kolk writes, "Our brains are built to help us function as members of a tribe" (2014, p. 78). He suggests that almost all mental suffering has to do with difficulties in creating satisfying relationships and in regulating arousal. The standard medical focus on drug administration to treat a par-ticular disorder diverts our attention from how our problems interfere with our functioning as members of our tribe.

Believing in energy influence and energy-sensing communication is extremely relevant to mother-baby communication – during pregnancy, birth and afterwards. It allows pregnant and labouring mothers to sense and interpret the prenate's cues and be aware of the psychobiological connection that guides mother and baby through gestation and birth (Sansone, 2004). I recall a Himba woman saying, "When the baby moved in my belly, I knew he was awake and wanted to talk to me". Himba women sing and dance to communicate and celebrate the new life. This fine conscious sensory capacity allows them to attune with the baby – in the womb, during labour/birth and beyond – and to anticipate their needs by picking up their cues. Empathy is established early in pregnancy through an intersubjective field. An indigenous mother has a sense of relational presence with her child from the very first moments of conception and even before. She treats the baby in the womb as a partner for whom she is a guardian (Turnbull, 1983).

Many tribal cultures, including the Himba I visited, consider a child's birthday to be not when she is born, nor when she is conceived, but as the day that the child's spirit is heard by her mother. In fact, when a couple wishes to conceive a baby, the woman goes out into the bush and sits alone under a tree. Here she waits and listens until she hears the song (soul) of the child to whom she will give birth. The mother then teaches the song to the father, so that the child's spirit is called during lovemaking. I have found that couples having difficulties conceiving a baby benefit significantly from creating a contemplative space around the baby's soul and a direct dialogue with the embryo and foetus. Unlike Westerners, our indigenous cousins believe their child to be conceived as soon as she is wanted, before the sacred act of intercourse that creates her. This is evidence that these spiritual beliefs help sustain the couple's fertility, thus affecting them physiologically. This is consistent with evidence of bioenergetics (Lipton, 2015).

In primal wisdom, compassion extends to all forms of creation and a grateful attitude towards nature is emphasised. Therefore, each individual – not only babies (including unborn), but also animals and trees – is respected as an agent. Individuals must be treated with courtesy and respect for their individual autonomy and there is no coercion. The spirit of generosity pervades each entity of the Earth and is manifested among humans by sharing with all entities. The world – both social and natural – is perceived to be generous and supportive. There is a deep understanding of interrelationship with the natural world and a sense of "expectations" to be met. Grass and plants expect to be harvested so as to sustain them and not to let them dwindle away (Kimmerer, 2013). A baby expects to be born naturally, receive constant affectionate physical contact, breastfeeding and attuned interactions. A baby has evolved needs which she implicitly expects to be met. We cannot neglect Nature and its beneficence. We need to understand it and cooperate with it in order to preserve it and ourselves. We need to promote co-parenting.

The Earth, like a Mother, is giving and provides all that is needed. The sharing of all entities is perceived as a gift and must be treated as such. "In a world where everything breathes with life, has motion, is intelligent with thought, and is kinsman, equilibrium can work only when everything is exchanged as a gift" (Martin, 1999, p. 62). This allows for the perception of the beauty of life, of its lyric. It is what makes a mother marvel at her baby who has been conceived or has just come into the world. This appreciation of Nature (including the unborn baby) as a gift enables us to catch the potential of non-verbal language, implicit preverbal processes and what is beyond the visible. Perception is the ability to see what is in fact there and to participate in the narrative of life. Perceptual stimulation allows for genetic expression, psychological and physical development; it is nourishment for the body-self. Within this view of openness to the world, harming others is forbidden, except for killing for food, which must be performed with respect for the life taken. "The world and its creatures are guests of the universe and of Mother Earth and should behave as guests" (Four Arrows et al., 2010, p. 12).

This sense of participation of all entities reflects in the care of the embryonic soul of the developing child, thus in an openness towards the unborn and infant human life, which we can see in the Mbuti, an African tribe, as described by Turnbull in the *Human Cycle* (1983). The act of intercourse between an Mbuti husband and wife is filled with joy: it is sacred because it is Nature's creative act that results in life. In the last few months of her pregnancy, the woman goes off on her own, to her favourite spot in the forest, and sings to the child in her womb. She talks to her child in a clear, informative, reassuring and comforting way, while rocking herself, sometimes with her hands on her belly. She tells her child of the forest world into which it will soon emerge, repeating simple phrases such as "the Forest is good, the forest is kind; Mother Forest, Father Forest". There is a sense of relational presence in the womb interweaving with a grateful attitude towards nature. Mbuti see their life as beginning the moment they were wanted, and throughout their childhood detailed knowledge of their earliest beginnings is passed on. The infant was conceived in love and joy, and that is how it is born.

The first man who had an insightful idea of what was to become evidence after four centuries – prenatal influences on human personality – was not a physician, but the great Italian artist Leonardo da Vinci. In his *Quaderni*, Leonardo describes the intrinsic relationship between a mother and her unborn child, "the same soul governs the two bodies . . . the things desired by the mother are often impressed on the child which the mother carries at the time of the desire . . . one will, one supreme desire, one fear that a mother has, or mental pain has more power over the child than over the mother, since frequently the child loses its life thereby" (Leonardo Da Vinci, *Quaderni*). A passage from the Bible also portrays the mother-baby prenatal lifeline and how the unborn baby is responsive to any maternal emotional nuances and changes of energy in her body: "When Elizabeth heard Mary's greeting the baby leaped in her womb, and Elizabeth was filled with the Holy Spirit" (Luke 1 p. 41).

The peculiar emotions of wonder, aesthetic profundity and spiritual intuitions about human life that many women begin to experience during pregnancy may be also the result of documented activity in the changing brain and have an evolutionary history (Hoekzema et al., 2017). The feeling of bliss and spiritual cultivation may serve as an antidote to stress (to protect the baby) and physiological co-regulators for both mother and baby while preparing the mother for a wider perception and understanding of the baby's world. In this way, mother and baby can also share the same sense of delight, marvel and curiosity. The pregnancy hormones transform a woman's brain and may make it more open to bodily intuitive wisdom and imaginative possibilities, enabling her to pick up the baby's cues and meet her needs (attuned responsiveness). It is a human work of art. Chronic stress, anxiety, depression and all mental suffering disrupt this human psychobiological adaptive system, in which mother-baby intersubjective engagement is the foundation of healthy development. Being able to rely on inner resources and body wisdom is crucial to heal mental suffering and build a fulfilling mother-baby bonding.

In Western societies, pregnancy and childbirth have lost their sacredness, their very natural essence; they become difficult and often a source of stress and depression instead of joy and fulfilment. This puts parenting at a great disadvantage. I believe that human beings' loss of connection with the environment – both natural and social – is at the basis of this dramatic change. A consequence of the human being ceasing to be part of the ecosystem is also the change in food chemistry in recent years, another major threat to our health, particularly regarding brain functioning and mental health (Crawford & Sinclair, 1971). Maternal nutrition, in particular omega-3 fatty acids provided by nature through fish, seafood and seaweeds, plays a crucial role on the unborn's brain development. Living far away from their marine sources has caused health impairments through evolution.

Ignorance and disregard for the essential relatedness of all life has created serious ecological problems on our planet, which have undermined our health and created a major crisis in the history of humanity. Nature is our Mother. When we live cut off from her, we get sick. Some of us live in apartments, very high above the ground, surrounded by cement, metal, electric energy and other hard things. In many societies we cannot see trees and the colour green is absent from our view. Unborn babies never hear bird songs, benefit from pure air or sense the mother embedded in nature. Our children and we adults never touch the soil with our fingers; we do not grow lettuce and other natural foods anymore. That is why we need to become aware of this situation so as to eat organically, go out regularly and be in touch again with Mother Earth. From this, a collective, wiser, more profound attitude to pregnancy and child-rearing will follow, nourishing the seeds for healthier generations.

Animal nature

The obstetrician Michel Odent suggests the term "symbiosis" instead of domination of nature. This would lead to an increased capacity for cooperating with other living creatures, particularly microorganisms, which are the foundations of all ecosystems (2015). It all started 10,000 years ago, when our ancestors started to dominate Nature, instead of cooperating and taking advantage of what Mother Earth can offer on a day-to-day basis. This major crisis, commonly called the Neolithic Revolution, had several facets: domestication of plants and animals through agriculture and animal husbandry, regulation and control by the cultural milieu of human physiological processes related to reproduction (genital sexuality and childbirth), and canalisation of the universal transcendent emotional states. Today the domination of Mother Earth has reached a point when, to survive, humanity must urgently change direction.

Cooperating with nature could improve our understanding of the laws and wisdom of nature, including our body wisdom and processes such as birth and bonding, in order to work with them instead of repressing them. We need to begin from the important role of the Mother, including the *mammal* aspect, which is necessary to understand human nature. We need to focus in particular on the preconception, conception, prenatal and perinatal period and childbirth and bonding, since these critical phases are highly influenced by mindsets and cultural conditioning.

Primal wisdom embraces animal nature as something good. Alienation from animal nature, including our mammalian nature (securing uncomplicated birth, responsiveness, attunement, breastfeeding) leads to disorder and harm. In contrast, our Western view tends to denigrate animal nature, viewing it as something to be controlled and suppressed in humans. The neuroscientist Jaak Panksepp writes that we can be quite certain that all mammals share many basic psycho-neural processes because of the long evolutionary journey they have shared. He points out that it is our ancient animal heritage that makes us the intense, feeling creatures that we are (Panksepp, 1998). He says that by understanding the neural basis of animal emotions we will be clarifying the primal sources of human evolution. Panksepp explains that of course, because of our richer cortical potentials, the ancient emotional systems have to interact with a much vaster cognitive universe.

A human mother can reflect on her own feelings, emotions and experiences. For instance, she can reflect on her reflections while writing them down. She can create art and practise mindfulness. This makes a human foetus's development more susceptible to her influences and less tied to genetics than another mammalian foetus's development.

Reason, developed from our most recently evolved cortical brain, is not then a quality that distinguishes us from other animals; rather it situates humankind on a continuum with them. In some circumstances, such as labour and bonding, the neocortex needs to be inhibited to let the primal mammalian brain fully function (Odent, 2015). In evolutionary terms, the neocortex equipped baby mammals to form attachments to their mothers and help get their mothers to bond with them. But it also continued to equip grown-up mammals to bond with babies and to form multifaceted relationships (Carter et al., 2001). This means that mammals' brains were designed for the formation of relationships in ways that the brains of other animals are not. But our modern lifestyles may have led to hyper-stimulation of the neocortex, which seems to have become unable to harmoniously work with our mammalian brain. Modern obstetric practices constantly interfere with the delicate synchronicity of mother-baby bonding formation that has evolved over 99 per cent of human history.

Appreciation of beauty and sacred as part of living

In primal wisdom, reverence and appreciation of beauty are integrated in everyday life. This virtue allows for attending pregnancy, birth and a baby with a sense of wonder. Reverence involves awareness that "one is always in the presence of the sacred" (O'Donohue, 2005, p. 31). "Only the blindness of habit convinces us that we continue to live in the same place, that we see the same landscape" (p. 34). "Humans may have greater capacities than other animals for enjoying the beauty of Nature, apprehending not only the grand totality but the subtleties, for instance of a single flower" (Narvaez, 2014, p. 238). They can sense the value of the details for the wholeness, leading to an intuition of holiness – the sacred.

Interestingly, some Asian and African tribes notice a heightening of spirituality in women during pregnancy and consider it very important in maintaining the health of the mother and child (Maidan & Farwell, 1997). Engaging with the sacredness of the feminine enhances and heals our lives. This tendency to turn to spirituality is noticeable in many pregnant women of our Western societies as well, although it may be curtailed by the demands and stress of modern lives. This orientation towards spirituality during pregnancy, and even before a contemplated conception, is consistent with scientific discoveries about long-term changes to brain structure triggered by pregnancy (Hoekzema et al., 2017). According to these findings, a decrease in the volume of grey matter may imply a fine-tuning of connections in regions of the brain involved in social and relational processes (attachment) linked with the ability to empathise. Therefore, these changes may relate to an increased activation of more refined areas of the mind (right brain) in charge of wisdom and boost a mother's ability to understand and care for a child. There may be an evolutionary purpose, in that these brain changes may be to prepare the pregnant mother to trust her intuitive wisdom, enabling her to attune to her baby's needs and feelings. It is about openness towards unborn and infant human life.

During my pregnancy, led by an intuition of sacredness, I often immersed myself in Nature either through walking meditation or by sitting under a tree. My widened perception allowed me to savour the view of the intertwining mountains of different heights and shapes, the blossoming trees and the infinite variety of colours. I perceived my baby as an invaluable gift of Mother Nature, of God. I felt connected with the sun, the sky, the tree and all wonders of the universe. The intelligence that created those wonders was the same force that conceived my baby. I felt as one thing with Nature. I felt God around and inside me. I had a sense of knowing that this state of bliss was sensed by my content baby and influenced her development. This practice of enriching the mind and nurturing the spirit can be a powerful way of improving our well-being but also of communicating with the baby. This sense of connection and synchronous unity with all life put me in touch with the innermost essence of my *being*, as well as my baby. This true essence is fearless, full of magic, mystery and enchantment. My space with my baby felt like dilating in a peaceful landscape, leading me into the sacred. The stillness and slow rhythms of the natural world ultimately support the body to recover its health and wholeness.

The mindful state seems to create a receptive presence of mind to whatever arises (O'Donohue & Siegel, 2006). In a mindful state we may start to notice the holiness in everything that is around us: the fragrant bloom of a daisy or the laugh of a mischievous child (O'Donohue, 2005). My breathing expanded and so did the conscious feeling of my unborn baby's soul and presence. I inhaled the pure fresh air to let the oxygen run through my bloodstream and the placenta to nourish all her organs. Like most of us, pregnant mothers may breathe far too shallowly, thus failing to take in enough oxygen to run the pregnant body at an optimal level. Our relationship with our body and its rhythms, how much we feel in control, defines our sense of agency (van der Kolk, 2014, p. 331):

> In order to find our voice, we have to be in our bodies – able to breathe fully and able to access our inner sensations. This is the opposite of dissociation, of being "out of body" and making yourself disappear. It's also the opposite of depression, lying slumped in front of a screen that provides passive entertainment.

While in wisdom, the mind is aware that all has energy, is changing, moving, alive and does not cling to a particular manifestation (McGilchrist, 2009), our medical/healthcare system tends to constrain a mental condition in a diagnosis, often generating labelling and stigmatisation. Contemporary psychology has realised that excessive psychiatric approach to human suffering ends up being schematic and unable to detect the changing processes leading from normality to pathological conditions: personal discomfort, emotional dysregulation, muscle and postural tension as self-defence. Healthcare practitioners' trainings generally reflect the Western intellectual analytical mindset rather than embracing intuitive wisdom. Intuition is the ability to know something immediately, without verbal explanation or conscious reasoning (Orlinsky & Howard, 1986). Prenatal, perinatal and postnatal mental healthcare providers should nurture a mindful state, enabling them to inspire a sense of sacred in pregnant mothers. Recall that the mindful state expands our attention and perception to whatever arises. Unfortunately, these vital relational visceral sources of mental health and well-being are seriously undermined by the current mental health crisis. We need an innovative model for how to challenge a ruthless system lacking a humane approach, and the climate of fear and intimidation it engenders. At the cutting edge of holistic medicine, we are called on for our connectedness to all of creation and most especially to ourselves. This sense of connectedness also allows for compassion towards every other being and ourselves.

"The agile brain/mind is mesmerised by the beauty of the earth, of the energy field all around us that enliven all things" (Narvaez, 2014, p. 238). Beauty is about marvelling at all things in the present moment. A sense of beauty emerges from deep knowing of the presence of a thing and its true nature. (O'Donohue, 2005). It is what makes becoming parents marvel at the miracle of pregnancy and the creation of a developing baby. For indigenous cultures, beauty is a central value that encompasses harmony and congruence. It is a facilitating force for a healthy pregnancy, uncomplicated birth and fulfilling parenting. This is the place where indigenous teachings and healing arts (embracing contemplation, music, dance and ceremony, Earth medicine) meet with modern Western holistic approaches.

Here the core problem of life may reside, affecting parenting and child mental health and well-being today: if we are not fully ourselves, truly in the present moment (hardly to achieve in our modern stressful societies), we miss everything, the real sources of happiness and well-being. "When a child presents himself to you with a smile, if you are not really there – thinking about the future or the past, or preoccupied with other problems – then the child is not really there for you. He is not seen or felt. The technique of *being alive* is to go back to yourself in order for the child to appear like a marvellous reality. Then you can see him smile and you can embrace him in your arms" (Thich Nhat Hanh, 1991, p. 43).

2   The human work of art

The importance of surrender and ego detachment for perceiving the whole

An aspect of wisdom is letting go and surrendering to divine energy. Bourgeault (2003) contrasts bracing (self-protection, shifting to the I-Ego, resisting) with softening, opening and yielding (relational connecting and shifting to wisdom). This capacity for surrender is a driving force in a labouring and birthing woman and in a mother's capacity for reverie. Spiritual practice is about learning moment by moment not to do anything in a state of internal brace or reactivity (Bourgeault, 2003). This self-regulating ability is crucial for parents to be able to pause, breathe and not react to their child's impulsive behaviour but understand what is behind it. Silence is an important part of wisdom practice. Clarity of mind is often expressed through silence. Resting with a bodily and sensory presence is a state that allows quick understanding, intuition and insight. It is a state of grace, of not needing anything else. In my work with mothers and babies and my own motherhood, this has become a sort of benchmark – if all goes well, mother and baby find themselves in a kind of cocoon of peace and love that allows a deep connection. This state of body-mind is present during breastfeeding, which deactivates the mother's own stress response; her amygdala emits less CRF (corticotropin-releasing factor in response to stress), removing anxious, fearful feelings; whilst the prolactin generated by breastfeeding provides a feeling of tranquillity. Breastfeeding facilitates the mother's ability to calm her baby and to manage his stress. Once established (this may not always be easy to achieve in our modern society and with modern obstetric practices), breastfeeding can be a powerful source of co-regulation for the mother as well as the baby. This is why it is so important that this state of calm and grace is promoted in the process of becoming mothers. This internal state manifests through the mother's posture and body language, which are the manifestation of the way she regulates her emotions (self-regulation).

While in Western culture the self is a psychological entity, in primal wisdom the self is psychophysical. Therefore, muscular tensions have not only a mechanical function of postural organisation but also a psychosocial meaning, as they become signals of bodily presence (Ruggieri, 2001). It is as if the body told the self that it is present through its muscular tension and level of perception. The body provides stability and safety to the self. Therefore, the mother's body and the way it organises her tensions, movements and gestures provides the baby with a sense of safety, which teaches her how to regulate her emotions.

When we practise letting go, softening to openness, then we can develop conscious, co-regulated and socially engaged behaviour (Bourgeault, 2003). This is especially difficult for those who are under high stress, were neglected or abused, and thus not nurtured in their childhood and have learnt to build defences against others to protect themselves from the adverse consequences of trauma. This can be a major problem in parenting, preventing parents from opening their hearts, being present, receptive and responsive to their babies' needs and mental states. The therapeutic, clinical or mentoring relationship needs to be infused with openness of the heart and a meaningful connection. Such a compassionate approach from healthcare providers can facilitate in parents the compassionate caring relationship they need to develop with their unborn babies and infants.

Most wisdom-related practices involve learning to subdue the thinking, ego-driven intellect so that one can be fully aware. Thinking inhibits the system for communicating energy. When the sensory energy system can soften and widen perception, thinking can become more fluid and heart-driven. Ego detachment facilitates the ability to access the receptive attention, the energy and relationships in the present moment and particular context, acting accordingly or in harmony with it. Wisdom acknowledges the power of mood, nuance and the form in which it is expressed, thus its body-mind state of dependence. This energy/vitality or mood state shapes the quality of the mother's interaction with her sensitive unborn and born baby; it is the emotional nuance of a touch, a holding gesture or facial expression, to which the baby is very sensitive and responsive, that, when occurring repeatedly, affects gene expressions.

Detaching from ego means drawing attention to the "greater whole", which "leads to selflessness or abiding interest in the welfare and success of others" (Four Arrows et al., 2010, p. 65). Wisdom practices emphasise the most ancient power, most important belief of all beliefs: the power to let go of what our intellects cling to when our souls say, "No, there is something better. The earth is kin, and its ways are grace" (Martin, 1999, p. 14). When we genuinely let go and widen perception, we discover that each one of us, the whole Earth, is connected and synchronous, contributes to the orchestra of beauty and participates in it and even creates it. Our prenatal and perinatal healthcare services would benefit enormously from this well-being-sustaining view and approach to the client/patient, based on the awareness that every practitioner, every member of the community is in a communal visceral narrative, contributes to the well-being of a pregnancy and is thus influential in the parent's and the child's well-being. The dominant approach is characterised by hyper-specialism, tribalism and intellectualism, and the stress of long working hours, which tend to lead us away from real needs and connection, as well as wisdom practice.

Letting go of fear and intellectualisation

In wisdom, freeing oneself from fear is a primary, ongoing practice. It allows people's lives to flow in a narrative. "Fear takes human back in phylogenetic time to unreflective self-protection" (Narvaez, 2014, p. 243). It interrupts the flow of life and hinders connection. A mother who is too concerned about her baby's weight gain, feeding times or reasons for crying is unlikely to connect with her baby's feelings. Those who have experienced trauma tend to shut down from their bodily feelings that once caused so much pain, because they are too overwhelming. They get stuck in the fear they experienced because the fight/flight response has been thwarted. Their bodies are frozen due to inhibiting muscle tension, which like a shell, prevents them from feeling and connecting with the world. The traumatic memories become dominant in PTSD (post-traumatic stress disorders) because it is so difficult to feel truly alive right now. "Traumatised individuals become hypervigilant to threat at the expenses of spontaneously engaging in their day-to-day lives" (van der Kolk, 2014, p. 5). "Trauma compromises the brain area that communicates the physical, embodied feeling of being alive" (p. 5). The ongoing practice of letting go of fear (e.g. in mindfulness/ wisdom practices and yoga, or indigenous dances) concurs with scientific discoveries of methods and experiences that utilise the brain's own neuroplasticity to help mental sufferers feel fully alive in the present and deeply engage with relationships as well as every moment of their daily lives. This occurs by allowing the body to have experiences that deeply and viscerally contradict the helplessness, automatic defensive behaviour, rage and collapse that result from trauma and chronic stressful experiences. This is why talking therapies, when they rely on the intellect only and not on the body's resources as well, are usually ineffective.

Our society, with its problems of mental ill health, criminality and socioeconomic contrasts, generates intrinsic fears and anxieties in its members. Our ancestors' flight-fight response was designed to attack or flee a concrete threat (e.g. a snake or lion) but in our modern society we are often in a chronic physiological state of alarm (anxiety) due to an "unknown" psychic threat. When a threat cannot be attacked or avoided, it causes chronic tension or freezing. Think of a labouring woman in fear and the inhibiting effect of fear on labour and birth outcome and bonding. The high rates of complicated births and their impacts on the baby's well-being tell us a lot. It is known that fear and anxiety enhance levels of adrenaline, which inhibits the release of oxytocin, making labour and birth longer and difficult (Odent, 2015). Oxytocin also facilitates bonding and fosters the mother's and the baby's well-being. Very often this modern attitude is embedded in the midwife or any other birth partner. The level of adrenaline released by a midwife in a birthing place is an important issue, since adrenaline is contagious and easily transmitted to the labouring woman.

I recall the studies of brain-to-brain non-verbal communication (Schore, 1994, 2001a, 2001b), or those on the role of the "mirror neuron system" (Rizzolatti & Craighiero, 2004). This means that when we are in an emotional state, we activate the same part of our brain as this person. As I learnt from my visit to the Himba, if an indigenous woman leaves the village to give birth in a quiet place and with another woman who is just *present* and *connected*, it is because primal wisdom intuitively considers and respects these delicate dynamics. But it is also because the path to good birth has been written deeply in our DNA for millennia by nature's wisdom. We have always known what and how to do it. But fear and the hyper-stimulation of the intellectual brain that characterises our modern culture, as well as medical staff, interfere with this wise natural programming.

Whereas in wisdom traditions the transmission of knowledge occurred through wisdom practice and collective mirroring, today it mainly occurs through explicit, conscious, verbal, rational processes involving the left hemisphere. Hyper-stimulation of the neocortex, or intellectual brain, is not a good ally in birth and bonding, as it appears to have an inhibitory effect on the physiological process of giving birth and bonding that we have evolved (Odent, 2015). This could also alter the flow of hormones sustaining the earliest attuned mother-infant interactions, which are precursors of the capacity for empathy. Maternal sensitivity expresses in the ability to implicitly read infant's non-verbal right-brain to right-brain visual-facial, auditory-prosodic and tactile-gestural emotional communications, which involve the right-brain hemisphere (Schore, 2012). This capacity relies on interpersonal attunement, intuitive wisdom, self-trust and not intellectualisation or instructional guidebooks. Excessive stimulation of the neocortex can also interfere with our evolved capacity to attune to our own needs and others', for instance by hindering a midwife's intuitive capacity to understand and respect a labouring or nursing mother's need for a quiet non-interfering environment.

Think of modern parents' overprotective attitude towards their children and how this restricts the child's range of possibilities of experiencing his or her being. Indigenous children learn to overcome fear from a very young age (Four Arrows et al., 2010). Fear is challenged and managed by taking risks for the good of the family and community, which develops a child's self-confidence and social consciousness.

The way forward is through the conscious development of qualities born from abilities associated with the "heart", such as care and compassion, and replacing judgemental reactivity or fear with more kindness. While the brain may think, the heart deeply knows and often provides answers that mental speculations cannot. Research has greatly expanded people's understanding of the heart's role beyond being an organ that pumps our blood, but also able to send important information throughout the body and have profound influences on our brain. Heart rhythms are reflective of people's emotional states and implicit processes, and they offer a unique window into the communication between the heart, the brain and emotions (McCraty et al., 2009). Another study found that positive feelings of love, care, appreciation and other uplifting emotional qualities long associated with "heart" and wisdom induced a highly beneficial physical and emotional state called physiological coherence or "heart coherence" (McCraty et al., 1995).

The abilities fostered by wisdom practices can improve emotional self-regulation and self-empowerment skills. Researchers have found a correlation between deeper connectedness between people and increased heart-based coherence. They recorded a number of instances in which a loving mother's brain waves synchronised to her baby's heartbeats and where happy couples' heart rhythms synchronised with each other when sleeping together (McCraty, 2004). This coherent communication between mother and baby reflects not only a physiological/emotional synchronisation or co-regulation but also in the mother's mindful holding of her baby. Her muscular tension while rocking, singing a lullaby or holding her baby organises in the baby the psychophysiological foundations of human relationships (Persico, 2002).

Psychophysiological coherence

The coherence of the physiological heart and muscular tone can be nurtured during pregnancy and around the period of birth through body-self awareness, wisdom and heart coherence guidance. This can prepare parents to attune with their babies and understand them prior to birth, which leads to the possibility of heart-to-heart and touch/holding biocommunication or synchronisation between mother and baby, but also between two other individuals or more. Through the in-arm experience and affectionate touch, the baby has his first bodily experiences of the pleasure of emotional and social relationships. It is the "mutual perceptions" of muscular tension and energy – such as the mother's containing arms and the baby's own visceral responses – that shapes the gestures, movements and the quality of vitality and holding. These highly communicative experiences are on multiple levels and reciprocal. On the basis of these early experiences, the baby learns to develop trust, a style of intimate relationships and attachment with meaningful people. Surrounded by other sensitive caregivers, the baby develops a mindful personality and mindful gestures and movements. This may also suggest how the interweaving dynamics influencing a baby's sleeping pattern develop. Difficulties in the baby's regulation and sleep may be linked to parents' difficulty in mindfully holding and rocking consequent to their disconnection with bodily feelings or emotional shutdown leading to frozen muscular tension (Persico, 2002). Movements, touch and holding may be rushed, unconfident or frozen, rather than slow, firm, carefully attuned and reassuring.

Our mindful relationships are embodied in responsive faces, gestures, touch and coherent energy, which create an attuned physical synchrony (or asynchrony) (van der Kolk, 2014). Wisdom traditions are aware of the embodiment and relational aspects of the mind. If indigenous cultures develop a strong sense of rhythm, capacity for attunement and social cohesion, it is because they acknowledge the subtle relational dynamics from very early life onwards. The healing power of the community is expressed through music and rhythms fostering the flow of life and feeling of being alive.

When the Himba showed us the primal foot-tapping movements, dance and singing they perform when a baby has been conceived or to celebrate any other important life event, I could see how they use these practices as tools to physiologically regulate and maintain social ties. It was astounding to see the vitality shining through their rhythmic movements and their faces becoming attuned. There was an agile expressivity that movement and dance naturally induce. This use of dance among indigenous cultures creates a communal synchrony or resonance. All cultures have dances and art, which respond to people's need for stress relief. In fact, dance and movement therapy allow the body to express itself, release tension and occupy a space. It is enriching as it values the individual's unique experience that manifests through the body. Even a lullaby is a dance important for an infant's development and differentiation, as it regulates her emotion and muscle tensions and has a soothing effect.

This psychophysiological model overcomes the psychiatric categorisation of illness and focuses on the posture and body as the result of an individual's subjective story and the way they organise their emotional and muscular tensions. Educating the body to the expressivity of dance and art is not about a beautiful performance that is merely physical but the growth of the personality, and in the mother-infant dyad, the growth of the relationship. The goal of dance, as conceived by our indigenous cousins, is not to create a beautiful product but to allow the body to express itself and its inner potential, re-balance and restructure. Dance is also a narrative and often works during pregnancy. It can draw out a pregnant mother's positive resources and create an embodied narrative, telling the preborn a story with its sequence of events. Dance can educate towards the unfolding of mindful movements, so important in handling with an infant with responsiveness.

Over a period of sharing the Himbas' life, I could see the links between the communal resonance, the capacity to naturally connect with me and my family despite the language and cultural diversities, and the attuned physical, emotional synchrony indigenous babies spontaneously develop. All these rhythmic practices shape a human being who is a coordinated whole of rhythms. Practising to become attuned provides parents and children with the visceral experience of reciprocity, which is a source of joy, vitality and well-being. We also feel physically attuned and experience a sense of connection, joy and being alive when we play together freely and laugh.

One of the most revealing discoveries of my experience with the Himba was seeing children content, self-regulated and self-motivated even while doing nothing or just curiously interested in us. We seldom see this in the hyper-stimulated over-scheduled children of our societies who become unable to be bored and be curious about human relationships. The ever-demanding pressures we have in today's society to keep our children entertained and all the attractions of the Internet have diminished our capacity for boredom, which is crucial for developing an "internal stimulus" that then allows true creativity and reflection. I recall boredom making me write from a very young age. I kept a diary, filling it with observations, poems and short stories. I ascribe these early beginnings to becoming an observer and writer later in life and to my young daughters doing the same in moments of boredom. Boredom is a chance to discover what truly interests us, contemplate life, be in the flow of life and be imaginative (Phillips, 1998). The capacity to do nothing, to be bored, can be a developmental achievement for the child.

The human work of art and implicit processes

Wisdom acknowledges the existence of energy fields behind the visible and considers human beings capable of moving from the purely physical to the purely energic. This is a fundamental capacity for connecting and understanding human needs and *being* as a whole. One of our human purposes is to move subtle energy from the latent realm into the physical realm, providing nourishment and immortality for the physical world.

In 1996 it was discovered that when an individual is in a state of heart rhythm coherence, their heart radiates a more coherent electromagnetic signal into the environment that can be detected by the nervous system of other people and even animals. It was found that the heart generates the strongest magnetic field in the body, approximately 100 times stronger than that produced by the brain (McCraty, 2015). This field can be detected several feet away from the body with sensitive magnetometers. The heart's electromagnetic field provides a plausible explanation of how we can *feel* or *sense* another person's presence and emotional state independent of body language and other factors. This is a key aspect of coherent mother-baby communication and co-regulation (through heart and breathing rhythms) prior and after birth. "The heart's intelligence by its very nature is inclusive, and heart coherence activates higher centres of the brain that experience compassion and the desire to help others develop their higher potentials" (Childre et al., 2016, p. 99). Accessing our natural wisdom or heart intelligence can create an energy field of unconditional love and harmony, helping people realise that we are all interconnected on Earth. Wisdom abilities, such as compassion and love, can bring all of us together coherently and make us thrive.

An aspect of primal wisdom is seeing things as they really are. It is important that babies are seen for what and how they are and not according to adults' expectations and agendas, in order to be understood and responded to sensitively. Dewey (1960/1933) describes the type of relational attention: "To grasp the meaning of a thing, an event or a situation is to see it in its relations to other things; to note how it operates or functions, what consequences follow from it; what causes it, what uses it can be put to" (p. 135). Receptive attention embraces the sensory communication system and heart intelligence and is essential in parenting. It is more likely to lead to eco-mindful morality, attending to and allowing an understanding of the whole picture and including detaching from ego-self (Narvaez, 2014).

Keeping the harmony between the visible and invisible worlds is a human work of art (Bourgeault, 2003). As human beings, we are "artisans of energy" whose cosmic role is to use energy consciously and constructively, keeping the fragile homeostasis of harmony between the visible and invisible worlds (Bourgeault, 2003). Human beings co-create the physical world through what they do and cultivate (e.g. prayers, meditation, songs, movements, dances, art and stories), which is a reflection of their inner or invisible (and perceptible) worlds.

From prenatal life, parents mould their children's predispositions through an interweaving of their *being* and *doing* – their beliefs, intonations, and quality of movements while holding their baby, gestures, facial expressions – and by keeping the fragile homeostasis between their child's behaviour (the visible) and physiological state (arousal/energy). My daughter Gisele revealed her awareness before birth in many ways. I would talk to her, recite a rhyme or simply contemplate about her and I knew she was engaged and was having pleasurable experiences, even if in a rudimentary way. I regularly listened to my favourite classical piano music and she learnt to respond more and more in rhythm with the music. Her movements changed from jerky to increasingly fluent with the maturational processes and her habituation to music. Gisele was born very curious, making eye contact and particularly interested in people. In my work with pregnant mothers and indigenous cultures, I have often seen this link between a mother's cultivated sense of relational presence in the womb and the baby's early awareness and capacity to attune.

Perceiving energy and acting accordingly or in harmony with it, an essential characteristic of wisdom, is highly relevant to parenting, caregiving and the infant-parent relationship. Babies may cry when their parents' energy in anger is translated into the movement and quality of their in-arm experience. Wisdom acknowledges the power of mood, energy and aliveness, the form in which it is expressed and is passing. What is happening these days shows that parents, human beings in general, have been greatly misusing their powers.

During pregnancy, an indigenous mother sings the same song she sang before conception (to the soul of the baby) to the baby in the womb, reassuring the baby of her place in the natural world. The baby is therefore introduced to the natural world. The pregnant mother has a sense of relationship with her child and is very focused on the life growing inside her. She senses how the child is affected by her actions and thoughts and behaves accordingly. The Himba baby is perceived as a sentient being, able to send cues with his motions. When the child is born, the mother is already in a reciprocal relationship with him. Our ancestor mothers teach us that maternal consciousness is about practice. In our Western world, there are almost no opportunities to practise it. These traditional beliefs show that having the baby in mind (mental representation) enhances maternal consciousness of the baby and can physiologically affect conception, pregnancy, birth and parenting.

It is interesting that indigenous and Aboriginal cultures have been aware of the influence of the conceptional environment for millennia. Prior to conceiving a child, couples hold ceremonies to purify their minds and bodies. As Church (2009) pointed out, every minute one million cells die and one million are born in your body, and your thinking and beliefs affect their health. This primal wisdom resonates with today's increasing acknowledgement of the importance of preparing the womb as an environment by enhancing prospective parents' well-being. Epigenetic studies provide evidence of how maternal experiences and mental states even before and during conception influence genetic expression over generations (Weaver et al., 2005, 2006).

Celebrating the movement of energy: songs, ceremonies and dances

From time immemorial, human beings have used communal rituals to cope with stress. Ancient Greek theatre seems to have developed out of religious rites that involved dancing, singing and reacting to mythical stories. Among the indigenous peoples, daily ritual songs, collective ceremonies and dances celebrate the movement of energy from life to death and back, as the universal activity of creation guides every aspect of living. Singing and dancing are tools for sharing knowledge. Social amusement such as jokes, as well as dances and songs, keep social interactions and moods positive. Indigenous dances and ceremonies, in particular those around conception and childbirth, through rhythmic movements, teach us the function of the rhythm in maintaining social ties and community life (Goodridge, 1999). They release tensions and regulate emotional states. Myths, stories and dreams are treated as alive and influencing well-being; visualisation is an "active form of meditation" (Four Arrows et al., 2010, p. 59). At the same time, stories allow us to lose self-consciousness and disappear into the mysteries of the Earth to discover the meaning of kinship through multiple levels of understanding (i.e. allegorical, spiritual). All these activities imply a wisdom-based way of knowing, requiring the whole being, in which body, mind and heart are prepared and integrated. They are not just activities; they are gateways of perception and tools for expressing the full potential of being. It is surprising how little research exists on how these collective activities affect the mind, brain and body and how they might prevent or alleviate trauma.

Theatre and drama are based on the properties of these creative activities and are integral parts of the treatment of trauma and other conditions (van der Kolk, 2014). van der Kolk (2014) describes how by playing a character, his son gained a chance to experience deeply and physically what it was like to be someone other than the learning-disabled, oversensitive boy he had gradually become due to chronic fatigue syndrome. Making a valued contribution to a group gave him a visceral experience of confidence, power and competence. The acted character became a new embodied version of himself, leading to the creative adult he is today. Our authorship or sense of agency relies on our relationship with our bodies and its rhythms. "In order to find our voice, we have to be in our bodies – able to breathe fully and able to access our inner sensations" (van der Kolk, 2014, p. 331). This is the opposite of dissociation, of being "out of body" and losing yourself.

Acting involves thoughts, desires and emotions but also breathing, the heart and movements, and each of these dimensions has its own rhythm. Traumatised people are terrified to feel deeply and to connect with their bodily sensations. They are afraid to experience their emotions because emotions lead to loss of control. In contrast, theatre offers them an opportunity to embody emotions, give voice to them, become rhythmically engaged, taking on and embodying different roles. Theatre involves releasing blockages to discover and telling the audience your own truth, exploring your own experience on stage (van der Kolk, 2014). Through acting and embodying different roles, traumatised people get in touch with the complexity of the human condition. Prof Vezio Ruggieri (2001), founder of the "Psychophysiological Theatre" in Rome, posits that we can imagine a human being as a coordinated mind-body whole of expressive rhythms. The wisdom-based way of self-regulating and knowing resonates with contemporary science, which is focused on the modalities through which different dimensions – imagination, emotions, movements, words and music – are connected to form an experiential unity.

Through storytelling and other interactive and creative activities, our indigenous cousins intentionally practise receptive attention and are aware of the importance of slowing down and taking time to notice all appropriate cues and make the right decisions, considering different perspectives (Kohn, 2013). This became clear, for instance, from the Himba's mindful slow-paced movements and social interactions, in particular with babies, contrasting with the hurried jerky movements of modern "civilised" humans. In this way, implicit knowledge (intuition, insights) cooperates with executive functions in sorting things out. Sacred knowledge is written deeply within our bodies and conveyed in gestures, not in words (Bourgeault, 2003). Indigenous cultures use contemplation and reflection, which are known to improve insights (Clark, 2008). These capacities are crucial to pay attention to bodily cues from unborn babies and children, as they react to our behaviour. Their reactions tell us whether we have upset them and need to stop. Therefore, attending to bodily cues is crucial to responsiveness and attunement.

Liedloff (1986) tells us about an Amazonian father who built a playpen in the jungle to protect his very young son. When he put the baby in the playpen, the baby felt his autonomy trapped, and he screamed with horror. The playpen was unsuitable for human babies. The father respected his son's reaction and accepted the failure of his experiment without question. He listened to the energy force that guided human behaviour and met babies' never-changing needs for two million years, still endangered by our highly developed intellect. But modern parents are subject to huge pressures – work, economy instability, running around and moving very fast – which disconnect them from embodiment and do not favour raising children. Parents do not actually know that they need to have the time to slow down with themselves and their children in order to observe, notice, mirror and respond.

Listening to music and speaking rhymes during my pregnancy strengthened the connection with my baby and sharpened my receptive attention and ability to pick up her cues. I discovered the fine power of musical sounds to penetrate the body and depth of the psyche and induce energy movement with healing and communicative effects, especially if combined with wisdom or mindfulness practice. Regularly listening to my favourite piano music shaped my daughter's sense of rhythm, love of playing piano and composing music, as well as her mindful personality. It created a blueprint. I recall her rhythmically dancing without music on (rocking side to side) while sitting up at four months old. It was as if she was performing the pieces memorised in her body during gestation, to which she had been regularly exposed. This possibility is strongly supported by Alfred Tomatis in his book on the power of sounds and their effects on development in intrauterine life (1991). The memory of sounds is also a memory of physical contact and energy in the womb, as sounds emit vibrations in the form of energy fields, especially if they have an emotional content. From an early age, Gisele manifested a capacity to attune with and understand others' feelings, write imaginative stories, mind-read or read beyond the visible and a curiosity about human development. She has always been open to meaningful interactions and affectionate contact.

Music contains an element that transcends verbal communication: spirituality. In his book *Alla Ricerca Della Madre* (In Search of the Mother, 2016) Prof Lucio Zichella writes about a son who lost his mother during birth, and whose mother lives in his recollection of the music she enjoyed playing on the piano during pregnancy. The embodied memory of musical sounds influenced his predisposition, his love of music, and opened him to perceiving the energy and catching its potential. Throughout his life, he felt an intimate need to perform on piano the pieces the mother had played (and he had heard) during gestation. These pieces seemed to be vividly present in his visceral memory. His constant search for his mother manifested in an obsessive bodily narrative, driven by the violent rupture of the mother-child continuum by her death. It generated anxieties that only music could soothe, inducing a psychophysiological regulation. Music almost re-established that missed continuum. The role of music documented through individuals' memories of musical pieces to which they were exposed during gestation resonates with ancient wisdom.

Music is an essential component of primal wisdom and well-being among all cultures, as it celebrates rhythm, fine non-verbal sensory communication, movement of energy and spirituality. Among some indigenous cultures, detailed knowledge of their beginnings is passed on to children throughout their childhood, including singing the same song to which the child was exposed in the womb (Turnbull, 1983). They are aware of the capacity of music to be stored in the body and maintain a safe continuum or recreate one when it has been broken.

3 Integrating primal wisdom with the modern Western worldview

From preconception to parenting and beyond

Exploring the contrast between primal wisdom and the dominant Western worldview can provide a key to understanding the dysfunctions in our society and why humanity has reached a major crisis. In a study of 9,508 adults who had completed a standardised medical evaluation and responded to a questionnaire about adverse childhood experiences, more than one-half reported difficult childhood experiences and household dysfunction, including stormy divorces, neglect and abuse, which affected their health and were even leading causes of death in adults (Felitti et al., 1998). The effects of trauma, including prenatal and birth trauma, are long-lasting, ranging from anxiety to post-traumatic stress disorders to physical illness. The latest scientific discoveries teach us that neurobiology is interpersonal. The brain is a social organ that is affected by the environment, particularly by the psycho-emotional environment. But by focusing solely on the role of family and parenting in childhood trauma and consequent brain changes, we miss the bigger picture. Society and culture play a significant role, as they are embedded through mechanisms of perception and create mindsets (way of thinking) that guide our behaviour, posture and gestures (including parenting), and become psychophysical reality (Ruggieri, 2001). If I fit in a social system, I need to perceive it, elaborate it, form a representation and connect it with other brain functions.

Genes are expressed thanks to perceptual stimulation from the social environment, thus experience, without which there would be no development of the body and mind. Infants deprived of sensory stimulation die. Spitz (1945) and Spitz and Wolf (1946) studied institutionalised children in orphanages and hospitals. The institutions were poor quality and staff rarely interacted with the children. They found that one-third of institutionalised children died before the age of one year. The other children failed to thrive and showed signs of "anaclitic depression": apathy, withdrawal and helplessness. Spitz compared children living in an orphanage with others living in a penal institution where they were cared for by their mothers. Although physical conditions in the orphanage were better, the children did not develop properly. Within two years, 37 per cent of the orphanage children were dead, whereas five years later, all the "prison" children were still alive.

While we know from research about the consequences of adverse childhood experiences in leading to addiction and suffering later in life, and what we all need to flourish, society is not putting this knowledge into practice (Mate, 2003). A lot of work has been done on the prevention and healing of trauma, but still we are not applying that knowledge in the mainstream. Gabor Maté points out that there are powerful forces in our society benefitting from not implementing the findings. Science exists within a social, political and economic context. Information is presented to the public according to the institution's orientation, a particular intellectual perspective, or those who influence policy making and so on. Thus, information is fragmented and incoherent, separates the mind from the body and soul and curtails the wholeness of being. In our Western culture, signs of mental illness, when we are suffering from severe fear, anxiety or depression, are seen as separate from other signs, such as irritable bowel syndrome, skin conditions, arrhythmia or asthma, which are seen as indications that our body and organs are not functioning well.

Now with new breakthroughs in our knowledge about the interconnectedness of the brain and the body, it is becoming clear that a mind/body division is no longer useful or valid. We are learning that the brain is an organ that is interwoven with the whole body and its system and influenced by the social environment, and how the body and its organs are constantly influencing the brain (Porges, 2011). The dense and complex system of interconnectivity defies categorisation and separation. Because it is all connected, those symptoms always defined as "mental" are indeed part of our bodies. As Peter Levine says (quoting D. H. Lawrence), "The body-unconscious is where life bubbles up in us". Wisdom practices foster mind-body awareness and an integrated state of being.

Then we need a society that coherently embodies what we intuitively know and what research has reaffirmed in accordance with old-age wisdom. For instance, if society supported mothers' as well as children's basic human needs for attachment and connection as early as gestation and even before (as small-scale societies have done for 99 per cent of human evolutionary history), we would promote a more integrated state of being in both of them and have fewer traumatised adults and much less suffering. Parents, prenatal and perinatal practitioners, medical students and psychiatrists, teachers and policy makers should all become aware of the crucial importance of meeting children's relational needs from as early as gestation. Most physicians never hear the word "trauma" or "attachment" in their education and have no understanding of it. They do not know the importance of relationships for brain development or complex interconnectedness between the brain, body, mind and soul.

We are not meant to be disconnected

The essence of trauma and consequent mental suffering is disconnection from ourselves, from our body and emotions and from other people (van der Kolk, 2014). Trauma is the shutdown of the bodily sensations and emotions. But our true nature is to be connected. It manifests from the very beginning of life: conception. There would be no human being without connection. The human species, like any species, could not have evolved without being grounded in the body. We would not have evolved if mothers had not felt safely connected with other members of the community to share childcare (Hrdy, 2011). Therefore, we are not meant to become disconnected. Disconnection is the result of a certain way of life, a certain style of parenting and thus certain childhood experiences that cause too much pain to stay connected, so disconnection becomes a defence. In all traditional and African indigenous societies I have visited, the connection and reciprocal support among members of the small community appeared to be the very element supporting parents' and children's well-being.

Supported by anthropological studies, my insights lead me to suggest that wisdom-based knowing can be used as a baseline model to explain the roaring rates of maternal and infant/child health issues today and inspire new ways to reconnect and heal starting from parenting and as early as pre-conception, gestational and birth period. I will have the pleasure throughout this book of presenting the reader with the findings of modern science that confirm the intuitions of age-old wisdom. "In pre-agrarian societies, wisdom is fostered from the beginning of life with companionship care and a society that provides support for basic needs throughout life" (Narvaez, 2014, p. 251). Because we have become so hyper-intellectual, so dependent on spoken and written language, we have neglected our energy-sensing communication system, our intuitive wisdom, heart intelligence, which has been our primary way of knowing for millennia. Our Western culture has emphasised the role of the left-brain hemisphere – rational, linguistic, explicit reflection processes – as dominant. But a new paradigm shift acknowledges the right-brain affective processes operating at levels beneath conscious awareness as dominant in development and psychopathogenesis (Schore, 1994, 2001a, 2001b). In addition to the limited analytic intellect is a vast realm of mind that includes psychic or extrasensory abilities – intuition, wisdom, a sense of unity and aesthetic, qualitative and creative capacities. These heart faculties are operating best when they are in concert.

Neuroscientist J. B. Taylor (2008) had a stroke in her left hemisphere, which left her with a right-hemisphere dominance that opened up a new way of perceiving reality, one very similar to the indigenous way of knowing. She could perceive all things having living energy, had no judgemental attitude, connected with the present moment and did not feel tight to her past or fearful of the future. She says,

> My right mind . . . honours my life and the health of all my cells . . . and it doesn't just care about my body; it cares about the fitness of your body, our mental health as a society, and our relationship with Mother Earth.
>
> (p. 141)

Quantum physics has come up against the objective limits of rational knowledge itself. Paul Davies, one of the most respected writers on physics and cosmology, makes this point very clearly in his book *The Mind of God* (1993). He reminds us that the challenge is to regain what he calls a "mystical" way of knowing. The rational mind by itself can see no more than self-cancelling parts. Accessing the underlying coherence beneath the surface chaos requires a different way of knowing. Davies clearly heralds the direction in which the Western mind may be travelling towards a renewed sense of dignity and coherence and a perception of divine purpose and beauty. It is a vision containing not only our minds but also our hearts and souls and attained by yielding of our whole being into the intimacy of knowing and being (Bourgeault, 2003). Interestingly, for the ancient Israelites, the word used for this kind of Wisdom-based knowing – *da' ath* – is the same word as for "knowing" a partner in sexual intercourse. Experiencing this underlying coherence requires self-giving and bearing the wounds of complete vulnerability, which is a major issue in traumatised people.

In any culture, people's imagination and expectations shape child-rearing practices, the children's predispositions, the sort of adults they become, the way they experience pregnancy, birth and parenting and the type of culture adults create for their children. It is through their resources – time available, interest, attention, imagination, creativity, passion, spirituality, love, moods and forms of vitality – and the way they treat their children (from gestation) that parents convey messages, which are perceived and stored in their children's cellular and visceral memory. These messages shape their self-perception, self-esteem, values and life purposes, in a kind of blueprint. Perceiving implies the formation of representations in the brain; it means representing the world.

Epigenetics is showing that trauma changes DNA through generations, unless the trauma is healed or moved beyond. These changes can be transmitted from the mother to the unborn and infant and across generations (Weaver et al., 2006; Yehuda et al., 2016). Children absorb and learn what they see and feel, especially from their caregivers. And so children, even unborn babies, can experience the mother's anxiety, low mood, or bliss or the emotional and spiritual states induced by the practice of mindfulness/wisdom. Early relationships between mothers and their infants can influence health across the lifespan, for better or worse. We see later on that the father and his relationship with the mother play an important role in child development and health. A study shows a possible link between increasing depression symptoms in mothers and cellular damage in their infants, which may increase their vulnerability to the early onset of poor health outcomes (Berens et al., 2017). Early adversity becomes "biologically embedded" in dysfunctional physiology involving body systems. The silver lining is that infancy is a sensitive developmental period when human beings are especially responsive to their environments. Fostering positive nurturing experiences between infants and their mothers – as well providing scientifically supported and compassionate caring services for mothers experiencing depression or other mental disorders – may allow infants to move towards a healthier life trajectory.

Primal wisdom cultures teach us that constant affectionate physical contact with a baby is critically important for a child's healthy development. Scientists have known this for decades. How often an infant is touched and held and the related feeling of connection and being felt can leave lasting effects not just on behaviour and growth, but all the way down to the molecular level of the DNA (Moore et al., 2017). The pleasurable experience affects the epigenome – the biochemical changes that influence gene expression in the body. This underscores the importance of feeling connected through physical contact, especially for distressed infants. The potential physiological benefits to infants sleeping in proximity to their caregivers, especially in the first year of life, and to breastfeeding, so biologically entwined to co-sleeping, have been described (McKenna et al., 1994; McKenna & Bernshaw, 2017). Breastfeeding and infant-parent co-sleeping have been both designed for adaptation by natural selection over millions of years of human evolution. Because human infants are born neurologically immature, develop slowly and remain dependent for a long period of time, continuous contact and proximity to the mother served to maximise the chances of infant survival and thus parental reproductive success (Konner, 2005). Feeling connected is hence a human biological necessity.

I will explain later on how a human foetus, during maturational processes leading to and preparing for birth and life outside the womb, already has a psychobiological identity designed to connect, influenced by the stimuli of the internal environment (maternal psychosociobiology – her emotions and behaviours also conditioned by her external environment and culture). This environment contributes to forming the baby's implicit (visceral) memory and nervous system regulation preparing for birth and life outside the womb.

In our society, children (and their parents!) are influenced by the media and the content narrated by those who create the media: their worldviews and interests shape children's perceptions about social and moral life, representations of it and behaviour (Oliver, 2005). The knowledge that used to be transmitted through real meaningful human interactions and shared experience through generations is now passed on through social media, virtually. This may create a distorted perception of self, other and the social and moral reality. How is this reality going to affect their parenting?

Furthermore, media, the use of electronic devices, the demands of our work-centred materialistic culture and consequent stress have considerable influence on politics, institutional policies and the distribution of resources, including the prenatal and perinatal healthcare professionals and services – all of which have led us away from the implementation of wisdom (and fostered human virtues). This has indirectly influenced families and children, including the way of conceiving them. For instance, today working parents have very limited time to provide the constant affectionate physical contact and responsive relationship babies expect to develop healthily. The quality of that little time is often impaired by the stress of long working hours, preoccupations and media interference, often as early as from pregnancy, leaving no time for contemplation or relational engagement. This lifestyle restricts imagination and perception, and imagination gives us the capacity to envision new possibilities and become freer of our genetic heritage.

The heavens of imagination

Imagination widens perception by opening the senses and heart, and thus enriches our experience. In turn, perception opens up the heavens of imagination. Imagination fosters creativity, problem-solving, frees us from boredom, alleviates our pain and stress, enhances our pleasure and enriches our most intimate relationships. Without imagination there is no hope, no chance to envision a better future and no goal to pursue. Inspiring people who lead by example to bring real change have strong imaginations, which open them to many possibilities. Imagination is what led an Australian senator to breastfeed in Parliament, clearly leading by example. Although it may have not been the best environment for such beautiful moments between mother and baby, that gesture was a creative strategy to generate a synergic movement. Isn't breastfeeding in public something that our indigenous cousins have done for all our human history and are still doing? It was interesting to see the humane, alive expressions of the politicians attending the meeting, who commonly appear angry or tense. This is called the oxytocin effect or heart resonance! We know that oxytocin is responsible for our feeling of love, social connection, trust and generosity; the social scientists call it the "molecule of social cohesion", which means that when this hormone is running high in individuals and society, society comes together and harmonises, rather than fragmenting and falling apart (Kok & Fredrickson, 2010). Who knows if by being exposed to this and similar gestures of human connection, policy makers' focus would more often shift towards better investments in childhood and families?

Imagination allows us to evoke in the body, e.g. in the muscles, an activity that we perceive in ourselves, just as an external stimulus does (Ruggieri, 1991). Professor of Clinical Psychophysiology Vezio Ruggieri explains that it is because of the relationship between imagination and perception (body process) that imagination can influence physiological processes. Therefore, imagination can be used as a powerful source of well-being and healing during pregnancy, birth and bonding. For instance, if we believe that trees can provide a healing energy, without wondering whether this could be true or not, what does seem to be true, is that when we believe it and do something about it – for example by sitting close to a tree in order to calm down – then we do indeed feel calmer. I quickly learnt the self-regulating homeostatic function of these beliefs and imagination during my visit to the Himba. Believing in the soul of the child before conceiving it boosts the couple's fertility. Indeed, our beliefs affect our cells, physiology and health (Lipton, 2015).

When we imagine something, the image can trigger sensations in the same way as an external stimulus. For example, inducing imaginary relaxation in a pregnant or birthing woman can have the same effect as inducing it with an external stimulus. If a mother imagines talking to her unborn baby and believes he is listening, or cradles him with rhythmic deep breathing, this has a physiological effect on her and the baby. Her mental representation of the baby evokes real bodily sensations of pleasure or relaxation that are passed to the developing baby. The Italian word *sentimento* derives from "*sentire*" (sensing), which links directly to the sensory experience.

Art therapies aim at widening the spectrum of imagination and perception, and that of experience, freeing us from genetic determinism, repeated patterns, and inhibiting blockages used as self-defence (Ruggieri, 2001). Those who have experienced trauma may use excessive muscle tension to block painful sensations felt during the traumatic event. Therefore, transformation occurs through a therapeutic approach including valuation and reorganisation of posture and movements, such as freeing the parent's gesture of holding the baby and rendering it mindful and attuned. Parents' inner worlds, love and all emotions become manifest through their posture, breathing, movements and other body language, which convey their way of being in the world and relating to the baby. Babies sense the quality of their caregiver's gesture and posture, its vitality and mindfulness – if it is tense or relaxed, full of vitality or apathy, approaching or avoiding – and this sensory experience shapes their spectrum of perception and mental representations.

Hypnotherapy, shamanic work, sound work and mindfulness can have the same effects. Scientists have discovered that being surrounded by birds and hearing their sounds is good for mental health and an antidote to depression (Cox et al., 2017). There may be calming or curative elements at work here, but it is also true that imagination is a powerful healing source. If we can use our minds to enter positive states and hold positive beliefs, these can in turn contribute to a form of nourishment or healing. This is what indigenous mothers have done for millennia to prepare mind, body and soul for conception and welcome the child into a healthy womb.

Securing the foundations of human connection before birth

Creative imagination enriches our resources and, under favourable social circumstances, enables us to use them. It enables a pregnant couple to nourish a relationship with their developing baby. Imagining a relationship with the unborn baby changes the representation of pregnancy, with the perception of the baby as a sentient being rather than an inert organism. These processes shape a prenatal mother – baby attachment leading to emotional availability. Emotionally available parent-child relationships are a good indicator of the quality of interaction and supportive of child health and development (Barfoot et al., 2017). We know that long before birth, the quality of a mother's prenatal attachment towards her unborn baby is essential for development (Branjerdporn et al., 2016). This finding is supported by clinical evidence as well as millennia of indigenous maternal experiences. The meaningful interactions on which prenatal attachment is based provide an intersubjective ground as the material from which the mind is created. Studies suggest that our capacity to empathise with others may be mediated by embodied prenatal and perinatal mechanisms, that is by the activation of the sensorimotor circuits underpinning our own emotional and sensory experiences (Ammaniti & Gallese, 2014).

The other is present in the self-experience from conception – without the other there would be no self. Therefore, the prenatal self is a visceral self on which mental processes are built through an intimate communication between mother and baby and meaningful others. The body is the "very basis of human subjectivity" and we have to take bodily manifestations and wisdom much more seriously than we have so far (Shaw, 2004). The narrative of interactions with my preborn baby will show this entanglement of the body. To further sustain the function of prenatal engagement, findings consider the quality of foetal-maternal interactions as psychobiological precursors to adaptive infant development (Novak, 2004).

Alfred Tomatis describes the foetus's sonorous experience, in particular listening to the maternal voice (its timbre, tone and emotional nuances) as an organiser of his hearing system and listening (1987). My work with mothers and infants and my first pregnancy experience led me to the insight that *in-utero* perception of meaningful music and maternal voice may play a role in child development. In particular, it may regulate the baby's nervous system and muscle tensions and shape a rudimentary sense of rhythm through her sensorimotor responses to the melody. We know that the baby's responses to sonorous stimulation are intentional and conscious, even though it is a rudimentary intentionality. The memory of sounds is also the memory of physical contact and energy in the womb, as sounds emit vibrations in the form of energy fields, especially if they have an emotional content.

The American psychologist Evelyn Thoman proved the social nature of interactions inside and outside the womb and how motion and emotion work in synchrony from prenatal life (Thoman & Graham, 1986). She documented the vital importance for premature babies to *continue* to be close to human stimulating rhythms, which they have developed within the womb. The Italian clinical psychologist and psychotherapist Gaetano Persico has written a book entitled *La Ninna Nanna: Dall'Abbraccio Materno Alla Psicofisiologia Della Relazione Umana* (The Lullaby: from In-Arm Experience to the Psychophysiology of Human Relationship), describing how the quality of maternal holding, including her embodiment and forms of vitality (e.g. muscular tension) during pregnancy, contributes to shaping our physiology and future ability to self-regulate and deal with relationships (2002).

Elementary mirroring mechanisms fostered by mother-baby intersubjectivity may play a role in children's development and emotional attunement with their mothers long before birth (Ferrari et al., 2016). During a 33-week scan while I was listening to my favourite musical piece, my baby looked content, seeming to attentively perceive the music and tune into my emotional response to music. Observations suggest that when the unborn baby hears music, she responds to the maternal emotional response to it and the related biochemical mediators (Zimmer et al., 1982). Investigators have explored whether the propensity to socially interact and engage is already present before birth, suggesting that the unborn baby is a sentient being, responsive to maternal communications (Carter Castiello et al., 2010). Prosocial and love capacities emerge easily from companionship and care, where since conception the environment signals "all the way down" that the child is welcome (Emerson, 1996; Lake, 1979). This energy state is transferred to subsequent generations.

Clinical accounts argue that parents' anxieties and stress may harm the vital intersubjective bonds, birth and development, suggesting that bonding before birth is vital for growth and development (Ammaniti & Gallese, 2014). It is plausible, if we consider the baby's essential need for meaningful connection, that poor prenatal connection between mother and baby, along with pollutants contained in the air and processed food and nutrients deficiency, may be a contributing factor in the brain disorders responsible for autism spectrum disorders that affect an increasing number of children today. In the last decades, the mother-baby intimate space has weakened, mainly due to a technological stress-driven culture, with adverse consequences on prenatal attachment, birth outcome and maternal and infant health. This provides a foundation for assessing and improving prenatal attachment and intersubjective engagement through wisdom practice, or related mindfulness, to harness the power of our body-mind for personal transformation.

Scientific and clinical studies and insights provided by indigenous wisdom practices depict an unborn baby as a sentient being. This can change the way we relate to pregnant mothers and their developing babies. A more humane approach to pregnancy means using empathy, compassion and deep listening, so as to foster these right-brain to right-brain communication virtues in the mother and child.

By practising wisdom, we can re-sculpt our mental pathways and break free from the mental patterns that hold us back from living life, therefore pregnancy, birth and child caregiving to the fullest (Siegel, 2009). We can rewire our brain for greater happiness and well-being through our mind. Siegel argues that the connections between wisdom traditions, attachment theory, mindfulness practice and well-being and integrating the functions of the prefrontal cortex as a window into wisdom, kindness and compassion are striking. The functions of the prefrontal cortex are body-self regulation, attunement with others, emotional integration and balance, modulation of fear, flexibility of response, receptive attentiveness, engagement with life, insight, intuition, empathy and morality, all fostered by wisdom practice and all essential for healthy development (Siegel, 2007). Mindfulness practice expands our capacity for engagement, compassion, affective empathy, receptive attentiveness, relational attunement, imagination, sense of humanity, reciprocal communication, intersubjectivity in the moment, right-brain affective communication and emotional regulation. These are all age-old wisdom capacities that benefit prenatal attachment and the mother's and child's well-being.

Few things are as meaningful as conception, pregnancy and being a part of our children's childhood because they concern the future of our humanity. What is the point of climbing the steps of our professional career having missed the enjoyment of pregnancy, or our children's first steps? What is the point of being a famous businessman if your child doesn't even know his father? What is the point of having a baby and sending him to nursery at the premature age of just a few months, depriving him of the meaningful one-to-one interactions and constant affectionate physical contact that make him a happy, positive contributor to his family and our society?

People may become so addicted to a certain way of life that it can be difficult and painful to change, and our governments do not help, as they are influenced by the mindset themselves. But we need to rediscover the ability to use our powers and mitigate the effects of trauma or cultural conditioning. We need to believe that change is possible through wisdom and mindfulness practices. We need to reclaim the joy of waking up every morning full of energy and exhilaration and decide to self-author our lives. We can then experience the ecstasy of an inspired pregnancy, birth and babyhood, hence an inspired life.

We need to live our children's childhood with mindfulness, joy and wonders. This is translated into a beneficial increase in our endorphins and oxytocin levels – our feel-good hormones – and the health of our cells (Lipton, 2015; Church, 2009). This has a collective resonance effect on our heart-related abilities. We need to take the time to attentively watch children grow and thrive. The best gift we can give our children is our empathic love. They need to feel more important than the fleeting rewards of our professional career. They need us to be fully present and connected with their experience rather than our minds to avoid being carried away by external instructions, fears or other effects of stress.

Are we losing our capacity for nurture and the essence of parenting?

If we do not work towards sealing the gap between the realm of age-old wisdom and the Western worldview, the incongruences in the prenatal and perinatal healthcare system are unlikely to be solved. The intersubjective nature of human relationships, from prenatal life, on which healthy growth and mental development rest, includes our mammalian caring skill, the care for our mammalian needs, and the care of our soul. The Western worldview has had to do mainly with intellectualisation, mentalising and the dominance of the rational, leading to amazing scientific and technological discoveries, but also leading us (and parents) away from human wisdom and fundamental virtues. Modern obstetric practices interfere with the unfolding of mother-baby mammalian wisdom. Stress and mental ill health have undermined mother-baby intersubjectivity ever since conception and gestation. Parenting begins at conception and is rooted in our culture, politics, family and early caregiving experiences. It is much influenced by communal creative imagination and the way we perceive children and families. For instance there is something incongruous and bizarre in the modern cultural attitude that it is fine to force children into independence prematurely, such as by putting them to sleep in a separate room at only a few days or months old, leaving them to cry, or leaving them in a nursery before they are ready.

Most people do not even notice how disconnected modern people are from each other, compared to cultures where the bond is still intact. For instance we know how in Mediterranean cultures people learn and receive support from one another, but we are not aware of the connection between these phenomena and how our bonds between each other and with nature and the divine have been torn asunder. In one UK town, Frome in Somerset, there has been a dramatic fall in emergency hospital admissions since it began a collective project to combat isolation (paper awaiting publication). The compassionate Frome project was launched by Helen Kingston, a GP (general practitioner) who noticed that patients were defeated by the medicalisation of their lives: being treated as if they were a cluster of symptoms rather than a human being who happened to have health problems. I hold that this unnoticed, epidemic disconnection is the source of much mental suffering, also reflected in prenatal and perinatal ill health. Disturbances in embryonic, foetal and child development are only the tip of a silent iceberg.

If in the US, the UK and other countries, children's emotional needs are far from being at the centre of policy making (unlike countries such as Finland, Holland and Canada), this may be partly because of politicians' upbringing and consequent insecure attachment style, which may lead to a harsh attitude. The national political focus on children's needs has been short-term, ephemeral, inconsistent and untrustworthy. In the UK, you may still go to a public place and read, "Children not allowed here", showing society's intolerance of children. Unlike traditional and indigenous societies, English and US cultures tend not to celebrate childhood. The UK has been accused of failing its children, as it came bottom of a league table for children's well-being across 21 industrialised countries (UNICEF, 2007). One of the key factors seems to be parents' not spending enough time with their children and not involving them in their lives. Children's mental health in the UK seems to be far worse than 40 years ago. The rate of infant mortality and premature births is one of the highest.

Children's needs, happiness and well-being, from conception and gestation, should be at the centre of public and political attention because not meeting their emotional needs has serious implications for humanity and society. Their bereavement predisposes them to learning difficulties, mental health issues, aggressiveness, challenging behaviour and criminality (Anda et al., 2006). Therefore, parents' well-being and mental health need to be supported so that they can meet their children's basic needs and enjoy them. A comparison between primal wisdom and the Western worldview teaches us about the unchanging emotional needs of children in our ever-changing society. It took 99 per cent of human history to develop prenatal, perinatal and childcare practices that foster emotional, social and moral well-being (Hrdy, 2011). But the recent changes in our society have occurred too quickly for us to adapt without serious consequences for our health. Primal wisdom is a body of interdisciplinary knowledge that crosses cultures and historical periods, although there is more than one route to wisdom (Narvaez, 2014).

We need to turn to the wisdom of our ancestors and integrate it with our advances, when it comes to finding more humane child-rearing practices, since they foster healthy development and stability. Children of wisdom traditions are viewed with a much higher sense of integrity and are assumed to be competent, fully entitled members of society from a very young age. Cultures with more "progressive" unenlightened (according to Western standards) views of children tend to have harsher child-rearing practices. Historically, in becoming an object of study, childhood needed to be recognised as a unique stage of life; instead it was objectified and children were essentially removed from adult life. They became subject to inspection, management, control, exploitation and misunderstanding, at the expense of human connection. Describing the continuum from foetus to child and adult, Montagu writes, "We think we know that an adult human being is nothing like the foetus curled up in its mother's womb . . . we tend to believe that grown ups and children are two separate classes of beings . . . yet the truth about the human species is that in body, spirit, feeling and conduct we are designed to grow and develop in ways that emphasise rather than minimise childlike traits . . . we were never intended to grow 'up' into the kind of adults that most of us have become" (Montagu, 1986).

Imagination that includes relational being

Although creative imagination is emphasised in both primal wisdom and the Western view, the latter imagination is more focused on technical manipulation and innovation and change, not inclusive of intersubjectivity or relational being. As Einstein stated, "Logic will take you from A to B. Imagination will take you everywhere".

During the few thousand years since we left the way of life to which evolution had adapted us, human beings have not only altered the natural harmony of the entire planet, but also disrupted the highly evolved intuitive wisdom that guided our behaviour and sustained our well-being for millions of years (Liedloff, 1986). Much of this good sense, vital in guiding mothering and bonding, has been undermined recently as the rationale of science and technology has taken over. Mothers started to rely on instructive books and "experts" instead of their own intuitive resources, which are fundamental to connect with the baby and respond to their unchanging emotional needs and expectations. Natural-birth advocate and obstetrician Michel Odent reckons that pregnant women should not read books about pregnancy and birth as their time is too precious. He believes they should, rather, watch the moon and sing to their baby in the womb. In Victorian times, pregnant women were advised to be exposed to the arts, visiting art galleries, telling stories to their unborn babies, singing, believing that education began in the womb. I always felt my unborn daughter benefitted from my being embedded in nature, in a landscape covered with snow, listening to birdsong, with the waves warming the seashores or my favourite piano music and writing my pregnancy memoir. Our innate sense of what is best for us has been dominated by the intellect, which knows little or nothing about our real needs. The Western tendency is to escape from natural wisdom, and from trusting our mammalian caring competence, which for 99.99 per cent of our history has secured natural birth, extended breast-feeding, fulfilling parenting, empathy, trust in shared childcare and infant/child well-being.

Although the constant closeness between mother and baby has for many million years been a source of health and well-being, human beings evolved with a particular type of care provided not just by the mother and father but by a forging community (Hrdy, 2011). In these communities, children were often nursed by their mothers, grandmothers and other members of the community, which secured the continuity after nine months in the womb. These practices were transmitted through generations by default, securing their epigenetic consistency. For an unborn baby and child, having his or her needs met was facilitated by the support of the entire community and mother's nurturing mental state. The mother's intuitive embodied wisdom and mammalian instinct, and her reflective understanding of her baby unfolded as a matter of routine, undisturbed by modern medical interference, media influence or social isolation. These are the conditions that make a human being and are shared by all mammals, although humans are much more sensitive to social care. It is in the word "we" (from conception and beyond), in the collective reference, that interdependence of humans lies. And we need to recognise this to have hope in the birthing of a new healthy humanity.

The Northern European cultures have, in the name of "civilisation" and "progress", gradually destroyed the tribe/village/extended family or community and replaced it with the nuclear family and its disastrous consequences. The consequences are immense, leading to overwhelming pressures of isolation, particularly for mothers, who often end up bearing total responsibility for their children. A mother's perception of low social support or isolation during pregnancy and the perinatal period leads to depression, anxiety and other forms of psychological disorder (Priel & Besser, 2002; Hagen & Barret, 2007). At the same time, our sudden unprepared exposure to the needs of an infant – for suckling at the breast, being lovingly held, being constantly in the presence of her caregiver – who expresses them vocally and physically when these are not met, may stir up our buried memories of our denied needs as infants, plunging us into deep pain and psychological suffering. These patterns are likely to be transmitted through generations if the real need is not addressed and the trauma is not healed.

Girls in our cultures also get far less nurturing than required and suffer the consequences of failed bonding, which will affect their own motherhood. We are already living through a crisis of touch. People hug less. As humans feed the illusion that virtual devices can substitute for real time in affective tactile interactions, they also become more and more in need of touching and hugging. The neglect of this fundamental need (not just infants' but also adults') is seriously threatening humans' well-being. I have been advocating nurturing touch in my classes and therapy for many years in these times when we are literally in danger as a society of losing touch with ourselves and with one another.

To decide how a baby is to be treated is not a matter for the reasoning capacity. But women often call on instructive books to find answers. We have distanced ourselves so much from this long-standing intuitive knowledge that we rely on research to find out how we should behave towards children, ourselves and one another. But parents need to go back to their reliance on their body wisdom and whole being. The experts and practitioners are so restricted by the knowledge they get during their training that despite their failure in discovering the key to happiness and well-being, they keep interpreting the problems from a "reasoned" perspective and ignore what reason cannot understand or control (Liedloff, 1986). We even expect to heal through the intellect. Practitioners may expect a mother affected by a mental condition to heal by introducing a good "technical adviser" into the alien territory of the unique mother-baby subjective experience and their needs, rather than applying heart-based and relational qualities. With beautiful insight, Jean Liedloff explains that of course, our ability to reason is suitable for other businesses but not those areas that for many million years have been managed by the more refined and knowledgeable areas of the mind called "intuitive wisdom" (1986). While the conscious intellect can consider only one thing at a time, the intuitive mind can perceive what is behind the surface, the invisible and the wholeness of it.

I believe it is possible to heal the adverse effects of the predominance of the intellect and reasoning, including birth trauma and perinatal mental ill health, by reconnecting with our authentic human virtues, fostered by our more refined and insightful areas of the mind. These areas of the right-brain hemisphere are the site of wisdom, intuition, insight, affective empathy and compassion. They integrate body, mind and heart qualities. A right-brain to right-brain communication shapes an attuned relationship between mother and child and is the foundation of secure attachment (Schore, 1994, 2001a).

Birth as the unleashing power of wisdom

Due to the dominance of medical control and technical advice, our hospitalised birthing practices induce stress in mother and child by interfering with their animal instinct, the physiological process of birth and their psychobiological bond, providing a sensory shock (bright light, rushing, separating a baby from the mother, handling the baby roughly). This is aggravated by the fact that birth-related professionals are often under stress themselves. Birth is a sequence, a mother-baby partnership, an embodied narrative that needs to unfold through a free dance. It is a continuum that is an imprint, or a sensory experience of how we are in this world and do things, of wisdom. In the US, circumcision is widespread in medical practice, traumatising babies. The kind of impressions a baby stores in his body leads him to trust or distrust the world.

Primal wisdom finds its security in the natural world and the undisturbed continuum of development from intrauterine life, whereas the Western worldview finds it in innovation promoted by ego, intellect and technology (Narvaez, 2014). While the 3D scan mistakenly detected the small size of my second baby's head and possible neurological implications, it was my obstetrician friend's experienced touching of my belly that proved to be accurate in sensing the normal size and reassuring me. Dr Yehudi Gordon retained the old-age wisdom of a birth practitioner. While primal wisdom implies human beings live in harmony with nature and bodily sensations, the West tends to distrust nature and dominate and manipulate it. To me, the denial of our natural body wisdom and relational being (especially with babies and children, but also with our partner, birth practitioner and the entire community) could explain why modern parenting is in a serious crisis and why we need to bring a new paradigm of parenting and well-being to the fore. This paradigm shift is based on an awareness of the unchanging emotional needs of children, including their prenatal needs. To change the world, we must first change the way pregnant mothers are treated and babies are being born.

The distrust in those far more refined areas of the mind in charge of primal wisdom may be a major contributing factor in pregnancy and birth complications, perinatal mental ill health and the failure of healthcare, as it hinders the practitioner-client/parent relationship of compassion and empathy. This lost wisdom is also reflected in how human beings are destroying the Earth and its resources. While industrialisation and technology have led to many improvements in our lives, we have distanced ourselves from our most fundamental human needs and the importance of birth and early life has been left aside. We do not make the connection between the quality of birth and childhood we had and the kind of society and culture we live in. Social media and the use of technological devices certainly do not facilitate any turning of the tide. The iPhones, Tweets and Instagrams are driving our children (and adults) away from practising the most fundamental human virtues and an appreciation of them. How are these young people going to be wise, connected and responsive parents? What opportunities of experiencing empathy are our children offered to become nurturing sociable human beings?

We need to find a way back to our best interests, integrating what we had with our modern sensibility and advances, beginning in the womb. Only this reconciliation can preserve humanity's well-being and prevent endeavours that are leading us astray. "The more a culture relies on the intellect to decide policy and rules, the more restraints on the individual are necessary to maintain it" (Liedloff, 1986, p. 39). The social and moral behaviour of a child develops through her or his exposure to expected influences and examples set by her parents and society. She perceives what is expected by her culture. This can create heart-related abilities and resonance of the heart in intelligence. When I visited the Himba, a young girl mindfully carrying a baby or witnessing other women in constant physical contact with their babies and breastfeeding was a common scene. This has a powerful cultural influence, as it provides a shared example that shapes caregiving physiology and behaviour. Learning is a process of fulfilling expectations that shapes the emotional regulation of the child as well as her social and moral development. In many Western societies, childhood is not celebrated and nurtured and this affects children's self-perception. If we want to prevent more damage to our society, we need to start from parenting, ideally before conception, to have an impact on children's well-being and the next generations.

The neglect of relational being in the Western worldview is a consequence of extreme individualism, while primal wisdom considers each self to be the agent and part of a common self (Narvaez, 2014). Narvaez pinpoints that in wisdom traditions, social cohesion and morality derive from reciprocal intersubjective relations with all entities. Compassion comes from Nature, being learnt through mammalian caring behaviour and its continuum from life in the womb and beyond, not from law or education. For the Western worldview, morality is external to the self and develops through coercion. In primal wisdom, all people are part of the common self and non-group members are welcomed with hospitality, whereas in the Western worldview, others are distrusted and tribalism and competition are encouraged. This may create huge gaps in the healthcare system, including perinatal and children's healthcare, as every agency or organisation operates as a singular entity and in a territorial way rather than cooperating. Rather than sharing knowledge and multidisciplinary mindsets, we have hyper-specialisation that prevents acknowledging the broad spectrum of reality and its interconnections. This is reflected in our maternity care, mother-baby units and perinatal and infant mental health. Policy making is also a reflection of this. In primal wisdom, there is a strong sense of sharing in a gift-based economy. So, each child is a community child, childcare is shared and everyone is responsible for his well-being. Giving is a source of power. In contrast, the Western worldview values private property, and the accumulation, not sharing, of resources represents power. Even a child is a private business.

A broader spectrum of reality

Wisdom-based tradition acknowledges a broader spectrum of reality that includes invisible energy, the non-manifest, the whole picture and the connections between its parts, whereas the Western worldview is focused on manifest phenomena through science, measurement and technology, and so it is reductionist. It follows that wisdom allows for a wide perception and multiple perspectives, including the intersubjective one, whereas in the modern dominant view, perception is narrow and materialistic. Therefore, wisdom is an essential part of the study of human development, including the prenatal and perinatal period, and is open to an interdisciplinary approach. It is reductionist to study human development and health merely through science. The rigour of scientific methods needs to be combined with the power of embodied intuition and other wisdom abilities.

The modern Western worldview, which is the cultural lens through which most of us perceive ourselves and the world, was founded in the surge of intellectual energy generated by the Enlightenment. Its American founders adopted the Cartesian "I think, therefore I am" as the pursuit of liberty and happiness. "This bias toward the individual, already deeply engraved in the American character from the earliest days of nationhood (and from there imprinted on the rest of the world), has been mightily reinforced in more recent history by Freudian psychology, with its foundational use of the term *ego*, to designate the conscious, functional seat of our personal self-hood" (Bourgeault, 2003, p. 64). In this view, we experience ourselves first and foremost as egoic beings, as individual selves. It follows that we suffer from mistaken identity. Our real "I", our being, lives far more deeply, in an inner form, and its real beauty and authenticity is conveyed in the quality of our embodied aliveness, in the harmony of our postural or muscular tensions. This quality of aliveness is the essence of our own life. It is simple enough to observe the difference between a child who is loved and cared for with receptive attention and a child who is neglected. An energic transaction occurs through the act of loving. The individual is embedded in the flow of a narrative with the other, from the very first moments of conception.

In wisdom, life is eternal and death is a transformation to new life, therefore there is no fear of death. By contrast, in our modern worldview life is perceived as lonely and limited. Primal wisdom individualises knowledge and relationships and recognises the unique subjective experience, whereas the Western worldview tends to abstract and make generalisations. This view delivers hyper-specialised knowledge, mainly based on technique, which hinders intuitive knowledge of the whole and its depth. This has a significant impact on parenting and mental health education and care, in which understanding of real needs and individualised care are vital and require sensitivity, intuition, attentive listening, connection, attunement and empathy. The Western worldview emphasises intellectual and book-based knowledge, whereas primal wisdom values intuitive knowing, deep, experiential, personal knowledge that tunes into a communal awareness, which involves a connection with every element and creature of the Earth, with our mammalian and intersubjective nature. This Western focus on intellect, reason, abstract and generalisation (left-hemisphere dominance) governs birth, parenting and mental health education today.

We can see how the emphases of each worldview can influence parenting, the way we value and organise child-rearing, our sociocultural and ethical orientations and ecological sensibility. Modern industrialised societies have distanced themselves from the prenatal and perinatal practices that made us human in first place and caused a global ecological crisis. Wisdom is about love, communion and commonality that fostered well-being early on in life, unlike the Western worldview that generates fear, safety and control as a consequence of learning and acting in accordance with abstract rules (Narvaez, 2014). If we want to restore well-being in our societies, we need to revalue wisdom. On being asked by the Pharisees when the Kingdom of God would come Jesus replied, "the Kingdom of Heaven is within you" (Luke 17: 21). Enlightenment is about realising the Kingdom of Heaven here and now, to look right through the physical appearance of things and respond to their innermost aliveness and quality (Marion, 2000). Marion argues that by "the Kingdom of Heaven", Jesus is actually referring to a state of non-dual consciousness that sees no separation between God and myself or between my neighbour and myself, between a pregnant woman's well-being and my smile or kind gesture towards her. This is the highest state of consciousness attainable by human beings while still in a bodily form. In my view, much suffering related to perceived isolation during pregnancy and the perinatal period is a consequence of the lack of this common consciousness.

Only the marriage of individual and communal wisdom practice can change mindsets, feelings and behavioural patterns due to the changes induced by regular practice in brain structure and functioning. This means that living well and healthily is only partly determined by our genes. Richard Davidson has suggested that a small percentage of an individual's affective style is genetically determined (Davidson, 2004; Davidson & McEwen, 2012). The rest is done by self-cultivation and self-location, including nutrition, lifestyle, relationships and a sense of community. These need to be regularly practised for the new parent's well-being, for a secure attachment and for the well-being of all of us and next generations.

The Western worldview has long been reflected in psychotherapy, behavioural and cognitive psychology. Currently science is exploring bodily-based emotions, subjective embodied processes and human virtues, and therapy is focusing on affective psychobiological states. There is a scientific, clinical and public interest in mindfulness practice and the related wisdom virtues fostered by it. "Affective processes appear to lie at the core of the self, and due to the intrinsic psychobiological nature of these bodily-based phenomena recent models of human development, from infancy throughout the lifespan, are moving towards brain-mind-body conceptualizations" (Schore, 2003b, p. xiv). Recent studies have focused on the embodiment of the mind since conception and gestation (Delafield-Butt & Gangopadhyay, 2013). Right-brain affective processes operating at levels beneath conscious awareness are dominant in development, mental illness and psychotherapy (Schore, 2012). Wisdom and mindfulness, and their psychobiological nature, have also become an object of exploration (Siegel, 2009).

The recovery of ancient wisdom in our contemporary world has been reflected in the discovery of quantum physics, which acknowledges the presence of an energy continuum running through all of creation, a fluidity of movement along this energy continuum, of divine consciousness at every level. Although the subtle energies cannot at this point be measured by science, we know they have a real impact on our physical world. These would include the energies of attention, will, meditation, prayer and love. Believing in this energy system is highly relevant to the mother-baby relationship and implicit communication as early as gestation. These energies of present attention are the ingredients conveyed through the loving between a parent and their child and in any love relationship. Now it is right here where spiritual wisdom and science come together. To the purely rational intelligence, this realm of psychic force is invisible; it does not exist or is pure speculation. But in the Wisdom way of knowing, this subtle energy is perceptible to the awakened heart and reveals a vast inner kingdom to be discovered and fulfilled (Bourgeault, 2003). It is a subtle intelligence illuminating the outward form.

The book *The Science of Meditation: How to Change Your Brain, Mind and Body* by Daniel Goleman and Richard Davidson highlights the intriguing dovetail between scientific data and ancient maps in relation to altered human traits (Goleman & Davidson, 2017). The authors recall an eighteenth-century Tibetan text advising that among the signs of spiritual progress are loving-kindness and strong compassion towards everyone, contentment and "weak desires" (Abboud, 2014). These qualities seem to match with an indicator of brain changes: activation of a set of circuits, those for empathic concern and parental love, and a more relaxed amygdala (centre of intense emotional reaction) (Klimecki et al., 2013). In many East Asian countries, the name Kuan Yin, the symbol of compassionate awakening, translates as "the one who listens and hears the cries of the world in order to come and help" (Thich Nhat Hanh, 2012). Most modern parents' approach to childcare is far from being this compassionate.

There is today a new paradigm shift from a divided brain, and dominance of intellect, reason and verbal language to a dual interdependent brain, embracing the dominance of the right brain and its wisdom-related functions. The shift is from a rational brain to an emotional brain, a linguistic brain to a social brain, explicit versus implicit energy, conscious versus unconscious mind (McGilchrist, 2009). A new focus has shifted from the postnatal versus the prenatal roots of mind and subjectivity (Ammaniti & Gallese, 2014). The right brain stores implicit processes – non-verbal for the holistic perception of emotional information, for social interactions and for affiliative motivations (Schore, 2001a, 2012). Expansion of the right brain, fostered by early experiences with caregivers through empathic cooperation, leads to adults with creative imagination and prioritising relationship. Interpersonal competence is the capacity to interact and communicate with others, to share personal views, to perceive the subtle energies, to understand the emotions and opinions of others and to cooperate with others or resolve any conflict that occurs. It is at the basis of affective empathy. Schore suggested that dysfunction in the development of the right hemisphere might affect infant mental health and interpersonal competence and thus lead to social difficulties in later stages of development (2001b). This finding raises the question: what are electronic devices doing to our children's brains and future capacities for interpersonal competence?

Implicit communication and body wisdom

The recovery of wisdom can also be seen in the therapeutic setting. Although technique and strategies are important, the quality of the therapeutic relationship, the acknowledgement of relational being, compassion and sharing, is the most robust aspect of a therapeutic outcome (Magnavita, 2006). Attention to the non-verbal, bodily cues and communication is encouraged by a wisdom-based perspective. "Without the non-verbal it would be hard to achieve the empathic, participatory and resonating aspects of intersubjectivity. One would only be left with a kind of pared down, neutral 'understanding' of the other's subjective experience" (Stern, 2005a, p. 80). With an intersubjective perspective, a more conscious processing of the non-verbal and bodily cues is necessary. This is particularly important for professionals working with pregnant mothers, parents and infants, as right-brain to right-brain intuitive communication governs their interactions and well-being.

The "second channel" of human communication, non-verbal and emotional, functions alongside that based on rational thinking and verbal communication, and it is much more important in human relationships than most people think (Buchanan, 2009). Non-verbal emotional communication, mental states that are in essence private to the self – self-awareness, intuitive wisdom, affective empathy and intersubjectivity – are all dependent on right hemisphere function, which is the first to develop, and may be shared between individuals (Decety & Chaminade, 2003).

Research suggests that when sensitivity and flexibility govern therapeutic interventions, it produces better outcomes than rigid application of principles (Castonguay & Beutler, 2006). Sensitivity is described as being susceptible to the attitudes, feelings or circumstances of others; perceiving very slight changes of emotions and bodily cues, which is in line with the wisdom-based way of knowing. Our behaviour and every action and gesture we produce have a quality of aliveness, a unique fragrance or vibrancy (Bourgeault, 2003). According to Bourgeault, our inner form, our real beauty and authenticity is conveyed in the quality of our aliveness, where the essence of our own being lies. This fragrance defines the quality of human relationships, in particular the mother-infant relationship, the triad including the father, their attunement, and is impaired by excessive stress and ill health.

Schore (2005, p. 845) describes the therapist's right-brain involvement: "the sensitive clinician's oscillating attentiveness is focused on barely perceptible cues that signal a change in state, and on non-verbal behaviours and shifts in affects". This intuitive wisdom allows a wider perception of what is "beyond" the verbal and the manifest. For example it allowed me to connect with indigenous mothers and quickly understand the meaning of their words by perceiving bodily cues that signalled shifts in state and affect. This occurred in fractions of a second, before our guide's translation. Any human relationship and even interaction, not just psychotherapy, is an inherently embodied process. We can see this clearly in the interactions between mother and infant. We need to take our bodily reactions much more seriously than we have so far because the body is the very basis of human subjectivity (Shaw, 2004). There is wisdom in the body. My narrative of the interactions between my unborn baby and me will show this exquisite embodiment of relational presence.

The intersubjective space between an empathic clinician and a client (e.g. the parent) includes more than two minds, but two bodies (Schore,

2005). This refers to any practitioners and mindfulness or wisdom facilitators working with pregnant mothers and parents. The therapist's practised sensitivity is the primary instrument brought to healing. In many ways, this sensitivity (wisdom in general) is akin to a musical instrument that must be carefully prepared, maintained, tuned and protected. Like the therapist, the prenatal and perinatal practitioner and anyone coming to interact with pregnant mothers (and fathers) need to attune their right brain and wisdom-related virtues to the other's right brain that is sensitively tuned to receive these communications.

Orlinsky and Howard (1986) argue that the "non-verbal preparational stream of expression that binds the infant to its parent continues throughout life to be a primary medium of intuitively felt affective-relational communication intuitively felt between persons" (p. 343). This kind of implicit communication also characterises the relationship between human beings and some animals, such as horses and dogs. This relationship can teach some people with mental disorders ways to deal with the fear that has been at the heart of their suffering (Equine Involvement Therapy). In fact, we can heal and learn from horses. The loving company of horses can rebalance the nervous system, freeing the sufferers from their anxious and unhappy state. Horses naturally release stress to conserve energy; they help and heal each other to create harmony with the herd and do the same for us when we are with them.

Wisdom, mindfulness and learning to acknowledge the beauty around us broaden our healing possibilities as they facilitate this attunement with horses, bringing a vestige of light into the patient's dark aspect. Interestingly, clients observe that how their connection with the horses has grown and the more they learn to be "in their body" through mindfulness practice, the more relaxed and peaceful the horses have become to them. We can imagine how a mindful mother, present in her body, can regulate and calm the baby's nervous system, freeing it from stress. As soon as you stop "thinking" too much, being too much in your head, or stop caring whether they will approach you or not, the horses approach you more. The connection between mother and baby works in a similar way. The key is to be really present, let go of your ego and the fear you feel about getting it all right and then the horses come to you. In the same way, a baby learns to relax and trust his caregiver.

Intuition, essential for a mother and any caregiver, is the ability to understand or know something immediately without conscious reasoning. Higher socio-cognitive functions emerge from intuition and insight, involving the right hemisphere (McCrea, 2010). These are key to understanding. One of my greatest revelations during my visit to the Himba was the strong relation between their regular practice of wisdom from early life and their strong intuitive ability, which facilitated our interactions, communication and mutual cooperation. Allman et al. (2005) posit that "We experience the intuitive process at a visceral level. Intuitive decision-making enables us to react quickly in situations that involve a high degree of uncertainty; situations which commonly involve social interactions" (p. 370). This fine ability is essential in parenting as it is the prerequisite for understanding a baby. Since it is cultivated by the Himba every day, as by all indigenous cultures, they were masterly at understanding my intention and willingness to share their culture before even explaining it with words.

There are similarities between an intuitive psychobiologically attuned primary caregiver (maternal intuition) and an intuitive therapist's or other practitioner's sensitive responsiveness to the patient's non-verbal affective communications, which are bodily based and intersubjective. Intuition is a spontaneous judgement process used in everyday life (Volz et al., 2008). As opposed to rational analysis, this fast, implicit, automatic cognitive process is defined as a "feeling of knowing what decisions to make, especially in the presence of uncertainty". It is what has allowed mothers to be responsive to and understand their babies for millions of years, a capacity undermined in the last few decades by the dominance of our technological materialistic culture.

This implicit primal knowledge does not presuppose conscious reflection or deliberation (Shotter, 1993). A responsive mother does not need to be an intellectual mother. Implicit knowledge is knowledge from within our relationships with others, and it determines what we anticipate or expect will happen next. It becomes visible only in the process of our interaction with others. It is therefore fostered in early life and by communal life. Implicit knowledge is embodied, and it relates to how people are able to influence each other in their being, rather than just in their intellects; that is, to actually "move" them rather than just "giving them ideas". The right brain is involved in the intuitive capacity. What is the relevance to parenting and thriving children? Within a preparatory prenatal and perinatal wisdom-based programme, prospective and new parents need to be inspired and moved by shared experience rather than merely being given instructions or principles. Because intuition is key to understanding, parents need to understand how to use it and other related wisdom resources with their children.

4 Raising children towards wisdom

The magnetic bond between child and mother, as well as the shared companionship with her mother, father and other caregivers in the community, provides a child with the earliest enjoyment and vital energies. Through the care given to her needs and love (as early as in the womb), the child learns to enjoy, prioritise relationship and perceive it as a source of pleasure, trusting that her needs will be met. To become a fulfilled human being, a child needs to develop key life skills such as self-esteem and communication skills and learn how to maintain her health and well-being, resilience, kindness, love and be inspired to achieve meaningful things by witnessing caregivers cultivating these abilities themselves. This learning is not a matter of reasoning – of discipline, punishment or acting according to abstract rules – but occurs through implicit processes fostered by cooperation, such as mirroring. It is about two human beings being connected. This social and moral learning involves our neurobiological and emotional development early in life (Narvaez, 2014). The right brain stores implicit processes of early life for holistic processing of emotions and social interactions and for affiliative motivations (Schore, 2001a, 2012).

Children need to learn human values from their parents through the way in which they are treated and cared for, starting from conception and gestation. If they are treated with empathy, compassion, kindness and respect, they become kind and caring human beings. They learn that violence is not acceptable. When children are not scared by punishment, they learn to trust their parents and openly talk with them when difficulties arise. Caregiving practices have long-term effects on psychosocial development in early childhood (Narvaez & Gleason, 2013). The kind of relationship between the parents also has an important impact on a child's socio-emotional and moral development. Through their interactions, they provide an internal working model to the child that is stored in the nervous system. In future, the child is likely to develop the same kind of relationships as they witness in their childhood.

When it comes to children, role modelling is crucial. Parents' wisdom practice lead to wise moral functioning in children. Capacities for an ethic of love emerge easily from companionate care, where from conception the environment conveys messages "all the way down" that the child is welcome (Emerson, 1996; Lake, 1979; Meaney, 2010). Through presence, reverence and loving attitudes, as early as conception and gestation, parents provide the optimal developmental niche, as the child learns the value of companionship, empathy and compassion (Narvaez, 2013). When the pregnant mother is surrounded by meaningful others, the child learns a rich intersubjective matrix from the mother's feeling of being emotionally supported and from other subtle ways. After birth, through a mindful community supporting parenting, the child expands his knowledge of the value of cooperation and mutual respect, on which a fulfilled working environment and peaceful society are based. In the chapter on professionals' interpersonal abilities, I describe how wisdom/mindfulness practices in early life shape professional empathy, interpersonal competence, morality and formation across the healthcare disciplines.

Through companionate care, "being with", the child learns to be in a common self, first with mother, father and grandparents, then with the larger community members, both human and animal. Studies show that, although having a responsive mother matters, infants nurtured by multiple significant caretakers grow up feeling more secure, empathic, independent, and orientated towards achievement. A vast literature attests to the fact that mothers with more social support are more responsive to their babies' needs, while the babies are also exposed to richer social stimulation, growing up emotionally more responsive, more resilient, learning language sooner and less likely to be abused by their mothers (Olds, Henderson, Tatelbaum, & Chamberlin, 1986; Olds, 2002, 2007). Children do best in societies where child-rearing is considered too important to be left entirely to parents (Coontz, 1992). In traditional societies, support from alloparents, which allowed our ancestors to evolve, not only improved health, social maturation and mental development; it was essential for child survival. Other researchers found correlations between a new mother's perception of low social support, postpartum depression and infant development (Miller, 2002; Hagen & Barret, 2007).

Children develop their full potential in a network of nurturing relationships in which school also plays an important role. Helping children develop kindness, companionship, empathy and compassion seems an obvious good idea, but today these valuable human capacities are left to chance, rather than cultivated, in our educational system, even in parenting. Many families of course instil these values in their children, but many do not. Programmes have been used in schools that encourage four-year-olds to practise mindful attention to focus on their body and feelings while interacting with other kids – particularly if that other child got upset – and to help each other and express gratitude (Flook et al., 2015; Davidson et al., 2012). Getting such programmes into school ensures that all children are given the opportunity to develop heart-based qualities, empathy and kindness alongside the traditional academic skills. "Kindness, caring and compassion all follow a line of development that our educational system largely ignores – along with attention, self-regulation, empathy, and a capacity for human connection" (Goleman & Davidson, 2017). Neuroplasticity tells us that brain circuitry can be guided through training such as the mindfulness-based Kindness Curriculum (centerhealthyminds.org), just as they can through the parents' practice and teaching of these human virtues.

A rich web of nurture and its lifelong effects

A rich social world of caring, playful companions leads to greater social perceptions and social skills. Early experiences become deeply embodied and inherited by subsequent generations. Darcia Narvaez (2014) posits that by providing responsive nurturing care to children, we support the development of our moral heritage, thus also social and economic stability. The rich intersubjective matrix provided by loving social care promotes a deep perception of the non-manifest and its energies. From conception and throughout gestation and the postnatal period, others are filtered through the mother's mind and physiological state sustained by social support. This is how common mindfulness helps to raise children who thrive. Babies, even in the womb, learn mindfulness through the mother's mindful state. My daughter's caring empathic nature has strikingly reminded me of this. And the mothers I have worked with have provided interesting insights of this primal learning, which has led me to the design of a PhD.

Moods and beliefs affect our behaviour, interactions and perceptions of action and energy behind the visible. The relational attunement and responsiveness are a source of relief and teach the child that fear is a passing event that is quickly subdued by surrender. She grows up self-confident since she learns, through early experiences, that life loves her and cares for her. She becomes able to give what she has received as she mirrors the way she is treated and the care and concern for all life that she perceives and experiences around her.

As Turnbull describes in relation to the Mbuti, in indigenous cultures *selves* develop in a supportive network of relationships, in a companionate culture characterised by sharing activity, resources and company (Turnbull, 1983). This is why I call for a community, including all prenatal and perinatal healthcare professionals, able to practise mindfulness and related wisdom, so as to develop human virtues that our Western healthcare system and culture unintentionally tend to violate. Midwives, doulas, obstetricians, psychologists, psychotherapists, paediatricians, neonatologists and so on are all involved in a child's development and well-being, and in our future generations. Knowledge of the secret life of the unborn and newborn baby has to become collective, through wisdom/mindfulness practice, resonating with scientific findings and personal maternal narrative. As parents, holistic practitioners and birth professionals, we play an integral role in "birthing" the next generations.

One very powerful way of consciously conceiving, raising and protecting our children, so that they can stay healthy and content, is to learn and practise the ancient wisdom practice of mindfulness meditation. This can boost fertility and foster conscious conception, pregnancy, birth and conscious parenting. As a result, children are raised to develop wisdom and resilience, as compassionate caring human beings who are physically, mentally and spiritually healthy. Preparing the environment of the womb as a sacred place, with nurturing vibrations, helps support a child's development from before birth. These children are likely to be creative, peaceful, confident, fulfilled, attuned with themselves as well as with other human beings and creatures of Nature.

Individuals develop capacities for action and perceptual capabilities within a rich network of nurture (Ingold, 1999). In this network, children are raised as companions, not as property, and each child is a community child. The child is respected and her needs are met as a matter of routine. There is no coercion and distress. Although the individual lives in a cooperative and collaborative way, at the same time there is high autonomy and authorship. As a result of such extensive support and acceptance, each member develops a small ego but an expansive "self", the common self (Ingold, 1999). This includes strong concern and empathy towards family and community members as well as creatures of the natural world. The development of big egos is prevented by all possible means as they are considered a danger. This cultural mindset influences the way children are treated, thus favours the development of empathy, rooted in early years, as early as before conception. If aggressiveness and mental disorders are likely to affect our genetic inheritance through methylation patterns (changes of expression of our genes), as epigenetics has found (Wahl & Metzner, 2012; Galea et al., 2011), so is wisdom and so are all related virtues. Evidence that epigenetic changes are reversible offers new opportunities for reducing the impact of adverse environments or practices on human health.

This social context and upbringing foster a higher consciousness that maintains awareness of "spirit" and universal connection (Turnbull, 1983). This is highly relevant to the mother-child relationship before birth. These virtues fostered by this social context and early childcare are picked up by the sensitive unborn baby in many subtle ways and through the mother's feeling of being socially and emotionally supported. After birth, the social network of interactions ensures the continuity of the prenatal experience. Examining the culture of the Mbuti of Zaire, Turnbull writes, "Those basic womblike qualities of protection, comfort, and the satisfaction of all needs, including affection, are always to be found somewhere. So in a very real sense the Mbuti child *is* always in the middle of its sphere/womb, for its sustenance moves wherever it moves, provided only that it does not move too fast" (1983, pp. 44–45).

This early shaping of social and moral heritage fostered by wisdom practice has huge longitudinal effects. We can see this clearly in small-scale societies such as those of our indigenous cousins. This building up of moral conscience during infancy affects the well-being of our society, as it is reflected in the network of work relationships and friendships and in inter-actions between prenatal and perinatal practitioners and expectant par-ents. It is at the root of policy makers' empathic and moral behaviour, and their focus on societal issues and decision making, for example whether they give priority to children's and families' needs and human rights. The way in which we were raised and treated as children, that is the cultural mindset with which we were brought up, affects our attachment style, our harsh or "connected" attitude. These factors matter to policy making and influence parenting and child-rearing. In Italy, Spain and other Latin cul-tures, childhood is very much celebrated, and children take part in adult life from a very young age and feel accepted, which shapes the way in which they perceive themselves. In the UK and the US, very young babies are usu-ally put in a separate room and left to cry, so that adults can carry on with their routines, with the illusion that this will foster independence. But what babies learn from this trend is to suppress emotions, as there is no one listening to them (Sansone, 2004). They do not learn reciprocity, empathy and valuation, the most essential aspects of human morality. This will affect their intimate relationships, their way of regulating emotions and the moral self of infancy.

As still happens in traditional societies, in small-band hunter-gatherer cultures, individuals gain great pleasure from social engagement – dis-played through playing, singing, dancing and storytelling. This was one of the most outstanding aspects of the Himba I visited. Their interest in human relationships and reciprocity, even with a stranger, is rare in industrialised societies. These shared activities help people stay in a posi-tive mood, which leads to more prosocial emotion and behaviour such as gratitude, generosity, compassion, forgiveness, empathy, humour and creativity. Studies show the infectious effects of moods on the people with whom we share our lives or members of the same group (Bradley et al., 2010). An energy field can form between individuals in a group, allow-ing flow, connection, and communication among all the group members. As more individuals within a group tune into each other's heart, this increases heart coherence, the group increases in social coherence and can achieve its objectives more harmoniously and effectively (McCraty & Childre, 2010). This group's energy is regulated by care and compassion, not by threat or force from others, and creates a positive disposition that can even improve physical health. Feeling calm and joyful, unlike feeling sad, angry or tense, can even increase your resistance to developing a cold (Cohen & Pressman, 2006).

One of the most striking revelations of my experience with the Himba was that all those activities involving social engagement – ceremonies, singing, dancing, playing and connecting with ancestors by gathering around the Holy Fire, as well as their prenatal and perinatal and childcare practices – foster a mindful way of living and being, including openness to new experience and transformation, appreciation of life, deep perception of the multiple layers of reality, connection with the present moment and awareness of invisible energy. These practices lead to proto-social behaviour such as empathy, gratitude, generosity, compassion and creativity, which are also foundations of the moral self.

Learning the flow of being and communication

In primal wisdom culture, any individual decision is made thoughtfully, after considering the effect on future generations. Indigenous people believe that their awareness of the child and their mind-body state at the moment of conception and during gestation affect the child's development and well-being. They set up ceremonies and connect with the child's soul before conception to influence fertility and well-being. This is consistent with the scientific discovery that it is not gene-directed hormones and neurotransmitters that control our bodies and our minds; our beliefs and representations are powerful mediators in controlling them and therefore also our lives and our health (Lipton, 2015). Accordingly, beliefs, wisdom and knowledge are not mere intellectual acquisitions but rely on implicit (body-based) affective processes of a psychobiological nature. A treasure in pregnancy, beliefs and wisdom are genetically transmitted through generations and form our embodied cultural heritage. It is clear from some Asian and African cultures how rituals and beliefs concerning the period preceding birth, even conception, sow the seeds for birth (Maidan & Farwell, 1997).

In wisdom traditions, there is a collective sense of contentment and well-being. An attentive observer can see it from their people's relaxed posture and gestures. There seems to be just the right arousal, modulating their movement, posture and social interactions. No one tries to control the other, but to creatively *be with* the other (Fry, 2006). This is a major challenge for modern parents, who tend to impose their agenda on their children rather than creatively being with them and engaging with them. But being with them is so important to create an attuned relationship with the baby. We need to tune the instrument before playing the music. Often stress alters the flow of communication and prevents parents from being present and connecting with their child. Attuned engagement allows for fluid sense-making and learning.

In the early months and years – including prenatally – the child not only senses patterns of action and behaviour in the way she is conceived, thought about and treated, but the "spirit", energy or *vitality form* with which actions and gestures are performed (if they are mindful, thus relaxed, at a slow pace, present, with wisdom, or with anger, depression, or an absent mind). To learn all of this, including the deeper invisible layer, the parent and child must cooperatively engage in a coordinating intersubjective communication (Trevarthen, 2005). During pregnancy, because of the intimate embodied relationship with her mother, the baby absorbs the subtle energy and vitality of the mother's thoughts, emotions and gestures and learns to relate and synchronise with it. Just as all cells, organs and systems of the mother's body communicate through chemical substances and changes. My daughter Gisele showed the ability to tune into our interactions and amazing awareness, probably learnt through her exposure to my favourite classical music, her responsive rhythmical movements, my mindfulness practice, yoga and our intimate communications. Some mothers have reported feeling their babies' jerky uncomfortable movements, even keeping them awake all night and leading to an argument with their partners.

Children who tend to be oppositional have likely not received the engaging cooperation with the parent at a critical time and consequently do not know how to cooperatively engage and surrender to the presence of the other. They have not learnt the attuned dance. When there is no pleasure, vitality contours or energy, cooperation and engagement are difficult.

When relational dysregulation occurs with the caregiver, restoring balance teaches the infant self-regulation and gives faith that when dysregulation occurs, things will be soon sorted out (Stern, 1985). This is an exquisitely embodied learning process. In contrast, when a parent is frequently not in tune, for example when she is chronically stressed or depressed, the baby does not get to practise the flow from regulation to dysregulation and back to regulation, which builds a sense of confidence, self-esteem and faith. The flow from being out of step to attunement also teaches the baby a sense that moods pass and attunement despite being out of step – the flow of human nature. This is so important for learning to accept and process unpleasant emotions. Sadly, too many children in the modern world are growing away from Wisdom. The many violations of babies' unchanging evolved needs and traumas of childbirth and childcare practices today foster many types of psychopathology. If we do not see them among wisdom tradition cultures, it is because of their very different social lives and the transgenerational heritage of nurturing practices.

Like every human virtue, the capacity for affective empathy and morality emerges from lived emotional experience (from biology and embodiment) and is deeply felt. The lived experience shapes how the brain and body work and how we function socially, intellectually, emotionally and morally (Narvaez, 2014). In the same way, the sense of cooperation and companionship develops from early experiences and play with the caregivers. When a child is raised with mindful awareness, she is likely to develop a mindful mindset. This view of social embeddedness includes Nature as well. Embeddedness in the natural environment of the local landscape builds a fundamental sense of belonging to a place and a relation with the natural world, which supports a deep sense of *being* and being at home.

Beyond attachment theory: embedded in multiple relationships

Our society has forgotten simple yet powerful sources of well-being. Studies have shown the benefits for mental health of living with Nature (Cox & Gaston, 2015). Watching birds near your home is good for your mental health. The vital bond with Nature could explain why one of the sweetest and most vivid memories of my childhood is of birds landing on our terrace covered with snow to eat the bread my Dad and I had left for them. We may realise that our strongest soothing memories in childhood are related to Nature/ outdoors. My husband was in boarding school from the premature age of five to 11 and recalls that his major source of joy and comfort was Mother Nature. I often felt a deep connection with my unborn baby while listening to birdsong and being immersed in Nature. I had a deep sense that she was sharing my bliss and felt well-being.

Narvaez (2014) proposes a Developmental Ethical Ecological Practice (DEEP), which an individual can take up for herself or with a couch or therapist. Narvaez proposes that we extend attachment theory beyond companionship attachment to include ecological attachment – the broader community of humans but also other entities, a deep bond to the natural world and a deep sense that Nature will take care of us. A DEEP approach is *developmental* since it aims at the development of awareness, perception, skills, and desires, and is *ethical* since it fosters moral virtue development. Beyond the concern for ourselves and the other that psychotherapy focuses on, Narvaez encourages us to bring that same attention and cooperation to our relationships with the ecosystems of our planet. She encourages us to ditch competing with Nature, since we and the world are one in dynamic relationship and we would only be competing with ourselves. Because the brain has plasticity, change is possible. Narvaez proposes ways to develop this re-alignment with our world that are very close to spiritual practices such as meditation and practising compassion. I recall recent articles in *Therapy Today*, which also encourage us to think beyond the therapy room and go into the wider community, the political and natural world (Totton, 2011; Taylor et al., 2014; Cooper, 2015). My view is that parenting, parent-infant healthcare (including psychotherapy) and policy making should regain this reconciliation with the world.

If we want to live wise, sustainable lives, according to our primal human essence, we need to make major changes to our lifestyle, worldviews and practices, in particular prenatal/perinatal and child-rearing practices, in which the roots of human development are set. But this takes some time. A new consciousness and way of being rooted in earliest life are not created overnight. If every individual begins to practise mindfulness and compassion, we will have more mindful and compassionate parents, who in turn will raise mindful children, thus influencing future generations and forming mindful communities. And we will have more mindful healthcare practitioners capable of deep listening, loving-kindness and understanding. Mindfulness, as the most ancient practice among all wisdom cultures, offers a pathway to change.

The primal worldview teaches us that the human is embedded in a social network from before birth, from conception, until well after birth. The other, the relationship, is present in the self-experience from conception – without the other, there would be no self. We are embedded in multiple relationships, beginning with our mother, who in turn comes from a line of cooperation (ancestors) originating far back in time, but is also one big cooperative unit of millions of organisms. This complex matrix influences pregnancy, birth, bonding and well-being. When I was pregnant for the first time, I cultivated an intersubjective relationship with my unborn baby that was a basis for bonding. Although I was living in London, away from the familiar community network of my homeland in Southern Italy, my ancestors' line of cooperation up to my mother was intrinsically (epigenetically) influencing my perception of social support, well-being and childcare practices. It was in my DNA, creating a nurturing biopsychological energy.

Therefore, a change can only occur through compassionate relationship and intersubjectivity, beginning from conception and gestation. The development of wisdom capacities, particularly in parents and children, is best fostered by a community of meaningful relationships. Within this community, prenatal and perinatal healthcare practitioners play an important role in mothering, alongside a mother's partner, friends, relatives, neighbours and others. Mothers play an important role in recreating society. A companionship culture nourishes harmonious biopsychological energy (Kupperman, 2010). It creates heart resonance and efficient cooperation rather than individualism and territorialism. When a pregnant mother receives emotional support (from the partner and members of the community), this translates into the production of feel-good hormones and a state of energy that benefits foetal and child development. This prepares the ground for intersubjective engagement, and eventually for communal imagination, from which eco-mindfulness and eco-wisdom can emerge and eco-parenting can positively affect successive generations.

The sense of inter-being in the flow of life

A deep sense of relationship with all entities is part of our human heritage and a source of well-being. If deep connection, companionship and care foster capacities in children that can lead to wise living, when early life has generated trauma and suffering the path to wisdom and well-being may have been obstructed. The development of our true self may have been undermined. How can human nature and essence be restored in adults? We do not have to go back to living like our indigenous cousins, but we can be inspired by them and integrate their wisdom to transform our self and pass the transformed seeds on to our children. We can foster communal and ecological wisdom and thus transform the world. We can start by nourishing the environment of the womb by practising mindfulness and eating mindfully, as this restores our inherited human nature and fosters a primal wisdom-based worldview. We can use the skills and tools that modern life has given us to further knowledge of alternative approaches through our imagination, and thus transform our being.

Being creative means not thinking analytically and logically. Conventional, logical, analytical thinkers tend to exclude information that is not related to the problem. They look for ways to eliminate possibilities. Parents with this mindset may not rely on their intuitions or use a range of responses to a baby's needs or possibilities or strategies to support their well-being. Creative people, practitioners and parents, have an inclusive mindset, which means including things that are dissimilar and "only apparently" unrelated. By generating associations and connections between conventionally unrelated or dissimilar things or subjects, they generate different patterns in their brain. These new patterns lead to new connections, which give creative people a different way to focus and to interpret information and experience. Albert Einstein once famously remarked:

> Imagination is more important than knowledge. For knowledge is limited to all we now know and understand, while imagination embraces the entire world and all there ever will be to know and understand.

This mindset will allow us to share our children's childhood with mindfulness, joy and wonder, to take time to attentively watch them grow and thrive, be open to understanding them, rather than anxiously applying conventional information. The best gift we can give our children is our empathic receptive love. They need to feel more important than the fleeting rewards of our professional career. They need us to be fully present and connected with their experience rather than our own minds to be wandering with fears. This same mindset should infuse prenatal and perinatal professionals' approach towards couples going through assisted conception, and mothers during pregnancy, birth and beyond.

> Wisdom seeing has always sought to change the seer first, and then knows that what is seen will largely take care of itself.
> (Rohr, 2011, p. 161)

This search is common to all mindfulness practices. When I visited the Himba and compared their lifestyle with our own, I realised how far we have stepped away from our species' typical behaviour and human essence. It seems that human cultural evolution in recent centuries has exerted a powerful influence, altering typical ontogeny (individual development) and perhaps even phylogeny (species development). We can see this in the high rates of psychological disturbances such as the Asperger's syndrome spectrum, developmental delays, learning difficulties, and even in the changing ways of giving birth, such as caesarean births and premature births. The French obstetrician Michel Odent, who advocates natural birth, foresees phylogenetic changes related to the increasing rates of caesarean births (2015). Processed food is also contributing to such changes. Social media and technology are likely to foster more and more bullying, abusive behaviour, as young people have fewer opportunities to practise their human virtues, in particular empathy, in real intersubjective engagement.

As human beings are sharpening certain skills with advancement of technology and specific learning, their emotional intelligence (so essential in parenting!) seems to be getting worse with evolution. Epigenetic inheritance may be altering the sense of empathy, morality and social skills, fostering social discomfort, contempt and oppositional behaviour, extreme self-reliance, obsessive-compulsive behaviour, dominance and hoarding (instead of generosity), pleasure for self (consuming), egotism, underdeveloped right-brain regulatory systems (nurtured in early life), a safety ethic and detached imagination. This contrasts with a mindful attitude to parenting, which is required for optimal child development. Darcia Narvaez (2014) suggests we need to move from a culture of isolation, detachment and control towards a culture of companionship, engagement, communal and wisdom-based ethics.

The implications of trauma and stress in early life: disconnection from the body and others

"In early life, the day-to-day experiences with caregivers, especially with mother, generate neuronal traces that form implicit memory that later underpin social life" (Narvaez, 2014, p. 257). Lived experience is the back-and-forth interaction between the activated senses and memory of related experiences (Ansermet & Magistretti, 2007). "Thus, the brain is a social dynamic organ whose neuronal connections are modified by external experience (life events) and internal experience (biological and psychic events), structurally and functionally creating a unique, singular individual" (2007, p. 6). This process of neural plasticity begins prior to birth (Partanen et al., 2013). My newborn daughter used to move her body in rhythm with the classical music to which she had been regularly exposed prenatally. She also looked content during her dance, showing a prenatal imprinting of the emotion associated with the musical stimulus. Other mothers have reported similar behaviour of their babies exposed to prenatal music listening. This could demonstrate the neural correlates of human foetal learning and memory of music or speech-like auditory stimuli. Partanen and colleagues have demonstrated a significant correlation between the amount of prenatal exposure and brain activity, with greater activity being associated with a higher level of prenatal speech exposure. Music can have the same influence as human speech on a foetus's learning. The learning effect can be generalised to other types of prenatal experiences.

Poor early experience leads to a non-integrative functioning of the brain and internal reality (Siegel, 1999). Siegel describes how the wisdom fostered by mindfulness practice can support integration of the brain and thus mind-body (2007). Prenatal exposure to chronic stressful life events is associated with a significantly increased risk of autistic disorders (AD), schizophrenia, depression, learning deficits, perinatal complications, immunologic and neuroinflammatory anomalies and low postnatal tolerance to stress (Kinney et al., 2008). This is because high levels of stress during critical phases of development can disrupt foetal brain development. This explains the value of the broad spectrum of benefits provided by mindfulness practice during pregnancy, ideally before conceiving a child.

Chronic stress alters the integrative functioning of the brain and our emotion systems but also our thinking and reasoning. For those who were neglected or abused, the perception of external reality and awareness of the present moment can be overwhelmed and distorted by internal reality (e.g. fantasy) (Freud, 1911). Trauma experienced in the past, unless healed, alters present attention, curtails full perceptions, and even movements, gestures and actions or forms of vitality (Stern, 2010). When too much stress has been experienced too early, our nervous and immune systems, our entire physiology, do not work properly, creating a predisposition to illness (Ladd et al., 1996; van der Kolk, 1987). There are ongoing effects on our capacity for self-regulation and social and moral functioning.

Relational trauma has the most significant implications on development because humans are social mammals who depend on social caring relations to develop into a well-functioning human being. Human relational nature manifests during prenatal development (Emerson, 1996; Janus, 2001; Carter Castiello et al., 2010; Ammaniti & Gallese, 2014). In fact, newborns already show a drive for intersubjective engagement straight after birth (Trevarthen & Aitken, 2003). This predisposition is particularly evident when a prenatal bonding has been nurtured. Multiple systems related to the stress response are influenced by early caregiving, with consequences on brain development and behaviour. These include the amygdala, the vagus nerve, gene expression and the LHA axis (Kaufman et al., 2000; Meaney, 2010; Porges, 2011). Chronic early stress or trauma increases the amygdala's capacity to learn and express *fear* and the incapacity of the prefrontal cortex to control it, generating a vicious cycle of fear and anxiety that in turn increases stress and dysregulation. The high reactivity linked to greater activation in the right prefrontal cortex in early life is likely to become a part of the personality. On a body level, the individual shuts down from his body sensations, which once were involved in the traumatic events, because reconnecting with them would be too painful. This impaired body-self awareness hinders the parent's capacity to engage with the baby/child.

In consequence, chronic stress and mental suffering (when not processed) hinders our sense of the present moment, our ability to be attentive and receptive, to trust others and to perceive the flow of life and its forms of vitality. We are more irritable, disconnected and less forgiving. We are more likely to develop a safety "fear" mindset, rather than being open to the unknown, with compassion, listening, connection and empathy. These tendencies do not support parenting and children's healthy development. They do not foster the well-being of a society and its relationship with other societies, including indigenous communities, group minorities, and Nature – the animals and plants around us – which can result in disrespect and maltreatment. I believe that this disconnection from our being in the natural world and community has led to a disconnection from our bodily feelings, thus our social mammalian nature, curtailing the deep journey through parenting and its fulfilment. This mindset may also be reflected in many parenting instruction-based courses available. The mindset that causes the problem cannot cure it.

Later I will describe how the wisdom abilities fostered by mindfulness practice support parenting and children's healthy development. They are vital for a mother to perceive a developing relational presence in the womb, to be attentive in picking up and interpreting the baby's cues and nuances, thus, to connect and be responsive. Thanks to the brain's neuroplasticity and ever-changing being, we can free ourselves from genetic determinism. We can overcome rigidity and repeated behavioural patterns through continued practice.

Adolescents and adults can self-create through a process of transformation, freeing themselves from psychological and biological determinism and reshaping their neurobiology (Ansermet & Magistretti, 2007/2004). By doing so, they can potentially prepare for fulfilling parenting, or a prenatal or perinatal profession, or just a contributing member of the community, either way making a positive impact on infants' and children's development. We can actively transform our being, creating new neuronal networks and making neural transmission efficient through our imagination and practice (Bear, 2003). Beliefs, thoughts and imagination are physiological events generating changes in energy and affecting muscle strength, movement, gesture (forms of vitality) and the experience of vitality (Stern, 2010). A ground-breaking study empirically proved what athletes and musicians intuitively already know: that those who only imagined exercising a muscle increased its strength as much as those who actually exercised the muscle (Yue & Cole, 1992). We can imagine how a mother may influence her unborn baby's predispositions and human traits through her mental states, imagination and interactions. When we can combine a daily formal practice (e.g. meditation) with the intention to be as mindful as possible throughout the day, we enable mindfulness to flow into our life and into our mental habits, offering the opportunity for transformation and growth.

This openness to letting *being* and brain be transformed by experience is of great significance to modern parenting in a world where humanity and the natural world are at high risk. Young people, the prospective parents, can enhance their well-being and caring abilities, their mindfulness through practice and influence their children's psychobiological well-being and wisdom, beginning in pregnancy and ideally before conception. This does not mean controlling their children's development but rather nurturing their being and inter-being to prepare a healthy environment in the womb and fulfilling relationships with the children. Humans are dynamic biosocial beings transformed by relationships and experience. This realisation is liberating as it teaches us to relate to our experience of living in a new way: to accept difficult emotions and mental states – our shame, our loneliness, our anger – with kindness and compassion, rather than resisting and wanting them to go away, because they can be transformed and are transient. The wisdom fostered by the practice of mindfulness offers a way to restore human nature to its full potential. The natural world, as well as the social environment, to which human beings belong, can contribute to human beings' transformation through cooperation, not competitiveness. Creativity and a comprehensive understanding of the complexity of human nature can open many paths to healing and individualise care. The relationship with animals, such as dogs and horses, and a bond with Nature, can also be involved in therapy or healing programmes.

A new way of thinking about parenting and health

In this perspective, mindfulness, as a way of being, is presented as the first grounding principle of fulfilling parenting and children's well-being. Being aware, attuned with oneself and the other, being present in the body and attentive, is the essential state of mind for a parent to "tune in" to her unborn's and her infant's needs. As parenting is a new unknown experience, and for most people challenging in our stress-driven society, it is important that the resources of one's individual and relational being are enhanced in the period before conception. Parenting is rooted in our culture, politics, family and early childhood experiences. Unresolved mental issues can affect our wholeness and consequently our relationship with our partner, with our baby and her development.

The overuse of the intellect characterising the Western view has influenced parenting education programmes. Many so-called parenting "experts" may be teaching parenting as a subject like math or English. But we know it is far from this. Conscious parenting is not an intellectual process but involves the senses, body wisdom and its implicit processes, other than just the reflective function. A wisdom or mindfulness-inspired parenting programme incorporates current knowledge of prenatal and perinatal psychobiological processes – pregnancy, labour, birth, breastfeeding, postpartum adjustment, the psychobiological needs of the preborn baby and infant, bonding/attachment, observation, attunement and mirroring. The study of human development has to include prenatal experiences, the birth experience, such as birth trauma and early bonding/attachment. This new paradigm is focused on the developing conscious baby from conception (and even before it) and the meaningful relationship between the baby and the caregiver, rather than on the parents, according to the old paradigm. A special focus of this mindset is "attuned interactions", which are considered in primal wisdom as well as some scientific studies and clinical observations to be the strongest predictor of maternal-foetal/infant attachment. This is also consistent with a study (M. W. Lewis, 2008) proposing an interactional model of maternal-foetal attachment, and with clinical observations (Janus, 2001). The enhanced awareness, attentiveness, motivational drive and sense of being in the present moment enable those becoming parents to connect with their preborn and infant. Evidence suggests the early infant-parent interactions lay an important foundation for the child's later emotional, social, moral and cognitive development and are undermined by adults' anxiety, stress and depression (Stanley et al., 2004).

When parents become aware that their preborn baby is a sentient being – able to feel, learn, communicate and relate to her environment – they also become more receptive to building a nurturing relationship. Would you communicate with a passive, unresponsive organism? An essential component of this mindfulness-inspired parenting programme, alongside prenatal and perinatal psychology, is to encourage a sense of community in the expectant parents, so as to reduce the potential adverse effects of social isolation on mental health and well-being in the prenatal, perinatal and early parenting period.

Daniel Siegel reveals how our ongoing experience creates an attunement, or resonance, with ourselves that harnesses specific social and emotional circuits in the brain (Siegel, 2007). He deems that mindfulness practice stimulates these "resonance circuits" to grow, transforming a moment-to-moment state of mindfulness into a long-term state of resilience (an essential human virtue, in particular for the process of adjustment to parenting). This physiological and mental transformation creates mind-body integration, or an integrated state of brain functions, which promotes well-being and positive affect and, more specifically, emotional balance; improved immune function; and an enhanced sense of empathy and self-understanding. If parents achieve this mindful state, their preborn babies and children are likely to naturally mirror these brain transformations and the state of integration. Therefore, through wisdom practice parents can achieve a sense of meaningfulness and deeper understanding, which affects the quality of their interactions with their children and on their development.

Offering the parents opportunities to nurture prenatal attachment is likely to protect them against childbirth complications and child development problems. The awareness of prenatal experiences and communication along the continuum of development from the prenatal to the postnatal period can be a protective practice *per se*. It favours a smooth transition to parenting that prevents many developmental problems, with significant reduced efforts and the costs of later intervention. Siegel teaches that when a parent and teacher see their own mind and their child's mind, they all thrive. Self-understanding and making sense of the past seems to be an important predictor of children's well-being (Siegel & Hartzell, 2003). Our connections with other people are important for our health and happiness and for the health of the planet.

Parents often lack confidence or feel left in the wings watching someone else become the "expert" with their baby, particularly those with premature babies or babies with medical or developmental issues in early life. By practising a wisdom-inspired programme, people becoming parents can begin to take an active part in their childcare and child development with confidence, intuitive wisdom, knowledge and a new way of being. By being offered effective practices, parents will be encouraged to consider nurturing their preborn baby long before birth to increase the chances of having a healthy and behaviourally adaptive child. These benefits will also turn to their advantage, since a healthy child contributes to shaping an attuned relationship, but also to a more fulfilled parent. Through mindfulness practice, we can achieve a richer sense of meaningfulness when caring for a child and a deeper understanding of the baby's non-verbal language, which benefits the interactions and thus her development.

This new model of mind-body nurture is aligned with a series of studies that supports the embodiment of mental processes and their foundations in prenatal rudimentary goal-directed sensorimotor experiences and shared mother-foetus experience, or intersubjectivity (Delafield-Butt & Gangopadhyay, 2013). The interlinking of the psychic consciousness and the body starts very early in life, possibly in intrauterine life, and a gradual process of delinking is linked to disease (Sansone, 2007).

There is increasing academic and clinical interest in implementation of training in relaxation techniques to attenuate potentially adverse consequences of stress, anxiety and depression; reduce pregnancy complications; and improve the labour and delivery experience (Nickel et al., 2006). But there is generally no emphasis on foetal-maternal interactions and bonding/attachment as prenatal psychobiological precursors to adaptive infant development. Therefore, these courses lack an emphasis on the whole process, or an integrative approach. A wisdom-inspired programme could expand the scope of childbirth preparation to include inner intuitive resources for mindful parenting.

This innovative mindset proposes a new psychology of the future that will be built jointly on evolutionary, neuroscientific and behaviourist psychology, incorporating affective wisdom, and on cognitive foundations in early prenatal and perinatal life (Panksepp, 1998). The lines of evidence may contribute to supporting a "new psychology" that recognises that the discipline must be grounded in neuroscience and wisdom and acknowledge the developmental continuum of prenatal and postnatal life. This integrative form of neuropsychology is still in its early stages. Primal wisdom and mindfulness can make important contributions to prenatal and perinatal psychology as an "interdisciplinary" field, which has recently attracted scientists, philosophers and practitioners from disciplines including paediatrics, obstetrics, clinical psychology, psychotherapy and neurology. Each of these fields is making important contributions to the knowledge of prenatal development and perinatal mental health, and the science is progressing, although the process has been incremental and fragmented rather than concurrent. For example we know that toxic substances and maternal emotional stress can adversely affect foetal neurological development and predispositions, but there is no consensus on what emotional or relational form these early injuries take after birth. Nor do we know what form is taken by nurturing prenatal experiences fostered by wisdom practice after birth. This book attempts to contribute to this understanding by integrating scientific discoveries with primal wisdom, as well as my maternal intuitive wisdom and intersubjective experience.

5 The art and science of mindfulness

In the West, we lack the traditions of cultivation and practice. Religion and philosophy have mainly been about theoretical teaching that has little or nothing to do with individual daily practice. The West has often mistakenly associated mindfulness practices with mystification or transcendence, whereas they actually teach self-discovery and self-cultivation in the search for happiness and health, through attentiveness, compassion towards oneself and others and practice that leads to changes in the brain.

In the last ten years, scientists have provided evidence of what mindfulness practice does to the brain and body, and the effects of this simple form of mental training on a range of psychological levels. Mindfulness training can be an essential tool to get people to take better care of themselves, change their lifestyles, mindsets and behaviours. Unconscious programming forming in earliest life can be changed by mindful repeated experience. By decoupling the cravings from the behaviour, mindfulness practice can create new habits. Prospective parents can improve their health and well-being, optimise the womb environment and sow the seeds for their child's healthy development.

However, if we want to improve perinatal and family health for a thriving humanity, our focus should not be limited to the parent-child relationship and well-being but expand to the environmental provision that supports such a crucial relationship. The qualities required by a fulfilling pregnancy, birth and parenting are those fostered by the practice of mindful awareness. In normal conditions, the physiological changes occurring during these important life events are designed to favour the development of the abilities involved in caring for the child. However, an environment that meets prospective and new parents' needs and promotes those human nurturing qualities such as empathy, attention and compassion is crucial for a child's healthy development. If these virtues and companionate care foster capacities in children that can lead to wise living and well-being, following significant adversities trauma in early life, the path to wisdom may have been obstructed. The science of toxic stress and the major findings of the Adverse Childhood Experiences (ACEs) study show that when children experience high stress levels (abuse and neglect), the impact on their brains and their bodies can be devastating, often leading to lifelong health and social problems which tend to pass from generation to generation (Felitti et al., 1998). The study found a strong relationship between the breadth of exposure to abuse or household dysfunction during childhood and multiple risk factors for several leading causes of death in adults.

Knowing about mindfulness, the science and wisdom behind it, and the potential to ensure safe and nurturing relationships and environments for children is useful not just to prospective and new parents as a route to fulfilling parenting and children's well-being. It is also relevant to all those who help them get along and grow, from family, friends, midwives, nurses and obstetricians to clinicians, educators, mediators, community leaders and policy makers. Mothers evolved to nurture a relationship with their infants from pregnancy supported by a community (Hrdy, 2011). It is self-evident that each person on the broad spectrum of these life paths is crucial in helping foster well-being in our society, just as each member's well-being is vital for the welfare of an indigenous community. If those at the helm have a full comprehension of the science and art of mindfulness, and its human virtues and strengths are reflected and replicated within systems, major benefits and advantages will ensue. A harmonious and felicitous combination of the mental virtues throughout any prenatal and perinatal organisation and service will lead to greater efficiency, as well as coordination between all the functioning elements of those systems, so that they work as a coherent whole.

I propose the practice of mindfulness as a very effective strategy in bridging the gaps within and between prenatal and perinatal care systems and between them and parents. It is, in fact, the most ancient, universal practice. On the one hand, when we have a mindful compassionate community, it is easier to foster mindfulness in prospective parents and future generations. On the other hand, the individual transforms culture and society through practice. Other and self are interwoven from the very beginning of life.

We need to make the science and art of mindfulness available to practitioners as well as parents, so that they can implement it in their practice and build a common ground. This would help refrain from an overmedicalised approach, which has been taking over globally. Today, more than 20 per cent of Americans regularly take psychotropic medications – chemical substances that alter brain chemistry and function, and ultimately emotions and behaviours. In 2010, the sale of such medications amounted to over $70 billion in the US and prescription rates continue to climb for both children and adults. Moreover, the list of negative side effects of these medications is overwhelming – weight gain, cognitive impairment, drowsiness, higher rates of diabetes, increased suicidality, sexual dysfunction, to name a few – a study suggests that long-term use of such substances may actually lead to increased disability over time.

Psychiatric drugs can be helpful in some cases, but they should be prescribed when truly necessary and with more awareness of alternative self-transformational practices such as mindfulness. My concern is that easy drug prescriptions reflect a cultural trend. The medical establishment often miscategorises healthy struggling and suffering as pathology, as we deny pain and suffering as an important part of human existence and source of transformation. It is often unaware of healthy alternatives to drugs, such as mindfulness practice, yoga, in particular breathing awareness, meaningful social engagement and compassion, equally effective in modifying brain chemistry and function and relying on the individual's resources. We need to develop an empathic, insightful and compassionate perspective to humanise care and therapy. The goal should be resources, empowerment and healing rather than "treatment" or cure.

The most ancient practice

Mindful awareness has been practised by all cultures for millions of years to enhance fundamental human virtues, such as empathy, attentiveness, awareness, engagement and cooperation. The Greek schools of philosophy espoused an ideal of personal transformation that remarkably echoed those of Asia. Aristotle posited the goal of life as a virtue-based *eudaimonia* – a quality of flourishing – a view that has continued in Western modern thought. In Aristotle's view, virtues are acquired by the ongoing practice of observing our thoughts, acts and experience, which leads to self-regulation. Other Graeco-Roman philosophical schools used similar practices with the same goal. For the Stoics, our awareness that our feelings about life events, not those events themselves, determine our happiness is key to well-being; we find equanimity when we can distinguish what we can control from what we cannot. This is echoed in the theologian Reinhold Niebuhr's prayer:

> God, grant me the serenity to accept the things I cannot change,
> Courage to change the things I can,
> And wisdom to know the difference.

For these Greek schools, philosophy was an applied art, and contemplative practices and self-discipline were taught openly as paths to flourishing. Like their peers to the East, the Greeks believed that we can cultivate qualities of mind that foster well-being. In the Graeco-Roman tradition, qualities such as integrity, kindness, tolerance, patience and humility were considered keys to fostering well-being. Both these Western thinkers and Asian spiritual traditions alike saw the value in cultivating a virtuous life via a similar transformation of being.

The term meditation, in Sanskrit *bhavana*, means cultivation, bringing into being. "Bringing into being" is also the Oxford dictionary's definition of creativity. The term for meditation in Tibetan, *sgom*, means familiarisation. In Buddhism, the term *bodhi* (in Sanskrit) expresses the ideal of inner flourishing, a path of self-actualisation that nourishes "the very best within oneself" (Dahl, 2016). "Mindfulness" meditation, as introduced by research clinical psychologist Jon Kabat-Zinn (1990), is based on the Eastern technique known in Buddhist tradition for 2,500 years as *Vipassana* meditation – often translated as "clear vision", in which you simply bring your attention to your breath, sitting or lying down, eyes open or closed. By breathing consciously in this way, you enter your body-mind system and emotions without judgments or opinions, releasing neurotransmitters from the brain to regulate breathing while creating an interactive flow between all systems.

Mindfulness is the awareness – of thoughts, feelings and body sensations – that emerges when we learn to pay deliberate and open-hearted attention to the moment-by-moment of the external and internal world (Williams, 2008). Mindfulness means attending to embodied experience in the here and now. It is presence in the body. It means being physically, emotionally and cognitively present to what is happening in oneself and the surrounding environment. The body is unable to live in the future. When we are worried or preoccupied, we disconnect from our bodily feelings. For a healthcare practitioner, being present with a parent-to-be means attending to their own bodily feelings and the parent-infant subjective experience in a non-judgemental way. This receptive attention promotes the same process between parents and infant.

The word *mindfulness* means compassionate and lucid floating awareness that witnesses whatever happens in our experience without judging or otherwise reacting, a sense of knowing what is happening in the external and internal world as it is happening. Perhaps the most widely quoted definition comes from Jon Kabat-Zinn: "Mindfulness is the awareness that arises from paying attention on purpose, in the present moment, and nonjudgmentally, to the unfolding of experience moment by moment" (2003a, p. 145). Most of us are more used to its opposite, times of *mindlessness* when we are not really conscious of what is going on, when we are liable to make mistakes and unwise choices.

The two words, mindfulness and meditation, are often used interchangeably, but they are not synonyms. Both involve heightened states of awareness. Both have myriad benefits. Mindfulness is about noticing the dynamic interplay between you and your environment, whereas meditation is about immersing yourself deep within yourself. The aim of mindfulness practice is to notice what is happening now and engaging with the present moment, rather than thinking about the past or the future, or being taken over by worries or racing thoughts. It is so important for parents to connect with their baby and understand his needs, as well as for practitioners to understand parents' mental states and needs. You can practise mindfulness while you are doing other things, like walking, eating, conversing, driving, breastfeeding, changing nappies and holding the baby. Developing a mindfulness practice is equivalent to paying attention to what is going on in the present moment.

I am not presenting one specific form of mindfulness here, but the overall concept of mindfulness and in particular its striking links with attachment and interpersonal neuroscience. The eminent psychiatrist Daniel Siegel argues that mindfulness can be cultivated by many means, from experiences within attuned relationships, including the therapeutic relationship, to educational self-body trainings that emphasise reflection, to formal meditation (Siegel, 2007). I discovered mindfulness and the importance of the therapist's presence and compassion several years ago through the healing relationship with expectant and new parents and their infants (Sansone, 2007). I have come to learn more about mindful awareness practice through deepened experience and my own educational and clinical applications, as well as by attending retreats and reading about the latest research in mindfulness and interpersonal neuroscience. The relational attunement experienced in the bonding with my baby also brought insights about my body wisdom and the beneficial qualities of mindfulness practice. A profound revelation has been sharing the life and wisdom of the Himba, the indigenous people of Northern Namibia, and discovering they practise mindfulness in every aspect of their life and as a matter of routine.

Studies of mindfulness and interpersonal neurobiology interweave and integrate knowledge from a variety of disciplines to find the common features that are shared by these independent fields of knowledge. Mindfulness practice, like cognitive psychotherapy, modifies the brain structure and functioning by modifying the neuronal synapses, leading to new alternative ways of perceiving, thinking and behaving (Siegel, 2007).

Boosting resilience and well-being: an antidote to pain, stress and depression

Today it has become almost normal to be stressed. It shows that you are engaged with the world, a sort of business card. We almost attribute rest to laziness. This adult attitude has affected children, and many develop mental issues or drop out of school in consequence of the pressure, as they cannot cope emotionally. We have got to a turning point where we need to create a new paradigm of *rest, being* and *presence*. Mindfulness practice offers a tool for managing stress and anxiety and helps to create this new paradigm. Mindfulness-based meditation interventions and other closely related meditation practices including loving-kindness meditation and compassion meditation have become increasingly popular in contemporary psychology (Hofmann et al., 2011). Combining ancient wisdom and twenty-first-century science, Mindfulness-Based Cognitive Therapy (MBCT) has proved to be a powerful tool to help prevent relapse in depression and the after-effects of trauma (Kenny & Williams, 2007; Segal et al., 2001). Mindfulness-based approaches in healthcare began in the US with psychologist Kabat-Zinn's pioneering research into mindfulness-based stress reduction (MBSR), which proved enormously beneficial for patients with chronic pain, hypertension and heart disease, as well as for psychological problems such as anxiety and stress (Kabat-Zinn, 1990). The improvements in health outcomes and the decrease in stress have been shown by other studies (Grossman et al., 2004).

At the same time, MBSR was being used in antenatal classes for both parents, with the aim of preventing the negative impact that high stress and fear have on maternal and neonatal outcomes (Duncan & Bardacke, 2010). A related approach using mindfulness for mothers has confirmed its potential to have a general positive impact on well-being, reducing anxiety, negative affect and stress (Vieten & Austin, 2008), which are often contributing factors in complicated birth, including premature births.

The potential benefits of mindfulness for pain are suggested by research carried out by Kabat-Zinn showing that it is helpful for people suffering from chronic pain, many of whom had not found pain relief in medication (Kabat-Zinn, 2003a). It shows that mindfulness can improve mood by connecting with the present moment rather than the constant fear their pain is "killing" them. With this new awareness, they can accept pain and carry on daily activities. Mindfulness meditation also appears to bring about favourable structural changes in the brain. One recent study found significant increase in cortical thickness in individuals who underwent an eight-week MBSR training programme and that this increase was coupled with a significant reduction of several psychological indices related to worry, state anxiety and depression (Santarnecchi et al., 2014).

The analgesic effect of mindfulness meditation involves multiple brain mechanisms including the activation of the anterior cingulate cortex and the ventromedial prefrontal cortex (Zeidan et al., 2012). The subjective experience of the environment is constructed by interactions between sensory, cognitive and affective processes. For centuries, meditation has been thought to influence such processes by enabling a non-evaluative representation of sensory events. Before they received meditation training, the group of people with chronic pain in Zeidan's study showed no difference in the way they rated the pain, whether they were focused on their breath or not. However, after their mindful meditation training, subjects reported a 40 per cent decrease in pain intensity between resting and breath-focusing. Also, looking at their magnetic resonance imaging (MRI) data, meditation seemed to reduce pain-related processing. The major difference was in the primary somatosensory cortex, a region associated with sensory-discriminative processing of information. This is significant as this area is presumed to play a role in the evaluation of pain. It seems that mindfulness meditation may work by allowing a better focus on neutral stimuli like the breath, therefore reducing the emotional response to the pain sensation, which amplifies the experience of pain. The anticipation of pain is also reduced by engaging the attention with the present moment and witness the unfolding of experience. Because of the changes brought by mindfulness, it is also used as a way of tuning in and preparing the system for the therapeutic work.

The meditation practices can teach the ability to quieten the system and access how to "be" rather than "do", which is essential to therapy.

MBSR emphasises that awareness and thinking are very different capacities. From the perspective of mindfulness, it is awareness that is healing, rather than mere thinking. Also, it is also awareness itself that can balance out all of our various thoughts and emotional agitations and distortions that accompany the frequent storms that blow through the mind, especially in a chronic pain condition. Mindfulness meditation is a practice that can change our selves both physiologically and psychologically in the search for happiness, something that current research programmes are demonstrating. This occurs through biomarkers, both on a chemical level, through the lowering of the stress hormone cortisol (Matousek et al., 2010), and re-forming of neural networks, reflecting for instance in expanded areas of the hippocampus involved in emotion modulation (Luders et al., 2013). Individual change will influence the change in other people and thus contribute to a small, though important, cultural change.

Pain associated with pregnancy and childbirth, often a consequence of maternal anxiety, depression and stress, has similar challenges. Mindfulness aims to change a person's relationship to the pain sensation as well as the thought of it, so that the experience of the pain is less likely to trigger a cascade of negative emotions, such as health concerns, which worsen the pain sensations and mental pain. Psychologist Dr Elisha Goldstein (2007) says that we need to be curious and non-judgemental about pain. Judging the pain only makes it worse. In fact, our negative thoughts and judgements not only exacerbate the pain, they also fuel anxiety and depression. Goldstein describes how our brains start brainstorming to soothe the pain and this creates a lot of frustration, anxiety, stress and a feeling of being trapped. These feelings can be overwhelming and damage our relationships, in particular parent-infant bonding.

It is encouraging to realise that learning to be in the "being" mode rather than the "doing" mode can have such profound effects. Mindfulness practice is central to the Buddha's teachings, which has now been accepted by Western teachers as a secular self-help technique. As a result of this secular appeal and abundant scientific findings, mindfulness is becoming widely used and accepted. Its appeal is growing, and more and more people are able to access this ancient wisdom.

The physiological wisdom of pain

Scientists have found connections in the brain between physical and emotional pain, which means that by learning to master our thoughts about the physical sensations, the whole experience becomes less all-absorbing, and we can reach a level of freedom enabling us to re-engage with life (Vastag, 2003). According to Melzack, it has been proved that human pain is not simply a function of damage and that the intensity and quality of pain are conditioned by previous experiences and by the ability to understand the cause and meaning of pain (Melzack, 1965). Therefore, giving full attention and awareness to pain might reveal that it actually peaks, drops and completely subsides. The culture in which we grow plays an essential role in how we feel pain and how we react to it. If natural birth represents the very first challenge for a baby, in that it prepares him for life outside the womb, labour pain prepares the mother for the great existential event and the great challenge of motherhood. The conscious appreciation of labour pain may be understood as a signal and as a defence function requested by the woman for herself and for her child. The emotional alarm, when on a moderate level, is meant to allow her to face the great event of childbirth and mothering. The total or partial suppression of labour pain or the conscious contraction induced by synthetic painkillers should be seen in this perspective.

Fear of childbirth (FOC), increasingly common among contemporary women, is still not well understood or support is not provided for in maternity services. A national survey reported disparity in the availability of services for women with FOC, with 47.3 per cent (n=52) of units not offering specialist support for women with FOC. Furthermore, there was variation in who ran the service and the type of service available (Richens et al., 2015). A UK prevalence study (n=545) found that the majority of women who presented with FOC had generalised anxiety disorders (17 per cent) or specific phobia (8 per cent) rather than tokophobia (0.03 per cent) – a specific phobia of childbirth or debilitating fear of childbirth that can be so intense that childbirth is avoided – when a psychiatrist conducted a Structured Clinical Interview (Nath et al., 2018).

Consultant obstetrician and Prof Lucio Zichella considers that when a pregnant woman learns that the conscious perception of the uterine contraction associated with pain is an expression of the maternal emotional charge needed to protect herself and her baby, she is enabled to accept it as an essential part of the labour process (Zichella, 2002). This consciousness is likely to reduce her pain perception. The pain does not vanish, but the relationship to it changes. Pain will not be perceived as an unknown monster but as an ally, "an expression of a psychobiological necessity". The body-self training, or practice of mindfulness, is particularly useful in preparation for labour, birth and mothering. Prospective mothers will learn to see the adaptive function of labour pain, the physiological wisdom of pain and thus of Nature as a subjective emotion vital to the unfolding of labour contractions. Mindfulness practice teaches mothers to be curious about the intensity of their pain and encourages them to let go of any goals and expectations. The idea is to engage with the pain just as it is and work out what we can learn from it and what we notice about it.

Unfortunately, modern obstetric practices often interfere with the delicate synchronised dynamics between mother and baby during pregnancy leading up to a natural birth. The changing culture of medicine is less and less sensitive to the birthing woman's inner physiological resources and the intersubjective reality of a mother and her collaborating baby. Mindfulness practice, in particular the body-self and breathing awareness, trust in the body wisdom, self-regulation and connection with the pre-born that it fosters, can counteract the medical control and minimise the risk of medical technical interventions.

My first labour offered me a first-hand experience of breathing as a strategy for releasing endorphins, quelling pain and trusting the body as the key to let the hormones do their job. Mindfulness preparation teaches a woman to use physiological responses to labour such as movement. Freedom of movement allowed me to assume positions instinctively to reduce resistance and compression and go with the flow of labour. A woman can protect herself from damage to her pelvis, her cervix and her perineum, while at the same time, protecting the baby's stress level. This wisdom is what previous generations of women relied on in the days before synthetic painkillers were produced.

We are dominated by a culture of fear and control. A tiny quantity of meconium detected in the amniotic fluid was what prompted the midwife to transfer me from the Hospital Home from Home Centre to the Birth Centre in my final stage of labour (nine cm dilation) in order to monitor the baby. Being tied up to a monitoring machine, kneeling, with my arms resting on the bed and thus being unable to walk disturbed the natural rhythm of labour. Walking back and forth had so far helped me maintain the flow of contractions, while at that point I started feeling trapped. Not surprisingly, after two hours the pushing phase had not progressed very far. I was aware that what was happening was being caused by the "monitoring", its loud sound, the inhibition of my body movement and my induced anxiety (rise of adrenaline). These were probably causing stress to the baby, who had stopped her final descent. My natural mammalian resources were being trapped by man's technological advance – a cold metallic machine. The hospital's need to prevent any minor risk "potentially" compromising health and safety was the priority.

I longed to tell the midwife that that was not what my body was meant to do just before entering the last phase of labour – move from position to position – which is best for both mother and baby. Yet, thanks to my mindful awareness practice during pregnancy, I never feared losing control. I never lost the communication with my baby or the connection with my body. With one only manoeuvre, the doctor was able to turn the baby's head slightly. With little energy left, I managed to effectively work through the coming contraction and help her out. Fortunately, I could rely on my body wisdom, confidence and sense of anticipation and elation, which had sustained my healthy pregnancy and prenatal bonding. These were my winning forces. The baby managed to find her way out. She was absolutely fine, emitting her first short cry of life. No doubt, the risk of foetal monitoring was a real threat in comparison to the "inexistent" risk of the tiny quantity of meconium. But what would have happened if I hadn't been able to rely on my "mammalian" endogenous resources? Or if I hadn't nurtured a prenatal bonding enabling my baby to maintain our psychobiological agreement on protecting each other to the very end?

There is evidence that foetal monitoring may cause foetal distress and that it frequently gives a false reading that can hasten "emergency" caesarean sections as well as having no reliable statistical advantage in predicting true foetal distress (Parer & King, 2000). The stress caused to the baby may prevent her from relying on maternal body cues necessary to help her progress in her own way. Because of the metallic beeping exposure, my healthy happy child for a period would suddenly manifest a brief reaction (nearly panic) when hearing a talking doll or any electronic toy. It was only when I recalled Gisele's birth story with her and made sense of her reaction that the reaction vanished. Gisele's personality predispositions had been shaped by a nurturing prenatal bonding, which gave her strong foundations to minimise the risk of intervention as well as make sense of the "monitor" experience. But imagine how a traumatic birth experience can affect a baby's temperament and a mother's well-being. Or if I had had low confidence and panicked; there would have been a different birth outcome.

The implicit attuned communication between a birthing mother and baby and the physiological benefits that they confer on each other during this interchange is so fundamental that it is clear that they were designed to continue the synchronic relationship they had maintained during pregnancy. But this relationship, as Montagu (1986) beautifully describes, is not understood by Western birth practitioners, the very people who have been elected the experts or authorities on the needs of mother and child in childbirth and beyond. Montagu argues that it is as if there were a conspiracy against mother and child to deprive them of their inalienable constitutional rights to human development. It is only by empowering women's *being* and *wisdom* and *humanising* birth professionals' approach to birth that the conspiracy can be defeated.

Pregnant women who undergo mindfulness training report that they become aware of the negative thoughts that worsen their intense physical sensations and learn to relate differently to them; they cease to be overwhelmed by feeling unable to cope with the pain, and less fearful of losing control (Duncan & Bardacke, 2010). Mindfulness practice is particularly beneficial for childbirth preparation. Many labouring women report feelings of being overwhelmed by pain, fear of not being able to cope or of losing control. These feelings, if excessively overwhelming, may cause complications, caesarean sections and premature births (Wadhwa et al., 2001). There are also women who seem to manage their pain without "pain relief" and have more positive, empowering experiences of childbirth than those who resist labour pain. Walsh and Leap have documented women's and midwives' perceptions of labour, confirming that the perception of labour pain is very individual. Women having a physiological uncomplicated childbirth tend to describe their experience as "going with the flow", "emotionally transformative" or "being present" (Walsh, 2007). They perceive the pain as an ally instead of an enemy. An understanding of the body and the breath creates the grounding in the mind and also allows for responses to come from a place of expansion rather than contraction.

We have learnt that regular practice can transform the brain (thus hormones, representations, behaviours, attitudes) through the formation of new neural networks and make it more resilient to change. Practising mindful awareness teaches us to bring conscious attention to previously automatic processes. Self is therefore experience-dependent. Psychoanalyst Gay Watson clearly explains that our suffering and psychological ill health arises from identifying with a permanent self, possessing it, and seeing our life and worlds through the lens of this concept, refusing to move with change and impermanence (Watson, 2008). Pregnancy, birth and parenting are a dramatic challenge to our capacity to change with the flow of experience while preserving our psychoneurological integration. When this challenge is perceived as an opportunity for growth rather than a threat, we significantly contribute to a healthy pregnancy and development of the baby.

A pregnant mother, just like everyone and everything else, belongs to something bigger than her own personal identity. She is part of the life force of the ecosystem. She is an expression of the wisdom of Nature. So is labour, a natural force, which a woman embodies while being subject to its power. This is a hard reality for many modern career women to accept, as they have been conditioned to excessively control every aspect of their lives, with the expectation that everything will follow as they intend. Besides this, the materialistic and medically orientated mindset that controls the birth industry in our modern world is unhelpful. It is important every woman learn throughout pregnancy that labour is not like that. It is about letting go of life forces, relying on the energy of sensory communication and becoming fluid like a sea wave. Labour involves letting go of expectations and fears and being present, so as to let the process unfold smoothly. Pregnancy and birth thus require an unresistant acceptance of a dynamic body-self, which mindfulness practice fosters.

Compassion and self-compassion

The idea that negative emotions are bad and positive ones are good is a Western cultural construct, a threat to well-being. We need challenging emotions, as they are key to survival. We just need to elaborate them. In the same way, dyssynchrony between mother and baby is normal, part of the life narrative, but repairing ruptures is important for development. It is how these things are dealt with that shapes the outcomes. Mindfulness practice trains the brain and body to notice the difficult emotions arising without reacting to them or being held captive by them. It can prepare us to confront depression with interest and curiosity and to take a perspective on our negative thinking. Mindfulness can help increase awareness of emotions, elaborate negative emotions and ruptures and increase life-enhancing emotional states during pregnancy, which sustain well-being and can benefit the life support system of a developing unborn baby and aid bonding. It is important to compassionately accept the wide range of emotions and body changes in pregnancy as important for the baby's healthy development. Mindfulness teaches a mother that, no matter how tough things may seem, feelings come and go and can be transformed. It acknowledges discomfort or pain and allows it to pass, reminding us that on the other side there is spiritual healing and growth. This is so important to face the transition to parenting.

Scientists have begun to unravel some of the benefits of compassion for our well-being as well as the transformations it brings about in the brain. Mindfulness practice can be an effective strategy to achieve this ability. Richard Davidson has studied the changes that meditation induces in the brain of not only experienced meditators such as skilled Buddhist monks, but also ordinary people after a period of practice. These changes translate into greater compassion towards family, friends and strangers, as well as sustaining positive emotions and well-being (Davidson & Begley, 2012). Engaging in compassion and loving-kindness practice has been shown to increase amygdala activation to suffering (e.g. distressing sounds like a woman's scream) (Lutz et al., 2008). When people were instructed to empathise with a video – to share the emotions of the people they were seeing – fMRI studies revealed circuits activating on parts of the insula – circuits that light up when we are suffering (Klimecki et al., 2013). But when another group instead got instructions in compassion – feeling love for those suffering – a completely different set of brain circuits activated, those for parental love of a child (Klimecki et al., 2014). These neural activations occurred in only eight hours of practice.

In an emergency situation, like a woman screaming in fear, the amygdala has extensive connections to engage other circuitries to respond. Meanwhile, the insula activates its connection to the body's visceral organs (like the heart) to prepare the body for active response (for example, increasing blood flow to the muscles). While the brain is primed to respond to human suffering, practicing compassion meditation makes one more likely to act to help someone. The brain seems primed to learn to love and help thanks to its neuroplasticity. Enhancing parents' compassionate attitude, thus their intense resonance with others' suffering, has huge benefits to their children emotional and social development. These children are more likely to be compassionate human beings, available to listen to and help people in need. Loving-kindness also fires the connections between the brain's circuitry for joy and happiness and the prefrontal cortex, an area involved in guiding behaviour (Weng et al., 2013). As previously mentioned, in East Asian culture, the name *Kuan Yin* is symbol of compassionate awakening, which means "the one who listens and hears the cries of the world in order to come and help" (Thich Nhat Hanh, 2012).

Several meditation practices aim to cultivate compassion. Gilbert (2010) developed compassion-focused therapy (CFT) and Neff and Germer (2013) developed an approach for non-clinical population called mindful self-compassion (MSC). These involve motivating people to care for their own well-being, to become sensitive to their own needs and distress and warmly understand themselves by engaging in activities such as compassionate cognition and kindness towards the self (Neff & Tirch, 2013).

It is much easier to be kind to others than to ourselves. Self-compassion is not a first instinct. We need to practise it. Early life patterns do not change completely. You can still be a reactive person in certain circumstances, but you can stop using self-criticism and accept the way you are. Change comes from acceptance. Compassion and self-compassion increase the motivation to learn. When a parent is judgemental and says to the child, "You are not worthy, I don't believe you", they are not motivating the child. But if they say, "I believe you, I trust you, you can take the risk", they foster the child's confidence and open him to learning experience.

Individuals who have experienced trauma or abuse may tend to avoid mindfulness because of unprocessed trauma. They shut down their bodily sensations and feelings to protect themselves against the pain experienced. But they may need to work through the painful feelings to release them first before being able to practise mindfulness. Existing evidence gathered in a review (Boyd et al., 2018) indicates that mindfulness-based therapies, including MBSR, are effective in reducing symptoms of post-traumatic stress disorders (PTSD).

A parent who was neglected or experienced trauma as a child does not need a therapist or mindfulness facilitator who merely applies a theory or technique but someone curious about their story, interested in listening with compassion and understanding. We need a trauma-informed compassionate care to improve perinatal and family health for a thriving humanity, since suffering does not concern only the sufferer but also the offspring. This means having the awareness that the parent or child we are dealing with behaves in a certain way because of a past trauma (including birth trauma) and that the behaviour can be triggered by it. This implies bringing a compassionate approach into our community. By bringing mindfulness into communication, through deep listening and loving speech, we improve our relationships. If there is no compassionate listening, there is not much understanding or true love. You may see a psychotherapist because nobody is listening to you. But even psychotherapists may not be able to listen, not deeply. Listening requires compassion for that person. To listen deeply we do not have to focus on words but on body language, movements, gestures, pauses and silence (Sansone, 2007, 2018a). Listening goes beyond verbal language, and the body gives us a lot of information about what is going on. This ability is particularly important for parents in understanding their children, but also for health practitioners in connecting with and understanding parents' needs.

Listening requires opening the heart and being non-judgemental, embracing others' suffering and being kind and compassionate. It requires the right conditions, which are certainly not favoured by stress. A study of bioenergetics on deep listening has found that the heart generates a powerful electromagnetic field in the body about 60 times greater in amplitude than the brain's electromagnetic field (McCraty, 2004). The author found that energy is not only transmitted internally to the brain but is also detectable by others within its range of communication. When someone is in a state of stress or anger, the magnetic frequency is very disorganised. Love, appreciation, care and peace equal to a state of coherence – a physiological state of magnetic balance. When we interact with another person, we know subconsciously or non-subconsciously what is going on emotionally in the other person, as we pick up the magnetic frequency of the heart. We sense when we are received or not, if we are judged or deeply listened. We can imagine how these energetic fields affect mother-baby sensitive communications. Mindfulness practice can foster awareness and co-regulation of this implicit intersubjective reality.

Through mindfulness and compassion practice, we can also achieve a richer sense of meaning, deep understanding and balance in everyday living, opening us to connecting with others and building mindful communities. Prospective parents and new parents can find this exploration extremely valuable. But also professionals in education, medical and mental health can find this exploration useful for helping others to alleviate their suffering and for promoting life-enhancing emotions.

This considerable evidence proves that mindfulness meditation is a long way from being a mystical experience, as often thought. It helps use the power of positive neuroplasticity to strengthen key psychological resources such as gratitude and compassion. Without being a long-term meditator, the practice of mindfulness or mind-body training can enhance well-being, as it can induce both short- and long-term changes to the brain. It can lead to long-lasting changes in perception, cognition and emotion, thus in our experience. The practice of meditation is used both to reveal our reality through concentration and insight and to transform it through self-reflection. Thus, mindfulness is a way of being. As Kabat-Zinn highlights, it is a way of life that reveals the kind and loving wholeness that lies at the heart of our human being, even in time of great pain and suffering (Kabat-Zinn, 2003b).

It seems that our contemporary Western everyday life takes us further and further away from this kind of thinking and self-reflection. We seek entertainment, not reflection; we flee from silence and contemplation. Technology has taken over and the television and computer surround us. Our stressful lives rarely leave space for contemplation of our reality and our human needs, or for free imagination of what might be. We are too busy doing to listen and reflect on ourselves, our bodily experiences, the links between our behaviour and early life experiences, our feelings for other human beings and the non-human world. From a very early age, children are subjected to the pressure of "doing" and are passively bombarded by computer games and television – i.e. by images – that may disconnect them from their feelings, imagination, experience. They have few opportunities to practise mindfulness or emotional intelligence. The attention and learning problems of many children are one possible consequence of this. Many of these children will be parents one day! Many parents find themselves beset by the pressure of everyday preoccupations, which lead to stress and a chronic sense of dissatisfaction with their lives. Parents' distress curtails emotionally available parent-child relationships, which are supportive of child health and development (Barfoot et al., 2017). Mindfulness and self-compassion help us see more clearly and deal efficiently with these pressures, thus develop the emotional availability and reflective function that are so important for fulfilling parenting.

The virtues fostered by the practice of mindfulness resonate with those described by the *Yin* qualities of the Chinese Taoist philosophy, which counterbalance *Yang:* receptivity as opposed to activity, listening as opposed to discourse, being in contrast to doing, cooperation rather than competition, connection and integration rather than analysis, expansion rather than conservation and a greater attention to feeling and intuitive wisdom rather than reliability on rational knowledge and science (Capra, 1976). Like any other aspect of our lives, pregnancy, birth and maternal and childcare have been dramatically affected by our culture, which has consistently favoured masculine values, or *Yang*, over feminine or *Yin.*

Meditation aims at making us stop and familiarise ourselves with our human reality, our emotions and impulses, and with the way our mind works, to encourage self-awareness and self-knowledge for the purpose of self-creation. By simply taking the time to isolate ourselves, we explore the healing power of silence and come to know who we really are, our predispositions and potential. Solitude and quiet connect us to our creative source. By practising it at the same time every day, even for just 15–20 minutes, a daily dose of silence will soon become a habit that you will never neglect. On a neurological level, meditation, by allowing long-buried thoughts and feelings to surface, can be a way of getting the biochemical of emotions (peptides and their receptors) to flow again, returning the body, and the emotions, to health (Pert, 1997). Neuroscience indicates that trauma, emotional stress and blockage can be stored at the cellular level and form our unconscious programming (Lipton, 2015). Therefore, when there are severe emotional issues, the practice of mindfulness may need to be combined with more in-depth psychotherapy. In these cases, it may be prudent – indeed a sign of self-awareness – to turn to psychotherapy.

Towards an open-hearted compassionate orientation

Fear and rage lead away from relational presence and other wisdom abilities. Desire (dopamine-driven seeking or euphoria) can also be addictive, as greed and envy can take over and move in a direction opposite to relational engagement. The more one has practised these emotions, watered its seeds, the stronger they have become. The stress response shuts down the ability to learn new patterns, to be open to the unknown. So it is important to find new effective ways to diminish one's reactivity. When the brain and body are calm, one can practise new ways of being, in particular relational presence, a key asset in parent-infant relationship. The practice of mindfulness leads to disentanglement from these emotions and minimises them by cultivating self-calming. Anger, anxiety and dopamine-driven seeking prevent us from experiencing ourselves, self-attunement and inter-attunement, which are foundational for parenting and secure attachment. Practising self-calming kindness and compassion meditation reduces concentration of the stress hormone cortisol and activates hormones (e.g. oxytocin, prolactin and serotonin) that promote prosocial behaviour (Jevning et al., 1978; Davidson, 1976).

An individual is made of different inside realities, seeds or layers corresponding to different emotions. We need to be the gardener of our seeds. Rather than fighting the anger, we can accept and befriend it, while watering the seeds of compassion and joy. This will allow the seeds of compassion to grow bigger little by little, thus weakening the seed of anger and changing angry behavioural patterns. Therefore, we can transform our behaviour from "me-first" actions to surrender to the common self. With persistence, little by little, we can change one's mindset from a safety ego orientation to an open-hearted compassionate orientation (Narvaez, 2014). Compassion for others requires a motivation to be helpful, capable of tolerating any distress feelings that arise, and capable of non-judgemental empathic connection with the suffering of others. There is growing evidence that practising and cultivating compassion for others has a range of psychophysical and health benefits (Keltner et al., 2014; Ricard, 2015). Compassionate goals were linked to feeling connected, low conflict and better mental health than were self-image goals. Indeed, the more self-focused, competitive and shame-focused people are, the more prone to depression they may be (Crocker et al., 2010).

Mindfulness presence allows you to be in the process and understand what is going on (e.g. in yourself, your partner, in his relationship with you, in your child, in pregnancy). Moreover, having the seeds of anger shouldn't nourish a sense of guilt, as seeds result from early life circumstances, e.g. trauma (abuse, neglect), school experiences such as bullying etc. In fact, very often an angry child has an angry parent. Then we need self-compassion through the realisation that seeds, like genes, are passed on by our parents and grandparents and are watered (switched on) by the environment and early experiences. There is considerable evidence that having a hostile and critical approach to oneself, in contrast to a supportive and compassionate one, is highly associated with vulnerability to a range of mental health problems, particularly depression (Gilbert & Choden, 2013; Neff, 2015). One way to think of self-compassion is an alternative to self-criticism and general negative self-evaluation. Neff developed self-interventions for non-clinical populations (Neff & Germer, 2013). Neff suggests:

> Self-compassion, therefore, involves being touched by and open to one's own suffering, not avoiding or disconnecting from it, generating the desire to alleviate one's suffering and to heal oneself with kindness. Self-compassion also involves offering non-judgemental understanding to one's pain, inadequacies and failures, so that one's experience is seen as part of the larger human experience.
>
> (p. 87)

The main way that self-compassion enhances positive well-being may be via increased self-kindness, common humanity, and mindfulness associated with a compassionate mind state, and the main way it reduces psychopathology may be via decreased self-judgment, isolation and over-identification (Neff, 2015). A study found that in patients with chronic illnesses, self-critical judgement emerged as the best predictor of depressive and stress symptoms, and the quality of life dimensions (Pinto-Gouveia et al., 2014). However, in patients with cancer, it was the affiliate dimensions of self-compassion that significantly predicted lower levels of depressive and stress symptoms, and increased quality of life. It was found that in recovery from psychosis, self-criticism was associated with increasing distress over psychotic experiences, whereas self-compassion was associated with empowerment and growth (Waite et al., 2015).

Self-reassurance/supportive/affiliate and harshly/fearfully self-critical ways of self-relating have different attachment histories and the resulting underlying representation of self and others (Gillath et al., 2005). A study of 197 students explored recall of early parenting of rejection and warmth, in relation to self-criticism and self-reassurance and their impact on depression. Parental rejection was associated with self-criticism and depression and parental warmth with self-reassuring and lower depression (Irons et al., 2006). There is also evidence that the physiological processes underpinning self-criticism and shame, compared to self-reassuring and caring, are associated with different brain systems (Longe et al., 2010). According to epigenetics, attachment history is passed on to next generations and affects parenting style, mindfulness, compassion and self-compassion. Training in these domains can significantly mitigate the adverse effects on children.

David Sloan Wilson, Distinguished Professor of Biology and Anthropology, has explored how the basic human needs towards goodness can be consciously nurtured and passed onto the offspring to create a better future for both humanity and the planet (2019). Sloan Wilson highlights that altruism, compassion, and everything we associate with goodness can evolve as a product of evolution, but only when certain conditions are met, that is when there is cooperation and altruism within members of the group. Furthermore, evolution can be a conscious process guided by humans to achieve an ethics of the whole world. The Dalai Lama stresses the importance of training the mind and nurturing to overcome destructive emotions and that such training needs to begin early in the way children are educated. The Dalai Lama calls for teaching children universal values, such as kindness, compassion and altruism, and cultivating our understanding of our shared humanity. Developing an open-hearted compassionate orientation creates a ripple effects since the way in which we behave towards others creates states of mind in others, facilitating a sense of safety (Gilbert, 2005).

Embodied presence, attentiveness and attunement

According to Eastern teaching, the deepest level of the mind is constantly in contact with bodily sensations, thus disproving the belief that meditation refers to a mystical experience. Mindfulness practice is about being present by "being in the body" and allowing each moment to be just as it is. A wonderful way to cultivate this is through breathing awareness and the body scan practice. With this practice, we gently and gradually move our attention through our body, paying attention to whatever sensation we notice from moment to moment. We may notice warmth, cold, tingling sensations, or the absence of sensations. Our mind will inevitably wander several times in the course of a session. The practice is just to notice and bring the mind back. In this way, we cultivate the mind's ability to be focused and present. At times, the practice may be pleasant and relaxing; at other times, we may become bored or feel agitated. We just notice and allow this. In this way, we cultivate the mindful attitude.

Through attention to sensations, we can train the mind to become conscious of bodily sensations and bodily processes, of its presence in the body. If proper attention is not given to the bodily sensations, then we are not going to the deepest level of the mind, as the mind is constantly in contact with bodily sensations and emotions. This process of consciousness has a physiological underpinning, affecting health, thus pregnancy and childbirth. By enhancing attentiveness, mindfulness practice can help during pregnancy, birth and parenting to connect with the unborn baby and infant and to communicate. In our society, pain in childbirth is often unwanted, but it is a physiological necessity in labour. In fact, it mobilises the woman's resources and enables her to focus and be present, notice and allow things, all qualities necessary for connecting with and understanding the baby.

The quality of parent-child interaction, from pregnancy (e.g. touching the abdomen in response to baby's movement or reflection on the baby), straight after birth and beyond, depends on the adult's sense of being present and awareness of their baby's needs and experience. This attentiveness and engagement with the present moment can be an antidote to anxiety and stress and prevent birth complications, caesarean deliveries and other kinds of intervention, and even premature births. Many studies have suggested that the early interactions between parents and their babies lay an important foundation for the child's later emotional, social and cognitive development (Stanley et al., 2004). Mindfulness practice positively engages with pregnancy, birth and parenting, as it encourages moment-to-moment contact with the flow of experience rather than constructs or concepts, which govern the West today. Nevertheless, while the West has mainly been concerned about pathology and cure, the East's focus is on prevention and practice to pursue balance and health and prevent illness.

The moment-by-moment interactions require focus and connection with the baby, thus empathy, and are undermined by an adult's preoccupation, anxiety or stress. Mindfulness practice provides a great opportunity to become aware of the habitual patterns of a preoccupied mind and their denial of the attention and connection the baby needs to thrive. Interestingly, babies and children can teach us about moment-by-moment experience, which their flexible brain can freely and fully absorb. It is because of this neuroplasticity that their brains need moment-by-moment interactions with a mindful caregiver, which create the neural relationships necessary for developing well-being (Siegel & Hartzell, 2003).

Neural changes resulting from mindfulness meditation may increase the efficiency of attentional control (Malinowski, 2013). Focused attention meditation is typically practised first to increase the ability to enhance attentional stability, and awareness of mental states with the goal being the ability to monitor moment-by-moment changes in experience. Mindfulness meditation may lead to greater cognitive flexibility (Kashdan & Rottenberg, 2010). Neuroscientists tell us that perception is never "the thing as it is". Mindful awareness does permit us to get as close as we can to clear vision, to a *grounded receptive state*, which allows mothers and fathers to connect fully with the feelings and experiences of their preborn babies. To be open to experiencing, we first need to be in a state of intentionality to receive (Siegel, 2007).

The same occurs in the therapeutic process. The state of right-brain receptiveness in a sensitive mother, expressed as *presence*, is the same as that of the sensitive therapist or mindfulness facilitator, expressed as "therapeutic presence". Both maternal and therapeutic presence involves being fully in the moment on a multitude of levels – physically, emotionally, cognitively, spiritually and relationally. Therapeutic presence involves being in contact with one's healthy self, while being *open* and *receptive* to what is poignant in the moment and immersed in it, with a larger sense and expansion of awareness and perception (Schore, 2012).

Coupled with attentiveness, intentionality teaches a pregnant mother to notice and interpret her baby's cues and behaviour in the womb. Awareness of bodily sensations, breathing, quality of voice, movements and gestures, can help create a mindful *in-utero* and in-arm experience for the baby. Dr Alfred Tomatis has studied maternal voice as an organiser of the baby's hearing system and ability to listen (1981). I recall how my unborn baby's movements in response to my favourite piano music became increasingly more fluent and rhythmic towards the end of gestation – due to maturational processes but also my increased intentionality and her familiarisation with the music. This suggests that, like maternal voice or music, any experience of presence may begin to regulate the unborn baby's early sensorimotor experiences.

Meditation can be practised anywhere, in your bedroom or in a spare room in your house, as long as it is a quiet place for mental and spiritual expansion. You can practise mindfulness in Nature – a short walk through the woods, or even a few minutes cultivating your garden will reconnect you with the wisdom of your body-self. This practice will gradually take you to a new way of living. During my pregnancy I loved reflecting under a tree or while walking around a lake in Southern Italy or through a London park, and found Nature calming and inspiring. It gave me a deep sense of inner harmony and an abundance of physical energy. It is a scientific fact that contemplation of natural scenes is favourable to our physical and mental health and vitality (Kaplan & Kaplan, 1989). In South Korea, a university programme offers prenatal forest meditation and therapy to reduce stress hormones, suggesting it can reduce medical costs and benefit local economies. Korean researchers using functional MRI to observe brain activity in people looking at a natural scene detected the activation of areas associated with empathy and altruism. But I also practised while lying down in my bed. Mindfulness meditation enables you to see and appreciate the beauties and pleasures of each moment of living, thus of pregnancy, childbirth and parenting. A mindful way of life integrates reverence and regard for beauty in everyday life.

In a quiet mental state, I could experience how events were unfolding naturally around me, without me trying hard to make them happen. I became aware of synchronicity and started seeing connections between creatures in nature, events and people, and seeing some meaning in them rather than mere chance. The beautiful concurrence of mindfulness and pregnancy taught me to see life as a universal dialogue, a network of interactions and relationships with the ecosystem unfolding smoothly. This is living in a creative way. The message is "take the time to reflect every morning on the good you will do for your baby during your day, connect with each moment of her life, and appreciate each interaction". Every prenatal and perinatal practitioner should convey this empathic message. It is a good that a parent does both for the baby and for the whole society. Maternal reflective function (capacity to have the baby in mind) and attachment security have been found to be predictors of the child's capacity to read people's minds and be empathic (Meins et al., 2002).

Mindfulness is about learning to live in the present and see with a whole-ness perspective. Due to the demands of our modern life, and also to the nature of human mind, especially if it was not fully nurtured in childhood, we spend much of our time taken away by thoughts and worries, not really conscious of what is going on and liable to repeatedly make mistakes and unwise choices. Everyday anxiety carries us away from our embodiment, interconnectedness, wholeness and the present moment. Mindful preg-nancy, childbirth and parenting are best seen as a *practice*, a discipline, in that we continuously observe and reflect on our behaviour and interactions with our baby. Every time a mother holds, hugs or breastfeeds her baby, if she does it with awareness and connection with her embodied feelings as well as the baby's experience, it is practice, leading to learning and under-standing. She is fully present, knowing that she is picking up her baby, the impact on her, and the wholeness of the situation implied. It means being in touch with feeling, smelling, touching, breathing, muscular tension, with everything is happening (Kabat-Zinn & Kabat-Zinn, 1990). When a mother is breastfeeding, or changing nappies, or singing to her baby, she is there in these special moments. And the baby knows she is present, connected.

It is the pregnant body, its wisdom, that is telling a mother what to do. When she is connected with her body and aware of her unborn baby as a sentient being, able to interact and communicate, it is her baby telling her what to do in the present moment, not what she has learnt in an instruc-tional book. This is when a synchronised or attuned communication is unfolding, and the mother's and the baby's mirror neurons attune to each other. This is when we do not do things automatically and our mind is not somewhere else, and if it goes away, we can bring our attention back. It is not always easy, as our minds are so easily carried away by our thoughts, wor-ries and anxieties. This mental activity affects our body language, such as breathing, muscular tension, and so our gestures towards our baby.

By paying attention to what is going on in a present moment in preg-nancy, labour and any aspect of parenting and a baby's life, we practise and improve in our mindfulness and prevent many problems related to childhood in recent years. And we learn from each moment of the baby's life as well as from ourselves and our evolving being. When we live in this way, we live with creativity and make our daily lives a work of art. This art of conscious living is indeed transmitted to the baby beginning in the womb.

Mindfulness and attachment

Mindfulness refers to a form of healthy or attuned relationship with one-self, which is a condition for attuning with the other, thus for feeling empa-thy. This kind of attunement is so relevant to parenting in describing how a parent focuses attention on the child's interpersonal world (Siegel, 2007). Receptive attention by both mother and father is fundamental for a baby/ child to have a felt sense of being received, seen, listened, accepted, valued and wanted. This kind of attention is not an intellectual process but involves an open communication sensory system and integrated mind-body. When a mother's attentiveness is steadfast and her heart and body open to receive, the child feels connected and regulated. When her attention is inconsistent or poor, a child experiences emotional disconnection and difficult self-regulation. However, the sense of here-and-now interaction (presence) allows the mother to notice the dyssynchrony and re-establish synchrony and repair, allowing the intersubjective dance to unfold. When the mind is wandering and not focused, it is hard to be present and connect with the baby's present need and enjoy our experience and inner world.

This focus on another person's mind and body cues, for instance those of a child, harnesses neural circuitry that enables us to "feel felt" by each other, which equals with a feeling of being vibrant and alive. Therefore, mindful awareness is a form of intrapersonal as well as interpersonal attunement. This feeling of being felt or "connected" may foster in the brain *neural integration* that promotes self-regulation and balance. Some scientists have proposed that the secure attachment between parent and child and the effective therapeutic relationship between clinician and patient promotes the growth of the fibres in the prefrontal area (Cozolino, 2002; Schore 2003a, 2003b; Siegel & Hartzell, 2003). The prefrontal area is integrative. This means that the long strands of the prefrontal neurons reach out to distant areas of the brain and body, thus allowing for integration. Integration can be seen as the pathway leading to well-being (Siegel, 2001). I view the attunement and mutual understanding and support between parents an essential as contributors to well-being in the parents as well as the child. We can understand how connection and empathy between healthcare professionals and pregnant/new parent is fundamental to promoting prefrontal growth and well-being in them. This shared feeling of integration has an impact on the parent-child relationship.

This relationship between parent and child is highly relevant to child development. When it is attuned, a child can sense being "felt" by the caregiver and has a sense of stability within the present moment. During the here-and-now interaction, the child feels good, connected and loved and the parent can resonate with the child's state. Attunement is therefore relevant to parent's well-being as well. It can be nurtured during pregnancy in many ways, e.g. through the mother's reflective function, communicative tactile games with the baby, melodic music listening, meditation and contemplation in Nature. Parent-baby attunement is the precursor of perinatal health. Over time, this attuned communication feeds the *regulatory* as well as *integrative* circuits in the brain, shaping the child's capacity for self-regulation and engagement with others in empathic relationships (Siegel, 2007). Siegel argues that the interpersonal attunement, the essence of a secure attachment, leads to the same mindful awareness outcomes.

By practising mindfulness, expectant and new parents learn how to be reflective and aware of their children and themselves, with curiosity, wonder, openness, acceptance and love. Mindfulness practice also teaches healthcare professionals with a concern for prenatal and perinatal health to be reflective and empathic towards parents and their babies, so as to resonate with their mental state and offer a reinforcing mirror that promotes an empathic parent-infant relationship.

"The capacity to integrate conscious attention with emotional experience may be fundamental to empathic experience" (Tucker et al., 2005, p. 707). The authors argue that the process of developing skills of attention and attunement would foster adaptive self-regulation. The self-regulatory prefrontal regions, which monitor and coordinate the activity of a wide range of areas of the brain and body, require for their development appropriate experiences with responsive caregivers. In other words, relational experiences promote the development of self-regulation in the brain. Repeated, positive, synchronised caregiver-child interactions organise the infant's capacities for self-regulation through the proper functioning of the orbitofrontal cortex, mesocortical and mesolimbic pathways (Feldman, 2007). The foundations for social capacities are formed during this time and include mentalising, empathy, self-regulation, the gaze and facial expression, the experience of social pleasure, sensitivity to stress in others and attention (Narvaez, 2014). Early trauma and neglect interfere with the development of these areas, in particular the right hemisphere, which shapes the human stress response (Wittling, 1997). If we consider mindfulness a form of internal attunement, or secure relationship with the self, it would also promote the healthy growth of the social and self-regulatory prefrontal regions.

Seven functions of the middle prefrontal region are associated with attunement in both mindfulness and secure attachment: body regulation, attuned communication, emotional balance, response flexibility, empathy, self-knowing awareness and fear modulation (Siegel, 2007). Mindful practice also appears to develop two other middle prefrontal functions: intuition and morality (Kabat-Zinn, 2003b). All these functions are fostered by ancient wisdom practices. The social neural circuits involved in this attunement include the middle prefrontal regions, insula, superior temporal cortex and the mirror neuron systems. These regions contain the *resonance* circuits and enable one's mind to resonate with the internal state of another as well as with her or his own internal processes. This is consistent with the findings concerning activation in the resonance circuits (superior temporal and middle prefrontal cortices) in mindful awareness of the breath (Lazar, 2006).

There are striking links between mindful awareness, secure attachment and right-hemisphere involvement outcomes. Allan Schore's work on attachment and development, which brings together neurological, biological and psychological studies, emphasises the fundamental role of the right brain in emotional regulation, healthy physiological and psychological development and healthy development of the immune system (Schore,

2003a, 2003b). Schore writes of non-conscious right-brain to right-brain communications (non-verbal) between parent and infant, which develop regulation (or dysregulation when it is poor) of the autonomic nervous system. The right hemisphere plays an important role in the development of emotional intelligence, creativity, empathy, autobiographical memory and self-reflection. Interestingly, interdisciplinary studies of creativity propose the right-brain hemisphere as the seat of creativity. The baby and young child need the mother's right-brain involvement in their interactions to thrive physiologically, neurologically and psychologically. She needs right-brain to right-brain communications to learn empathy; compassion; awareness of her own emotions, thus of others' emotions; and self-reflection and to develop autobiographical memory.

It is evident that the interpersonal attunement of secure attachment between parent and child corresponds to an interpersonal form of attunement in mindful awareness (Siegel, 2007). Both forms of attunement promote the capacity for intimate relationships, resilience and well-being. Studies of secure attachment and those of mindful awareness practices have strikingly overlapping findings (Kabat-Zinn, 2003b; Sroufe et al., 2005). Siegel found that these findings were also associated with the functions of the prefrontal cortex: regulation of body systems, balancing emotions, attuning to others, modulating fear, responding flexibly and manifesting insights and empathy. The practice of mindfulness seems to also promote intuition and moral behaviour, two other functions of the prefrontal region.

Attachment and mindfulness are both species-universal. Narvaez (2014, p. 70) writes:

> The *attachment behavioural system* is a species-universal programme that bonds child to mother. It collaborates with the adult's *caregiving behavioural system*, which under normal conditions is a species-universal programme that guides maternal bonding and caregiving. Both these species-wide programmes appear to be shaped during sensitive periods in the individual's life.

Both these programmes are promoted by the universal practice of mindfulness.

The use of a compassionate relationship-based perspective in prenatal and perinatal care relies on collaborative and attuned patterns of interaction between infant and parent. In an attuned parent-infant/child relationship, the infant provides cues relating to his feelings and/or what he needs (e.g. more or less of a sensation such as movement, sound or temperature), and the parent reads these cues and responds accordingly. Parental responsiveness can be conceived of as nature's "dose-control system", ensuring that the infant regulates the type and intensity of sensation (Whittingham et al., 2016). This is so important for learning to modulate painful sensations. Mindfulness training facilitates this process of self-regulation in both parents and infant. When this attunement occurs, the infant's active role in regulating the intensity and type of incoming sensation can assist with maintaining a calm and alert state, which is considered necessary to support learning and development.

Thus, fostering parental responsiveness through nurturing practices such as mindfulness can be useful for helping infants and children to achieve calm-alert neurological systems to support optimal learning and development (Barfoot et al., 2017). Mothers who have been trained to embody mindfulness or other nurturing strategies through their relationship with the baby during pregnancy can report this positive development outcome in their child. My own mindfulness interaction-focused pregnancy experience shaped the self-regulated caring nature of my daughter. However, evidence of the influences of this embodied primal wisdom on mother and preborn/infant is still required. Moreover, with the parent-child relationship being more attuned and the child more regulated, targeted developmental strategies shared with the parents to support the unique needs of an infant or child with developmental problems or delays are implemented, while remaining mindful of their child's body signals (Atkins-Burnett & Allen-Meares, 2000).

6 Transformation of human traits and being

Meditation methods such as mindfulness have helped many people find relief, not just from post-traumatic stress disorders (PTSD) but from virtually the entire range of emotional disorders. Yet mindfulness, part of an ancient meditation tradition, was not intended to be a cure; this method was only recently adopted as a cure for our modern dysfunctions. "The original aim, embraced in some circles to this day, focuses on a deep exploration of the mind towards a profound alteration of our very being" (Goleman & Davidson, 2017, p. 2). Goleman and Davidson define an altered trait a new characteristic of our being that arises from a meditation practice and persists after we meditate, shaping how we behave in our daily lives. This is when mindfulness becomes a state of being, a way of life. The further reaches of the deep path of meditation cultivate enduring qualities such as selflessness, equanimity, loving-kindness, loving presence, compassion and self-compassion and responsiveness. These are highly positive altered traits that benefit conception, pregnancy and birth, parenting, parental mental well-being, attachment, foetal and infant/child development and well-being. These altered traits correspond to remarkable positive alterations in brain, feelings, cognitions and behaviour.

Fostering well-being and human capacities in children through responsiveness and companionate care can lead to wise living. When early life has been marked by adverse experiences, or has generated trauma, the path to wisdom may have been obstructed. The development of our true body-self has been jeopardised. How can human nature be restored in adults so as to create an optimal uterine environment as well as provide a mirror to our children? We do not have to go back to living like hunter-gatherers to recuperate our human essence but instead integrate their wisdom – our innate evolved capacity for nurturing – into a transformed self and world. We can foster communal and ecological wisdom. We can use the skills and tools that modern life has given us to adopt new ways of being and thus further knowledge about alternative approaches. While there are skills to be learnt on this journey, a mindfulness facilitator conveys the sense that wisdom is already present in any individual and group, and his role is to support an environment in which mindfulness can grow and individual wisdom can emerge. The practice of mindfulness offers a way to restore human virtues to their full potential, when their development has been curtailed in early life or by subsequent traumas (Goleman & Davidson, 2017).

When I visited the Himba, I had tangible evidence of how we have stepped away from species-typical behaviour, especially in regard to prenatal/perinatal and childcare practices, and community engagement. It seems that human cultural evolution in recent centuries has exerted a powerful influence and has altered typical *ontogeny* (individual development) and perhaps even *phylogeny* (species development) (Narvaez, 2014). The increase in psychopathologies such as Asperger's syndrome, developmental delays, attention deficit/hyperactivity disorder (ADHD), learning difficulties, complicated births and birth-trauma-related disturbances and perinatal mental disturbances could be partly a consequence of this cultural change. Prenatal, obstetric, perinatal and childcare practices have been significantly affected by this cultural change. For example the increase in rates of caesarean births is anticipated to be leading to changes in our species (Odent, 2015). Processed food is depriving pregnant mothers of the natural nutritional intakes needed for mental health and healthy foetal brain development, contributing to perinatal mental disorders and child developmental problems (Gow, 2021).

Social media and technology, despite having brought amazing advances, may foster more bullying, abusive behaviour as children and young people have fewer opportunities to practise their human capabilities in intersubjective relationships, which are the foundation of future parents' responsiveness and precursors of a child's secure attachment. As previously mentioned, epigenetic inheritance of adverse experiences may be curtailing the sense of empathy, moral sense, social skills and emotion self-regulation, fostering social discomfort, reactive behaviour, extreme self-reliance, obsessive-compulsive behaviour, dominance, hoarding instead of generosity, pleasure for self (consuming), egotism, underdeveloped right-brain regulatory systems (involved in mother-infant communication, responsiveness, mirroring and attunement) and detached imagination.

Darcia Narvaez (2014) has explained earlier that we can move from a culture of social and ethical disengagement, hyper-intellectualism and safety towards a culture of companionship, intersubjective and ecological engagement, shared parenting and childcare, and communal and wisdom ethics, which recreates the community that has supported pregnancy and parenthood and has educated children into wisdom over millennia.

The central role of emotions and self-regulation

For centuries in Western culture, emotions have been undervalued and regarded in a controversial way and yet, when well developed, they may be our finest form of rationality (MacMurray, 1992). Well-trained emotions guide adaptive animal behaviour. Neuroscientist Jaak Panksepp writes that we can be quite certain that all mammals share many basic psychoneural processes because of the long evolutionary journey they have shared (1998). He points out that it is our ancient animal heritage that contributes to making us the intense, feeling creatures that we are. He adds that we can clarify the primal sources of human evolution as we come to understand the neural basis of animal emotions. Of course, because of our richer cortical potentials, the ancient emotional systems have to interact with a much vaster cognitive universe.

Emotional systems play a central role in human brain and dynamically interact with more evolved cognitive structures. Emotions change sensory, perceptual and cognitive processing and guide behaviour. Darcia Narvaez posits that moral development derives from earliest socio-emotional experiences with our caregivers. Yet, psychological theories often consider emotion and cognition as separate entities. Components of emotion systems (arousal, action tendencies, prospective motor control and intention) are generally placed in the brain stem, hypothalamic structures and cerebellum. The brain stem develops during embryonic stage and the networks are integrating across different areas of the brain (Panksepp, 1998). Highlighting the complexity of emotion systems, Panksepp writes that affective feeling links brain stem, paralimbic and prefrontal structures.

Emotions and cognition often overlap throughout the brain. In fact, many of the brain systems are involved in both domains (Panksepp, 1991; LeDoux, 1993). In the neuronal cortex, there is no distinction between cognition and emotion. Emotion and cognition work as a functional unity and are linked to behaviour (M. D. Lewis, 2005). There is no emotion without thought, and thoughts in general evoke emotions. Researchers conceive of earliest rudimentary goal-directed intentional sensorimotor activity of the foetus as the necessary foundation for developing more complex mental processes such as emotions, cognition and consciousness (Delafield-Butt & Gangopadhyay, 2013). In fact, Greenspan and Shanker (2004) propose that emotions arise from multiple factors, including physical experiences, signals from others and meaning-making. These components, rooted in prenatal life, later become the source of a child's linguistic and cognitive advancement and reflective capabilities. Caregivers' responses influence the infant's subjective experience of sensations (including pain), affect and cognitions.

Attuned responses to infant cues help the infant to organise his emotional and physiological experience leading to reflective functioning. Emotions and affect form "the source of symbols, the architect of intelligence, the integrator of processing capacities, and the psychological foundation of society" (Greenspan & Shanker, 2004, p. 46). This is why it is crucial to foster parents' well-being and responsiveness through nurturing practices from pregnancy and ideally before conception. Mindfulness practice and a mindfulness-oriented therapy promote both sensitiveness and reflective functioning fundamental for parents' responsiveness and leading to the child's emotional self-regulation. In particular, mindfulness-based interventions encourage awareness of emotions and body sensations, enhancing stress tolerance and reducing reactivity, all abilities improving responsiveness and understanding of an infant's needs and feelings, thus important for parenting (Hall et al., 2015).

Babies' emotions are embedded in playful relationships, which therefore shape neurobiological development (Trevarthen & Aitken, 2003). Early experience has profound effects on multiple biological systems involving emotions, cognitions and symbols. Our bodies (e.g. breathing and heart rhythms, muscular tensions and posture) carry the traces of our experiences. The kinds of emotional experience that the baby has with his caregivers, for instance whether pleasurable or traumatic, are "biologically embedded". While developing in another human body, the baby absorbs all the internal chemistry of maternal emotional/mental states (e.g. stress-hormone cortisol or feel-good hormones) through the placenta (Chamberlain, 2013; Lipton, 2015). These influence the gene activity of the developing prenate (Anacker et al., 2014; Serpeloni et al., 2016). In the prenatal and perinatal period of human life – the most critical one – patterns of self-regulation are being formed as a result of the brain's extraordinary plasticity. Emotions are essential for self-regulation.

By responding sensitively and mindfully to the baby's needs, the mother helps him acknowledge his own feelings and regulate them. The mother's mindfulness is essential for the baby to develop self-understanding and mindful awareness. By learning to respond appropriately, the infant and child learn to settle the biochemical, muscular and autonomic responses that have already been triggered (rather than reacting to them). But if the baby learns to suppress the emotional response, for instance anger, because his mother rejects it rather than accepting and containing it, his body and its various systems remain aroused and biologically stimulated. This interferes with the flow of information and it becomes more difficult to behave with flexibility. Failure of regulation can generate disturbances and later pathology.

Repeated, positive synchronised parent-child interactions organise the infant's capacities for self-regulation through proper functioning of the orbitofrontal cortex (OFC), mesocortical and mesolimbic pathways (Feldman, 2007). According to Porges's polyvagal theory (Porges, 2011), attuned interactions between parent and child help establish optimal vagal tone, which equals with proper functioning of the visceral organs controlled by the vagal nerve, which in turn is connected with brain centres. Having a history with chronic misattunement with one's caregivers predisposes people to difficulties in managing negative emotions later in life, which has implications in social life (Dozier et al., 1999). Sadly, poor affect regulation caused by early adverse experiences manifests itself through behavioural problems in the face of stress, such as temper tantrums and emotional withdrawal (Shaver & Mikulincer, 2002). Mindful awareness allows for integrative functioning of the nervous system through shared meaningful timing and gestures at the infant's own pace and without rushing. It follows that promoting parents' mental well-being and responsiveness through mindfulness-based practices has to be the goal of every prenatal/perinatal educational programme.

Experience, implicit memory and the biology of freedom

In early life, the moment-by-moment experience with caregivers, especially with the mother, generate neuronal associations that form implicit memories that later underpin emotional and social life. A blueprint of these experiences begins in prenatal life. Everyday living involves the interaction between the activated senses (present) and memory of related experiences (past) (Ansermet & Magistretti, 2007). This explains why trauma, especially in early life, can cause a shutdown of bodily feelings and memories and a disengagement with life. "Thus, the brain is a social dynamic organ whose neuronal connections are modified by external experience (life events) and internal experience (biological and psychic events), structurally and functionally creating a unique, singular individual" (Ansermet & Magistretti, 2007, p. 6). Poor early experiences lead to a non-integrative functioning of the brain and internal reality, which hinders mindfulness (Siegel, 2007).

Chronic stress affects not only our emotional systems but our thinking and reasoning. For those who were neglected or abused, the perception of external reality and awareness of the present moment can be overwhelmed by internal reality. Trauma experienced in the past preoccupies and interferes with present attention, curtailing full perceptions and even actions (van der Kolk, 2014). Early and ongoing stress hinders our sense of the present moment, attentiveness, full perceptions and trust in people. When stress has been experienced too much and too early, our physiological and immune systems do not work properly. There are ongoing effects on social and moral functioning. This undermines our capacity to be mindful and compassionate towards others as well as our self, and if we are becoming or are parents, it is likely to affect foetal development and well-being and have lifelong emotional and social effects. Chronic stress and mental illness hamper the ability to perceive, be receptive or feel the flow of life and see beauty. For a mother, this ability is crucial to feel and enjoy a developing relational presence in the womb, to pick up the baby's cues and nuances, thus to be responsive.

Thanks to the brain's plasticity, we can free ourselves from genetic determinism. We can overcome rigidity, negative thoughts and behavioural patterns through the right practice and support. We can self-create through a process of self-authorship, freeing ourselves from psychological and biological determinism and reshaping neurobiology (Ansermet & Magistretti, 2007/2004). A lot of people struggle for many years, unaware of their inner resources for change or with undiagnosed post-traumatic stress disorders (PTSD), which makes it difficult to create intimate relationships or a happy and fulfilling life. Others may be prescribed drugs for years, causing more adverse psychophysiological effects. We can actively modify our being, creating new neuronal networks and improving the efficiency of neuronal transmission through imagination and rehearsal (Bear, 2003). Parents can mitigate the effects of intergenerational corrosive patterns through nurturing practices as early as during pregnancy or before conception. Thoughts and imagination are physiological events generating changes of energy and vitality, perception and even muscle strength (Stern, 2010). As mentioned earlier, a ground-breaking study revealed that those athletes who only imagined exercising a muscle increased its strength nearly as much as those who actually exercised the muscle (Yue & Cole, 1992).

This openness to letting being and brain be transformed by experience in contrast with a rigid self, which is in line with ancient wisdom, is of great significance to modern parents, as they can enhance their well-being and caring abilities and thus foster their children's neurobiological well-being and wisdom. Humans are psychosociobiological beings, transformed by experience and intersubjective relationships from early life. The wisdom fostered by the practice of mindfulness counteracts the effects of mental disturbances and trauma and offers a way to restore human nature and essence to its full potential. The natural world, including human beings, can contribute to human beings' transformation through cooperation instead of competitiveness. Mindfulness can allow the recognition of the need for psychotherapy in more severe cases. When mindfulness and compassion permeate therapy, the path to transformation through the therapist-client relationship is open.

Techniques of mindfulness

Coping with difficulties of life or recovering from the consequences of trauma are a matter of resources. Resources are to a large extent built in early life, although they can be cultivated at any stage of human life through practice. When we devote our life to encapsulating the true essence of being, we know the joy and peace that comes from being one with our body, mind and soul. Mindfulness requires a considerable investment in time as well as courage, determination and self-honesty. The business of life can also sweep us away from our practice. Amid so much activity, it can be hard to find the time for the nurturing practice of not doing but being. It requires a strong motivation. Preparing for fulfilling parenting and offering the children the opportunities to learn all the abilities fostered by the wisdom of mindfulness can only be led by a profound heartfelt motivation. Connecting with a deep and personal motivation for practising, such as that of having an impact on children's development and well-being, not only sustains us over time, it adds an energy to our practice in the moment.

Mindfulness is one of the most important foundations of health and wisdom through ways of knowing that are cultivated by three self-calming techniques: deep breathing (including yoga), savouring states and meditation.

Practise deep breathing

Breathing allows our body to take in enough oxygen and promote its optimal heath. But most of us do not breathe properly. We undervalue the benefits of breathing properly. The physiological benefits of oxygen include eliminating toxins in tissues, cells and the bloodstream; increasing the uptake of nutrients; killing infectious bacteria; and boosting the immune system (Altman, 2007). The psychological effects include boosted energy and a calmer self-regulated nervous system. Breathing properly during pregnancy is particularly important, since the supplies of oxygen increase by 20 per cent. The enhanced body awareness also helps connect with the developing baby. You can build a habit of deep breathing during some daily activities (e.g. dishwashing, while on the train, driving, holding the baby and breastfeeding). It is important to engage the diaphragm while breathing in. Extending the exhalation as long as possible keeps the parasympathetic system (calming) active. Breathing practice helps you connect with your body by becoming aware of the breathing and body sensations, feelings and needs.

Belly laughing has similar effects on health. Laughing with your friends and at each other reduces stress, thus improves cardiovascular health (Provine, 2001). Humour that makes you laugh changes metabolism. When we laugh, our lungs, larynx and the intercostal muscles are engaged, and the release of endorphins elevates our mood and sustain our health. The bodymind needs the life-affirming, joyous experience of laughter. Breathing and states of mind and emotions, completely ignored by the Western medical model, play a significant role in pregnancy well-being.

The connection between the breath and the mind has been understood since ancient times, and there is evidence of this in yoga texts. Therapists who are now working in the evolving field of the body-oriented approach to treating trauma are increasingly acknowledging that an understanding of breathing techniques is essential. Breathing allows us to access the autonomic nervous system, and it is one of the few bodily functions that is under both our conscious and autonomic control. Breathing is related to feeling. Rapid breathing, not involving the abdomen as well, is synonymous with being scared or angry, and when we feel calm and relaxed our breathing slows down and we feel grounded and connected. Maternal breathing is involved in co-regulation of the baby's breathing and feelings (Sansone, 2004). Sansone describes in her book *Mothers, Babies and their Body Language* how babies are very sensitive to bodily changes and cues and respond accordingly.

Contemporary specialists in the field of trauma are acknowledging that an understanding of the body and the breath creates that grounding in the mind and allows responses to come from a place of expansion rather than contraction. Dr Bessel van der Kolk, a psychiatrist and one of the leading exponents of the body-orientated treatment of trauma, explains that learning how to breathe calmly and remaining in a state of relative physical realisation, even while accessing painful and horrifying memories, is an essential tool for recovery (2014). When you deliberately take a few slow deep breaths, you will notice the effects of the parasympathetic brake on your arousal. Practitioners should not forget the role of the body in trauma and mental suffering, how the body affects the mind and brain and how a mother relates to her infant. They should keep all these in mind for maximum healing. Talking is not enough to heal trauma. Mindfulness heals the brain, body and relationship when healing trauma. To understand how this works, we need to look at what happens in the body when we have experienced trauma.

If we have not received the nurturing we need immediately after the trauma and developed resilience by having had our needs met early in life, situations that remind us of the traumatic event or experience (even very vaguely) can trigger excessive release of stress hormones, including cortisol and adrenaline. These in turn increase heart rate, blood pressure and the breathing rate, preparing us to fight back and run away. It is our brain's amygdala, which van der Kolk calls "the smoke detector", which sends out the danger signal that triggers the release of these powerful stress hormones (2014). The amygdala is located deep within the temporal lobe of the brain and is a limbic system structure. That is involved in many of our emotions and motivations, particularly those that are related to survival. It is involved in the processing of fear, anger and pleasure and also responsible for determining what memories are stored and when they are stored in the brain. It is believed that how memories are stored and where is linked to how huge our emotional response was to the event.

Pregnancy, birth and parenting are a critical time that can trigger old memories related to developmental trauma (Sansone, 2007). If the emotions are not regulated, they affect the interactions with the baby and attachment process. Breathing awareness is particularly important for mothers, as babies synchronise to mother's breath and heart rhythm and pick up emotional nuances from them. Whether the mother is anxious and stressed or attuned, loving, present and engaged, the baby senses it through many bodily cues. Mindfulness meditation and yoga can help regulate and strengthen the capacity of the frontal lobes of the brain, in particular the medial prefrontal cortex, to monitor bodily sensations, which can allow the human system to regulate feelings when the amygdala sends these danger signals. All yoga programmes consist of a combination of breathing practices (pranayama), stretches or postures and meditation. Breath, movement or touch allow us to access and regulate the autonomic nervous system, which originates in the brain stem. Learning self-regulation is one of the keys to recovery and healthy relationships. Dr van der Kolk (2014) points out that by staying focused on our breathing, we will benefit enormously, particularly if we pay attention to the very end of the out breath, and then pause a moment before we inhale again. He explains that as we continue to notice the air moving in and out of our lungs, we may appreciate the role oxygen plays in nourishing our tissues and entire body with the energy we need to stay alive and engaged.

Savouring states

Mindfulness practice can foster life-enhancing emotional states, such as love, appreciation and gratitude, which sustain maternal well-being and can benefit the life-support system of the developing unborn baby and bonding. These states might be called *savouring states* (Bryant & Veroff, 2007) characterised by *low arousal*, which is linked to an embodied feeling of being alive and social contentment – a feeling of social safety. This is a state in which attention is relaxed, open and receptive – when one is ready to explore, or when, for example, one is sitting relaxing with a friend or holding hands (Gilbert, 2005), or when a mother is breastfeeding or staring at her baby with wonder. Scientists have found in several studies that just by staring at her baby, the reward centres of a mother's brain will light up (Barret et al., 2012). This maternal brain circuitry influences the syrupy tone in which a mother speaks to her baby, how attentive she is, even the affection she feels for her baby. It is not surprising then that higher levels of stress or depression involving the amygdala functioning interfere with this process and why mindfulness practice can help mitigate or prevent them. It can be beneficial in supporting those "savouring states" that are conducive of attachment.

Maternal affect and the quality of parenting experiences are related to the amygdala response to infant faces, which provides a sense of being seen and felt. This is *low-seeking*, high-arousal engagement, corresponding to awe-filled attachment, such as feeling connected with the cosmos, or enlightenment awareness of no-self (Coxhead, 1985). This feeling of connectedness is accompanied by a sense of deeper awareness, alertness and sensory enhancement. It characterises the mother's relationship with the foetus and developing infant. These are states flooded with neuropeptide opioids, oxytocin and vasopressin. I experienced these blissful states during my pregnancy, induced both by the pregnancy itself and a mindful attitude, including regular exercise, compassion and healthy eating.

Some Asian and African tribes notice a heightening of spirituality during pregnancy and consider it important in maintaining the health of mother and child. We cannot deny the physiological effects of savouring states on conception, pregnancy and birth. Having a first-hand experience of growing a baby inside my body led me to a savouring state of spiritual insights. These were indeed a powerful force in the positive outcome of conception and an important part of the baby's life support system. The mental and physical state of my pregnancy also made me more aware of synchronicity, defined by Carl Jung as "The coincidence of events in space and time as meaning something more than mere chance, namely, a peculiar interdependence of objective events among themselves as well as with the subjective (psychic) states of the observer or observers" (Jung, 1967).

I began to see connections between events, entities and people happening simultaneously and to value this awareness. This is something described by many pregnant women. I recall wandering with my husband David in Rome at two-months' gestation and perceiving everything as so magical and full of promise and meaning: the blue sky, the ancient high trees of Villa Borghese, the bird song, the majestic historic buildings, our peaceful walk, our love, our creature growing inside my body. I saw connections between these elements and others that I had not had the chance to see in my previous fast-paced life. My new mental state and changing physiology made me perceive beauty everywhere, everything in a new light, reflecting my sense of wonder and harmony with the environment. A sense of gratitude and universal empathy made me wish I could share this state with many suffering pregnant women. I was enjoying walking while consciously feeling my breathing and the oxygen nourishing my baby.

I thought of the benefits for a pregnant mum of seeing beauty – historical, artistic, humane or natural, or even unmanifest – rather than being endlessly restrained by indoor office hours or domestic isolation, as it is often the case in our technological work-driven societies. There were moments when I felt calm and profoundly at peace – flooded with a feel-good cocktail of pregnancy hormones – progesterone and oxytocin – and endorphins boosted by my mindful awareness. I never doubted that the creature inside me was benefitting from my life-enhancing emotions. It is a maternal intuition and a feeling of cosmic connection that guided me throughout the journey into birth and beyond, just as guided mothers for millennia.

Meditative states have been found to induce increase in serotonin (other than neuropeptide opioids, oxytocin and vasopressin), suggesting that serotonin should be called the "rest and fulfilment hormone" (Bujatti & Riederer, 1976). In these states of *enlightened presence*, the mind or minds can come to new understanding, insights, creative synthesis and a higher consciousness (Tolle, 1999). Such proto-social positive states, with all related feelings such as gratitude, awe and joy, are nourishment for the sentient developing baby, as well as for the relationships between the parents and with others. Women's perceptions and beliefs during pregnancy shape their physiology, which affects their internal environment in which their developing babies grow and influences the lifelong programming of their babies' systems (Weinstein, 2016). Therefore, women and girls need to be surrounded by an environment supporting their perceptions and beliefs and promoting their human virtues and caregiving behaviour.

Meditation

Meditation refers to myriad varieties of contemplative practices, just as *sport* refers to a wide range of athletic activities (Goleman & Davidson, 2017). Like for sports, the end results of meditation vary depending on what you actually do and how. The true goal of meditation has always been the deep path leading to awakening and enduring qualities such as selflessness, equanimity, loving-kindness, loving presence and compassion. This occurs through the interaction between the practice and the brain chemistry.

Meditation fosters calmness on the physiological level by decreasing signals to the amygdala (Lazar et al., 2000), an area of the limbic system, which is activated by intense emotions. The amygdala, or fear centre, warns us of impending danger and activates the body's stress response and nerve impulses that drive up blood pressure, heart rate, and oxygen intake – preparing the body for fight or flight (Roozendaal et al., 2009). In a study of positive emotions and social connection, half of the group was assigned to practise loving-kindness meditation (used in the Buddhist tradition) for around one hour per week for several weeks. Weeks after the study was over, those who had practised the meditation showed increased positive emotions (joy, love, gratitude or hope) and an improvement in vagal tone from the baseline (an index of physical health), an effect mediated by increased perception of social connections (Kok et al., 2013). The cardiac vagal tone indicates whether the vagus nerve is functioning properly. The vagus nerve is connected with our main organs and informs the brain about how they are doing. Results suggest that positive emotions, positive social connections and physical health influence one another and this is indicated by increased vagal tone. Kok and Fredrickson also found that the combination of meditation techniques, which induced positive feelings of love, goodwill and compassion for oneself and others, and the resulting higher vagal tone enhanced the perception of social relationships, which in turn increased the final vagal tone (Kok & Fredrickson, 2010). Thus, meditation boosts health, human virtues and the perception of social support.

In my relationship-based mindfulness programme, pregnant mothers practise loving-kindness meditation and sensorimotor tactile communication to foster connection with the developing baby. In this kind of practice, connecting with the baby becomes *play*, which fosters social connectedness. Expecting a baby can help parents rediscover their playfulness and thus prepare for communicating with their infant playfully. The first time I felt my baby kick in the womb, I touched my abdomen exactly where I felt her movement and called my husband to join us in a triadic communication. The baby responded with more kicking, to which I responded with more stroking. By being aware that we were communicating I was engaging the reflecting function as well. Sensitivity and reflection are the foundation of attachment. Over time, as a result of practice and maturational processes, the quality of kicking and patterns of motion, became more attuned with the quality of my touch. In the same way, the patterns of her movements in response to my favourite music became more fluent over time and in rhythm with music.

There are many ways to meditate. Typically, there are unfocused and focused approaches. In unfocused meditation, we attend to the thought that comes and goes. If our attention gets caught on a particular item or thought, we draw attention back to the flow. In focused meditation, we attend to a stimulus (a visual object, like a candle or a sound), a sensation in the body (breath when sitting still; touching the ground when walking, a baby's movement from the womb), a mental event (an image such as a mandala or practice wheel) or a self-generated sound (a chant). Common techniques include focusing on breathing in a certain way (focusing on the diaphragm or following the breath through the body and out) or on a mantra (a statement that can be given by a mentor or chosen by the meditator).

More active approaches are walking meditation, tai chi and yoga, which can also be practised in a meditative way. It is also possible to meditate with a focus on gratitude, drawing our attention to the good things that are generating positive feelings. Through storytelling, dances and ceremonies, e.g. singing to the soul of the child before conception and other creative activities, indigenous people intentionally practise receptive attention, fostered by mindfulness practice. This would explain why secure attachments develop by default among these cultures, as receptive attention is at the basis of responsiveness and attunement. This kind of attention is likely to lead to ecologically mindful morality and communities, thus to alloparenting and shared childcare (Narvaez, 2012). Activities such as dancing, community art, gardening, music listening, singing, playful exercise, can all have elements of mindfulness and are all ways to learn social pleasure. Most of these activities help nurture positive moods and prosocial skills around the time of conception, during pregnancy and beyond, which foster responsiveness and shared care. The Himba I visited used to gather around the Holy Fire in a meditative and gift-sharing way. They connected with the ancestors to show them gratitude for supporting human life. Positive emotions need to be accompanied by a communal connection and respect for others in our attention to life (Valdesolo & DeSteno, 2006). Feeling a connection with something greater than the self, keeping a cosmic view in mind and creating a state of gratitude promote prosocial behaviour. Practising compassion- and gratefulness-focused meditation can not only support pregnancy outcomes but also nourish a prenatal bonding.

Receptive attention and intersubjective connection

We are embedded in a network of relationships, not only with members of our species, but with all entities. If the same mindful attention we pay towards others we mindfully pay towards the natural world, we can deepen our understanding of life (Husserl, 1989). When I moved with my family to Australia to undertake my PhD, I was exposed to new sensual and spiritual engagements, new smells, trees' scents and tonalities of colours. I had tangible evidence of the impact of ecological connection on the human mind. Such wonders and their aliveness broaden our perception and make us more receptive. The mindful state seems to create a receptive presence of mind to whatever arises as it arises (O'Donohue & Siegel, 2006).

We are never isolated individuals, but from conception we interact with a biological, emotional and social environment. This interconnectedness begins in the womb, even at conception. After nine months' gestational synchrony, human mothers and newborns under natural conditions continue this interactional synchrony of sound and movement within the first hours after birth (Condon & Sander, 1974; Papousek & Papousek, 1992). The attention developed through the practice of mindfulness and wisdom opens the way to a prenatal-attuned relationship and prepares for continued synchrony after birth. Ideally with a mindfulness facilitator, this practice can mitigate the effects of trauma and mental challenges which undermine that foundational synchrony.

Relationships, like continued practice, can change and enrich us. By developing social skills and connecting with other creatures and people, parents learn to connect with infants. A crucial step towards developing wisdom and well-being is the restoration or development of capacities for reciprocal communication from the very beginning of life. But this comes from community support and cooperation and not from isolation. Limbic resonance or relational attunement leads us towards unconditional love and reciprocity (Lewis et al., 2000). Relationships, to be attuned, especially with babies and young children, require practising embodied emotional presence and slowing down. To get into sensing our self, we need to slow down. It takes time and attention to build a relationship. Practising making eye contact, greeting or smiling with your heart, observing and noticing and enjoying shared activities help to practise interpersonal flow. "Husserl said that as you pay gentle attention to things, their essential nature clarifies. Things are naturally *self-showing*; they *unconceal* themselves to you. They give you evidence of their existence" (Sills, 2009, p. 26). In the same way, when a mother pays attention to her unborn baby, the baby will be self-showing as a sentient being. "Breathing deeply and mindfully attending to others can put one in a state of receptive attention, promoting deeper connection" (Narvaez, 2014, p. 280). One of the aims of primal wisdom is seeing things as they really are. This type of relational attention is described by Dewey:

> To grasp the meaning of a thing, an event or a situation is to see it in its relations to other things; to note how it operates or functions, what consequences follow from it; what causes it, what uses it can be put to.
>
> (Dewey, 1960/1933, p. 135)

This attitude helps us to understand the impact of the first critical thousand days from conception on human health and their significance. Indigenous societies apply this attitude to the whole system of life, including the unborn baby's life. Receptive attention enables us to attend to the whole picture and detach from ego-self, separateness and isolation. Through storytelling, ceremonies and other creative activities, our indigenous cousins intentionally practise receptive attention and develop receptive intelligence. They take time and reflect on making the right decision, looking at a problem from multiple perspectives and considering the effects on future generations (Kohn, 2013). Their inter-relational mindset explains the flow of mother-child connection in traditional communities and how this inter-subjective primal space is jeopardised in our modern society. Mothers have evolved to nurture a prenatal and postnatal bonding supported by a mindful community and connection with the cosmos.

By developing social skills and connecting to other people and creatures, we can learn to connect with infants. Mindfulness practice helps prepare the ground to foster the presence and receptive attention required for the embodied intersubjective engagement between mother and infant that begins during gestation. Alongside mindfulness, we can use certain situations to practise interpersonal flow, intra- and interpersonal attunement. During my pregnancy, I listened to piano music, held deep conversations with my partner and meaningful others resonating with my experience and used rhymes for my baby and tango dancing to practise synchrony. These embodied rhythmic activities created a resonating space for my developing baby.

Practices that develop social resonance include joining a mindfulness group on a retreat, a musical group (singing or dancing) or creative writing or painting group, camping with others in the wild and volunteering to help those in need. These activities induce a feeling of connectedness and enrich the practice of mindfulness. Some of these activities are routinely practised by indigenous people. These cultures are aware that unborn babies need a relationship with nature and access its benefits through their mothers' experience but also about more direct forms of exposure later on. Before conception occurs, women go into the bush and call for the soul of the child until they hear it. Once the child is conceived in the hut, group dances follow to celebrate the meaningful event (Sansone, 2018b). I experienced during both my pregnancies the effect of my body-mind state, for instance induced by the forest, the birdsong and direct sunlight, on the baby, through the cues she sent me and my receptive attention. The mother's awareness of this intimate connection between the womb, baby, nature and herself makes the bonding profound. The father plays a significant role in nourishing this mindful awareness.

Receptive attention changes our being and connects us to others.

> by attending to someone else performing an action, and even by thinking about them doing so – even, in fact, by thinking about certain sorts

of people at all – we become objectively, measurably, more like them, in how we behave, think and feel.

(McGilchrist, 2009, p. 28)

Therefore, the maternal reflective function allows a mother to identify herself with the baby, thus read his mind and understand his needs. The world we create around us very much depends on attention. This kind of attention is not a mere cognitive function but implies embodied relational presence. It operates through the cooperation of implicit knowledge (intuition) and executive functions. If parents' attention is on their unborn baby, from conception, they will invest more time and energy in creating the optimal uterine environment – pollution and toxin-free, nutritionally and emotionally nourished. Attention affects the quality of parenting. In mindfulness, attention is a form of relationship and, depending on the type of attention – receptive or focused – encourages different values (Narvaez, 2014). *Receptive attention* notices the colours, smells, sounds, beauty and graceful movements around objects and people; our breathing and feeling; and a child's emotional nuances, bodily cues and her enjoying the present experience. The profound revelation about babies through receptive attention is essential for fulfilling parenting and child well-being. In contrast, *focused attention* categorises the object or person – how big? How often does a baby have to feed? The focus is not on *being with* the object but on understanding its mechanisms, not on being with the child and his experience or being in the moment. This kind of mindset assists when focused problem-solving is necessary, but it can be used in other situations and may come from an inability to enjoy being with and perceiving things as parts of a whole. It may prevent parents from living their child's experience with wonder and curiosity. It is evident that receptive attention leads to a very different world, interconnected and cooperative, one embedded in the flow of life (yin/yang).

Our current education system and many parenting courses, even the way in which children are brought up, are a reflection of a focused-attention mindset, which pulls the parts of the whole separately rather than interconnectedly. Receptive attention allows a parent or a teacher to be in the flow of the child's development, respect his pace and share his experience. One of the most outstanding aspects of the Himba I visited was the sense of interpersonal and ecological flow.

Practising mindfulness and attending to others lead to the development of receptive attention and human values shifting. Positive altered traits can benefit parenting and child development. Neuroplasticity offers a scientific basis for a way of creating those lasting qualities of being we find in yogis and monks with repeated training. The benefits of mindfulness practice go beyond the health spectrum, including human virtues of being and mindset shifting, which significantly promote parenting and attachment. By shifting attention (to breathing, bodily senses, gratitude, compassion and loving-kindness) we change our mindsets, the way we parent and care for children, and the world we create. It is therefore important to promote a mindful relationship-based approach across all layers of society, including policy makers, in order to achieve changes at all levels.

Wisdom is a state of being that includes the natural world and the whole system of life. It is a human responsibility to co-create the life of the Earth, as our indigenous cousins have been doing for millennia. We can set the roots of these positive intergenerational effects in early life, counteracting those of traumatic experiences or adverse childhood experiences, starting from securing mother-baby relationship *in utero*. Parenting has to be reconciled with the natural world and embrace our mammalian competence (eco-parenting). Loving Mother Nature is the clearest way to know and be reconciled with the human soul and essence. By doing so, we can affect our communities and render them places where human beings and other creatures flourish. When parents live mindfully and eco-mindfully, parenting and childcare are not tasks to learn but an unfolding of a flowing relationship with children, with alternating missteps followed by repairs. Parents do not need to be taught by experts what to do with their children but provide an environment where they are able to rely on the resources of their being. Mindfulness is not merely a solitary practice. The abilities are only fostered if practised in specific relational contexts. This is also the only way to develop and maintain more communal mindsets, which – like the village – significantly influence children's developing brain and well-being.

Accepting each moment as it is: an antidote to fear and reactivity

Learning the art of mindfulness is a journey, very often a lifelong journey. While the practice is not without its challenges, it can also be deeply nourishing and transformative to our experience of life, parenting and caregiving. Mindfulness simply means to be aware of – in touch with – the present moment by attending to embodied experience. And yet, in cultivating this simple innate wisdom capacity, we open up new possibilities for releasing stress, for connecting more deeply with each moment of life and relating to ourselves and others in new ways. Learning to live in the present is a way of practising beingness as well as inter-being (Thich Nhat Hanh, 1991). It helps us to accept and work through challenging emotions, unlike the approach of getting rid of things and fixing the problem. We tend to associate the so-called negative emotions with mental dysfunction, which may stem from our culture's overriding bias towards positive thinking. This is relevant to modern parents, who may find the acceptance of the complex range of feelings involved in raising a child challenging, with all its consequences on mental health and attachment. But difficult emotions are key to well-being, since when elaborated and transformed, they foster strength and resilience in both parent and child.

A natural entry into your presence is through your body – breathing and senses. You may start meditation by simply connecting with your intention to come home to presence, like your attitude of being friendly, relaxed and curious. Yet, mindfulness is not a practice limited to the meditation cushion or something to be done for just 30 minutes a day. Rather, it is a way of being that can come alive in all situations and all moments of our daily life.

In the mindfulness tradition, the mind is often likened to a monkey. Just as a monkey swings from branch to branch and tree to tree searching for a piece of fruit, the mind has the tendency to race from past to future and from thought to thought, often impelled by worry, craving and anger. If for one day we could observe our mind, we would likely notice countless states, thoughts and emotions passing through: anger, sadness, joy, feeling low, fear, worry, self-criticism, compassion and happiness. So much of the time we live in the world of thoughts and thinking, "in our heads". We even create education programmes and institutions (including pregnancy and parenting) that reflect intellectualism and disconnection from body feelings and heart qualities such as compassion and love. This mindset very much affects parents' well-being and relationships with children.

The mind can be a stormy place; then suddenly it can become bright and clear. Mindfulness means accepting the emotions and thoughts that come and go, even disturbing feelings (e.g. anger and fear) because typically it will fade away after 90 seconds if not encouraged by reactivity. However, when negative feelings are fed with attention, this causes a cascade of subsequent interacting effects. But by nurturing self-compassion, we can transform negative feelings. Mindfulness offers us a way to recognise each feeling as it arises. After recognising the feeling, calming it down and releasing it, we can look deeply into its causes, which are often based on inaccurate perceptions. Only our understanding of the causes and nature of our feelings will lead to their transformation. Nourishing mindfulness will lessen the fear, bringing stability and calm to the mind. By saying, "Breathing in, I calm the activities of body and the mind", you calm your feeling just by being with it, like a mother tenderly holding her crying baby. By feeling his mother's tenderness in her arms, the baby will calm down and stop crying and will be co-regulating (Sansone, 2004). The mother's mindfulness will tend the feeling of pain (Thich Nhat Hanh, 1991). A mother holding her baby is at one with her baby. If the mother is thinking of other things, worried or feeding anger, she is not connecting with her baby and the baby is unlikely to calm down. Then the mother has to look into the baby to see the elements that are causing him to cry and understand him. This looking will help her transform the feeling, be free and know what to do. By bringing tenderness and care to the situation, the baby will feel better. It is a deep communication involving body and mind, sensory because it involves sensing the energy behind what is visible, and reflective.

Donald Winnicott (1987) insightfully suggested that the mother's milk does not flow like an excretion. This flow is a response to a variety of elements: the baby's sight, smell, feeling and thinking. I recall the "thinking breast" described by Bion (1962), which I have replaced with the "feeling breast" or "mindful breast". The periodic feeding develops as an interpersonal flow, a communication based on a rhythmical exchange of cues, a song without words, or a dance, in which the infant's needs to be fed and comforted are met. Sadly, the fast pace of modern societies, interfering technology and stress hinder the sense of presence and attentiveness required by a receptive breast and body that intuitively sense and meet an infant's needs and understand his mental state.

Because we spend so much time in the world of thoughts (in our head), the practice from moment to moment allows us to come back to the here and now by grounding our attention in the body – breathing, senses, muscular tension. This allows parents to widen their perception and to notice their unborn baby's movements and cues from the womb and after birth. We can do this not just on the meditation cushion but also throughout our daily life. Whenever we walk, it can become a path for walking meditation if we can bring our attention to our feeling, our breathing and our sensations. When we cook or chop vegetables, this can become a mindfulness practice simply by resting our attention with our breathing as well as paying our attention to cooking or chopping. Indeed, all our daily chores can become mindfulness practices: brushing our teeth, showering, dressing, eating, changing nappy, holding the baby, talking to the baby, sleeping with the baby, breastfeeding or feeding and so on. Mindful eating is highly important during pregnancy. Studies suggest that improving the goodness and nutritional properties of food during pregnancy would not only improve the lives of their children but also of their grandchildren, benefiting the health of many generations to come (Lumey et al., 2007). But this is only possible by developing a mindful attitude to nutrition and the developing baby's needs.

Every moment is an opportunity to cultivate present-moment awareness, to live more deeply and savour the beauty of life, to live more authentically, more honestly, and to relate to our experience and others' with more kindness and compassion. When we live in this way, we discover that joy and happiness are available in the present moment and we water the seeds of transformation and insight – we contribute to epigenetic positive effects on future generations. Part of our suffering depends on our tendency to crave for things to be other than how they are, even to have a child different from ours. We feel rushed on a task, wishing we had not left things to the last minute. We do this often with our children. We have a habit of resisting or rejecting what is present and this can create mental states that increase our suffering, such as anger, frustration, fear or self-criticism. These feelings prevent us from appreciating and enjoying our experience, including pregnancy, parenting and our child's childhood. With mindfulness, we learn to approach each moment of experience with non-violence. With constant practice, the acceptance of the moment develops into accepting ourselves just as we are.

The relief and freedom that can come from simply accepting each moment as it is can be immense. It is a practice of "being with" and accepting that can deepen over time. We develop strength to embrace experience in its wholeness. Note that this attitude of acceptance and non-violence is not resignation. We do not resign ourselves to situations that cause harm to ourselves or others. Nor do we resign ourselves to mental habits such as depression or loneliness that hinder our well-being and creativity. Instead, we recognise it in this moment, this is what is happening (Tolle, 1999). I see it clearly. I neither ignore it, nor am I overwhelmed by it. I simply see. It is only by recognising that depression may prevent her from connecting with the baby that a mother can work on it and learn to connect with the baby's present feeling. This seeing in a non-violent, non-reactive or compassionate way is a profoundly different way of relating to our experience, through which we empower ourselves. This inner power and freedom enable us to make choices to lead by wisdom rather than by fear or reactivity. This way of seeing is the route to fulfilling parenting. It is crucial in a parent-infant relationship as it allows the infant to be seen and felt.

When we simply see and feel without reacting, we connect more deeply to each moment of the infant's and our experience and savour it, as Tolle recommends, "Use our senses fully" (Tolle, 1999, p. 52). Babies are born with a fundamental need and capacity for human connection and nurture, and connection is therefore a biological necessity, providing the infant/child (and adult) with a sense of safety (Porges, 2011). The fulfilment of this need shapes babies' healthy development – the capacity for emotion self-regulation, empathy, social relationships and resilience. Our connections with other people are important for our health, happiness and the health of the planet. When fear or rage undermines our sense of safety, it takes over the rest of the brain and our system, challenging our energies without our realising it (MacLean, 1990). By contrast, meditation states induce feel-good neurotransmitters such as neuropeptide opioids, oxytocin and vasopressin. Serotonin also increases in meditative states, suggesting that it should be called the "rest and fulfilment hormone" (Bujatti & Riederer, 1976). In these states of enlightened presence, the mind can come to new understanding and a higher consciousness. Eckart Tolle offers helpful guidance on enlightened presence, which can be applied in any situation:

> Use your senses fully. Be where you are. Look around. Just look, don't interpret. See the light, shapes, colours, textures. Be aware of the silent presence of each thing. Be aware of the space that allows everything to be. Listen to the sounds; don't judge them. Listen to the silence underneath the sounds. Touch something – anything – and feel and acknowledge its Being. Observe the rhythm of your breathing; feel the

air flowing in and out. Feel the life energy inside your body. Allow everything to be, within and without. Allow the "isness" of all things. Move deeply into the NOW.

(Tolle, 1999, p. 52)

Tolle suggests that through allowing the "isness" of all things, a deeper dimension reveals itself to you as an abiding presence, an unchanging deep stillness, an uncaused joy beyond good and bad. This is the joy of Being, the peace of God. Through this guidance, parents can come to a higher consciousness and understanding of their baby in the womb and beyond birth and immerse themselves in positive prosocial states, such as gratitude, awe and joy, which benefit pregnancy and the baby's development.

Paradoxically, it is this full embrace and acceptance of the present moment as it is that opens up new possibilities for change and personal growth, detaching us from thoughts that once had control over us and letting go of old behavioural patterns. With this new biological freedom, new human traits form and a more compassionate way of relating to others and to yourself can develop. New pathways are formed in the brain, opening up a healthier way of thinking, feeling and behaving (Goleman & Davidson, 2017). When we get fixed in some ideas of how we want ourselves to be, we get stuck. Much of our suffering depends on a fixed self. It is only through continued practice that we can free ourselves from genetic determinism.

The wise gardener, the rewiring of the brain and genomics

In the path of practice, a couple conceiving a baby takes the approach of a wise gardener – gentle, patient and persistent. The wise gardener prepares the soil, plants the seeds and waters them regularly. The prospective parents prepare their body-mind and thus the womb environment. However, the gardener also knows that he or she is only one of the causes and conditions that give rise to healthy plants and flowers. The others include the sunshine, the changing seasons and the work of the Earth. So, the gardener trusts that the sun will do its work, that the Earth will do its work and that Spring will come at the right time. She does not try to force her garden to come into bloom before time. She knows gardening is an organic process and that plants will produce flowers when the time is right. In the same way, a parent-to-be needs to water the seeds with love and patience to create a welcoming womb and trust that the baby will be conceived at the right time and inherit the seeds of love and kindness. He or she will exert a positive epigenetic effect on conception and human development and contribute to a new birth of humanity.

Meditation and mindfulness practice are just the same. We can think of ourselves as gardeners of the mind, engaged in the art of cultivating new habits of mind: habits of awareness, embodiment, attentiveness, joy, compassion and kindness. These habits form new pathways in the brain and affect the genome (genetic material). We are also learning the art of letting go: letting go of mental habits that cause ourselves and others to suffer. But, like the gardener, we cannot force this process or set goals to strive forward. If we strive for a particular outcome, then we lose our mindfulness; then we are feeding an idea of the future, attached to an expectation, losing the connection with present needs. This is the case for many parents in our modern society who expose their children to the huge pressure of adult routines and expectations from a very young age, often from pregnancy. It also applies to couples whose failed repeated attempts to conceive generate counterproductive stress.

We can only attend to each moment as well as possible and be gentle and patient as we practise. We need to remember that our practice is just to cultivate the soil and water the seeds. Cultivating mindfulness and meditation are a lifelong practice of rewiring the brain and influencing genes (Goleman & Davidson, 2017). It is naïve to think that one will see changes in how genes are expressed during just one day of meditation or mindful awareness. For instance, if we have inherited a gene that gives a susceptibility to a disease such as diabetes, we may never develop it if we have a lifelong habit of exercising regularly and not eating sugar. Sugar turns on the genes for diabetes; exercise turns them off. Sugar and exercise are "epigenetic" influences, just like neglect and abuse, or nurture, kindness and compassion, among the many factors that control whether a gene expresses itself.

Epigenetics has become a frontier of genome studies (Goleman & Davidson, 2017). Davidson showed that a mental exercise, meditation, could have beneficial effects at the genetic level. The mind can be trained to affect the body and its physiology. Pilot studies have found that meditation seem to "down-regulate" the genes responsible for the inflammatory response; mindfulness practice can not only lower the levels of pro-inflammatory genes but also lessen the feeling of being lonely, as loneliness spurs those levels (Creswell et al., 2012). An epigenetic boost was found in research using two other meditation methods. One is the relaxation response induced by silently repeating a chosen word such as *peace* as a mantra (Dusek et al., 2008). The other is "yogic meditation", where the meditator recites a Sankrit mantra, at first aloud and then in a whisper, and finally silently, ending with a short deep-breathing relaxation technique (Lavretsky et al., 2013).

Meditation and the mindful cultivation of the wise gardener may also have an impact on the telomeres. Telomeres are the caps at the end of DNA strands that reflect how long a cell will live. The longer the telomere, the longer the lifespan of that cell will be. Telomerase is the enzyme that slows the age-related shortening of telomeres; the more telomerase, the better for health and longevity. A meta-analysis of four randomised controlled studies involving 190 meditators found practising mindfulness was associated with increased telomerase activity (Schutte & Malouff, 2014). Another study found the same effect after three months of intensive practice of mindfulness and compassion meditation (Jacobs et al., 2011). The more present to their immediate experience, and the less mind-wandering during concentration sessions, the greater the telomerase benefit. A pilot study also found longer telomeres in women who had four years of regular practice of loving-kindness meditation (Hoge et al., 2013).

A study on long-term meditators (9,000 average lifetime hours of practice) found that comparing each to a non-meditator of the same age and sex, the meditators were breathing an average 1.6 breaths more slowly (Wielgosz et al., 2016). Science has long known that people with anxiety disorders and chronic pain breathe more quickly and less regularly than those without. And if you are already breathing fast, you are more likely to trigger a freeze-fight-or-flight reaction when faced with something stressful. This is highly relevant to the parent-infant/child relationship as some modern parents experience having a child as a stressful event. While chronic rapid shallow breathing reflects ongoing anxiety, a lower breath rate indicates reduced autonomic activity (thus better vagal tone), better emotional regulation, better mood and good health (Porges, 2011). These are physiological cues benefitting parent's sensitivity, parent-infant co-regulation and caregiving behaviour.

Emotions evolved as fundamental intelligence to guide behaviour and action, but in early life they must be trained well to do so. If they have not, due to adverse childhood experiences, they can be retrained thanks to the brain's plasticity (e.g. through mindfulness practice and/or mindfulness-oriented therapy). Neuroscientists have discovered that the brain is an organ of experience, that is it changes its structure and activity in response to experience, to what we repeatedly think, feel and do. This property of the brain is called neuroplasticity. Psychological and neurobiological plasticity allow the individual to use, instead of being used by, fantasy (Ansermet & Magistretti, 2007). This frees prospective/new parents and foetus-maternal experiences from genetic and biological determinism and opens up the perception of an underlying rich vibrant dimension that includes the spiritual magic imbued with Nature's influences on prenatal and perinatal development. The brain is an organ and meditation is an organic process. But the brain also monitors our body functioning and vice versa. Thus, experience changes our body experience and perception as well. Mindfulness rejoins body, mind and spirit in a wholeness that is at the core of health and well-being.

Most of us are victims of a kind of living that is not mindful, and the practice of mindful living and meditation can stop or mitigate this suffering and the transmission of it to our children and grandchildren by transforming it. Childhood exposure to traumatic events has a profound and disruptive impact on mental and physical health, including stress physiology. A study demonstrated that traumatic experiences in adulthood were more strongly associated with hair cortisol concentrations among mothers with a history of greater childhood trauma. Findings suggest not only that adult exposures affect hypothalamic-pituitary-adrenal (HPA-axis) functioning during pregnancy, but that childhood traumatic experiences have long-term consequences for HPA-axis functioning during pregnancy (Swales et al., 2018). Maternal HPA-axis dysregulation in pregnancy has consequences for both maternal health and for foetal development. Therefore, Swales and colleagues consider prenatal maternal HPA-axis functioning as a potential biological pathway underlying intergenerational consequences of childhood trauma. Prevention or mitigation of the intergenerational consequences of developmental trauma through mindfulness practices and mindset is of utmost importance.

Epigenetics teaches us that genes are influenced by our beliefs, habits, feelings, subconscious and consciousness, and we can affect our baby's genetic expression from conception and gestation. Our body's cells are always listening. What and how we think affects the health of our cells (Church, 2009). Church pointed out that every minute one million cells die and one million are born in our body and our mind influences this process. For example the seeds (or genes) of a mother's anger may have been transmitted by her parents. The practice of mindfulness can enable the son to see that his mother may have been a victim just like him. This remarkable insight can help him transform his inherited anger into something else while learning to be compassionate towards his mother (Thich Nhat Hanh, 1991). In this way, the epigenetic cycle is mitigated or even broken. The son can even suggest the practice of mindfulness to his mother and thus bring enlightenment to her and help transform her. When we look at our parents with compassion, we can see that our parents are only victims who never had the chance to practise mindfulness and thus transform their suffering. We can offer them peace and forgiveness. This will free us from adverse effects and benefit parenting and our children. This new way of seeing leads to gratefulness and appreciation of ourselves and our own bodies as a gift from our parents and their parents. We see ourselves as the continuation of our parents and our ancestors. We see clearly that the giver (our parents), the gift (our body itself) and the receiver (us) are one. All three are present in our body.

When we are deeply in touch with the present moment, we can see that all our ancestors and all future generations are present in us and influence us. We can see this in indigenous people, who live fully in their body and in contact with the spirits of the ancestors and the soul of the child before conception. They are aware that every element of the cosmos is interconnected. Death is not the end of life, birth not the beginning; they are both a continuum. Therefore, there is no fear of death. Prenatal and perinatal healthcare professionals who practise mindfulness are in touch with the present moment and capable of receptive attention and deep listening, and they will intuitively know what to do and what not to do for themselves and their clients (parents and children). They are aware of the cosmic wholeness and their psychophysiological influence on the mother-infant family dynamic system and well-being as an interconnected community.

7 Connection and empathy

Enhancing prenatal and
perinatal healthcare
practitioners' interpersonal
skills

When eminent psychiatrist and psychoanalyst Daniel Siegel asked over 65,000 mental health professionals face to face in lecture halls around the world if they had ever taken a course on the mind or on mental health, 95 per cent replied no. We can imagine what the scenario is for midwives and other birth-related professionals.

Recent evidence suggests that a significant number of women experience common mental health problems such as anxiety and depression during pregnancy. While at a moderate level, these mental states are a normal aspect of human life, when chronic and severe they can have adverse effects on prenatal development, birth outcomes, maternal well-being, mother-infant bonding and child development (Alhusen, 2008). Antenatal depression and perceived stress are often a precursor to postpartum depression, postpartum increases in couple conflicts and the quality of mother-infant attachment (Austin et al., 2007). One study showed that around 15 per cent of pregnant women experience serious feelings of stress, anxiety and depression (O'Hara & Swain, 1996). The long-term consequences of birth outcomes on maternal and infant mental ill health have recently been acknowledged.

New mothers' understanding and response to their baby's evolved needs and expectations are crucial to their development and well-being. Although mothers are biologically programmed to respond sensitively to their babies, midwives and other birth-related professionals are in a unique position to provide an enabling environment for this to take place. As we nurture mothers with love, compassion, kindness, so they in turn are more able to share all these virtues with their babies who in turn learn, through mirroring, how to nurture themselves and others. True human compassion is a chain reaction. Mothers have evolved to nurture a prenatal bonding and be nurtured themselves by the village for millions of years, that is for 99 per cent of human history (Hrdy, 2011). Supporting a woman through pregnancy, birth and the early post-partum period means supporting the early mother-baby relationship and human development, and this provides many opportunities for healthcare professionals to provide humane resonating mirroring, while exploring attitudes and hopes for their future parenting experiences. This environmental provision unfolds by default among indigenous, aboriginal and all traditional societies; it is not the case in the more complex modern societies.

Modern medicine merely relies on the cell, on matter, neglecting the benefits of listening and a trusting relationship between practitioner and patient/client. There is no welcoming of the client's inner world, of the soul. Conventional doctors listen for approximately eight to ten minutes, which prevents them from seeing the patient in their complex wholeness and understanding the core of the problem. Alternative medicine practitioners listen for one hour since they believe in trust and empathy as powerful sources of healing. Our society produces high levels of stress in parents as well as professionals and often drugs are prescribed as the quickest solution.

Since the middle of the twentieth century, a number of phenomena have been converging to suggest that something is going wrong. Humans are not who they used to be. Childhood experiences do not always support evolved needs, creating species-atypical outcomes (Narvaez, 2014). Knowledge is still fragmented and hyper-specialised, creating huge gaps within and between social services and maternity care, which is too often unable to meet human basic needs such as compassion, empathy, listening and connection, which form the basis of true "understanding" and healing. These capacities are never usually emphasised, taught or practised during professional training. The overall goal of this chapter, and the entire book, is to suggest ways of shifting towards greater relational attunement and communal imagination; first of all, by nurturing parents and children from conception onwards, and even long before conception, to set up the foundations of human wellness. We are at a turning point where humans are yearning for change towards an empathic and cooperative prenatal and perinatal care system able to meet fundamental human needs.

Unleashing the potential of prenatal bonding

My several years of observational study of the "dance of attunement" between mother and infant led me to some astounding discoveries in mother-infant communication (Sansone, 2004). My own experience of pregnancy and motherhood provided me with a vivid sense of the sacred link between maternal life-enhancing emotions and the reflective function, mother-foetus relationship and child well-being. I came to the discovery that attuned bonding can be nurtured during pregnancy and that parents can prepare for birth and the postnatal mother-infant relationship, thus preventing both maternal and infant mental health issues. Therefore, it is essential that prospective parents, as well as the community at large, become aware of the preborn as a conscious sentient being, who needs emotional care as much as healthy nutrients. The preborn is sensitive and responsive in their own way to maternal emotions, thoughts, consciousness, stress and the surrounding physical and social environment, including the birth scenario (Verny, 1981).

There is increasing evidence that a pregnant woman's placenta can absorb more than just nutrition and oxygen. If the stress hormone cortisol is transmitted to the placenta, altering brain development at a high level (Van den Bergh et al., 2005; Glover et al., 2010), positive life-enhancing emotions and communications, flooded with feel-good hormones such as endorphins and oxytocin, foster optimal development. Maternal love, like any feeling during pregnancy, translates into neurohormones, which affect baby's brain development. We are learning from epigenetics that feelings of ambivalence, rejection and neglect can have a tremendous effect on the child's genome. Recent scientific discoveries have suggested that changes in gene activity can be induced by environmental factors, such as the mother's mental states, emotions and their cellular substrate (Lipton, 2015). In his book *The Biology of Belief*, cell biologist Bruce Lipton discusses how positive thoughts "perceived by mothers before birth" allow preborn babies to "optimize their genetic and physiological development".

A great body of research over the last decade has provided evidence of the relational and emotional abilities of unborn children. From the moment of conception, experiences in the womb contribute to shaping a baby's brain and personality predispositions. Parents' emotional and mental states play an important role in the prenate's development. Parents thrive when they live in a calm and stable environment and supported by family and friends, and thus have more resources to nourish a healthy womb environment.

These findings contradict the common belief that people's genetic make-up is fixed and revolutionises the centuries-old nature-nurture debate following the Cartesian mind-body split. The parents' emotional state and consciousness, even around the time of conception, can unlock their creative potential and create a "field state" that may influence their developing baby's genetic predispositions (Emerson, 1996; Lake, 1979; Laing, 1976; Meaney, 2010). "It is biologically impossible for a gene to operate independently of its environment: genes are designed to be regulated by signals from their immediate surround, including hormones from the endocrine system and neurotransmitter in the brain – some of which, in turn, are profoundly influenced by our social interactions", writes Daniel Goleman in *Social Intelligence* (1995, p. 151). Goleman explains that just as our diet regulates certain genes, our social experiences also influence the switching on and off of genes.

Therefore, we are not our genes, but the expression of our genes. The environment can turn some genes on and some others off. Therefore, a child who is conceived in love, felt and seen with love and affection throughout gestation and welcomed at birth with love is going to be a very different person from one who is not wanted and cared for or whose mother is abused or under considerable chronic stress. The way we treat our children from conception on, and their mothers, affects human development and health and the welfare of society. So, building a community's mindful attitude and protecting the womb from chemical, physical or psychological toxins matter to everyone.

At a time in history when rates of perinatal mental illness and infant developmental problems are soaring, we must all work together, with synergistic compassion and empathy, to ensure every mother and father get appropriate and timely care to optimise their health and mammalian competence and to prevent the adverse effects of perinatal psychological distress. We need to look at the protective function of prenatal attachment and the importance of supporting this early relationship before birth, since it has an impact on the welfare of our society and economy. It is time for a new awareness that the prenatal and perinatal stages are the most crucial in human life and that the preborn child is already a psychological and relational partner to her parents, and through them, to society.

While parents and babies have evolved together to "communicate" with each other since time began, under the demands of our fast-paced technological society, parents may tend to lose their ability to "tune into" their babies' cues, needs and feelings. Many are losing their capacity to tune into their own human resources and wisdom. Stress, reflected in body language, such as gestures, movements and muscular tension (forms of vitality), affects the way of holding babies and the tone, rhythm and speed of voice while talking to them, hindering parents' attentiveness, presence and capacity to connect (Sansone, 2004). If parents can tune into the language (non-verbal) of their preborn and born babies and follow their communication lead, they are offering them the best start in life, reducing the potential for mental disturbances.

Prenatal and perinatal attunement, understanding and connection are the foundations on which a profound lifelong bond between parents and children can be established, as well as the foundations for social, emotional and moral well-being. Therefore, we need to protect this bonding by enhancing maternal (and paternal) mental states through a community support fostered by the practice of mindfulness and the promotion of prenatal and perinatal nurturing practices. We cannot promote maternal mental health without focusing on its foundations. A poor maternal attachment towards the baby can lead to postnatal psychological distress and mental suffering, as it makes attunement and understanding the baby's evolved needs difficult.

Through a communal mindfulness-based approach to prenatal and perinatal care, we can protect the human mother-baby co-adaptive system – that embodied creative dialogue unfolding during pregnancy and determining the term of labor and outcome of birth. A mindfulness-based integrated programme tackling the deep-rooted ignorance of the mind-body processes of the prenatal and perinatal period and mothers' psychological and emotional needs could be the route to cultural change and optimal maternity care. The practice of mindfulness is as important to the well-being of the mother, the preborn and the infant as the physical care that healthcare professionals routinely provide. Mindfulness should be built into the care that is delivered to both families with or without high risks and disadvantages.

Our primary objective as a society should be to create the conditions for birth and for the mother's and the baby's interactions and bonding to unfold undisturbed. We need to acknowledge that babies are born with a capacity and need for connecting and communicating with their caregivers (Trevarthen, 2006, 2009). This drive needs to be cherished and respected, not neglected as for instance when the baby is whisked away for medical checks or a midwife interferes to instruct the mother about how to breast-feed. Furthermore, even though we have evolved to be capable of intersubjective engagement from birth, striking evidence and my personal narrative later in this book indicate that the roots of this capacity for relational interaction are set during *in-utero* experiences. Motivated for social interaction and connection, infants are born with a capacity to communicate feeling and intention. When parents feel nurtured and so are receptive, thus are in a mindful state, these human capacities develop quickly through intersubjective reciprocal proto-communications. These parents tune into the infant's emotions through every form of vitality of their mental state – voice, touch, facial expression and movement (Stern, 1985). The attuned interactions channel and enhance visceral energy (Trevarthen & Delafield-Butt, 2013). They have a neurophysiological effect and have an impact on infant well-being. Early experience prepares the growing brain for capacities (or incapacities) for both self-regulating and socially attuning, thus for empathy (Siegel, 2004).

Early on in life, babies' capacity to communicate, connect and show compassion and love form neural pathways that support the development of positive relationships throughout life. This process starts in the womb, through a myriad of physiological cues exchanged between a mother and her preborn and influenced by the environmental provision. According to Schore's regulation theory, "Attachment is, in essence, the right-brain regulation of biological synchronicity between organisms" (Schore, 2003b, p. 41). Thus, attachment represents the neurobiological history of the mother-baby relationship (Narvaez, 2014). Our future capacity to tune into relationships, for empathy and compassion, is sown in early life experiences through our parents' capacity to tune into our feelings. It follows that it is extremely important that the whole community, including healthcare providers, is mindful towards couples and parent-infant relationships starting from pregnancy, thus creating the favourable conditions for a baby to thrive. For the mother, the caregiving behavioural system can be influenced by what happens during pregnancy and birth (Trevarthen, 2001).

This paradigm shift implies that we need to introduce mindfulness relationship-based training and prenatal and perinatal psychology for midwifery, obstetrics and all disciplines involved in prenatal and perinatal care, in addition to preparation programmes for prospective and new parents. Self-development, personal experience of life, attachment style and proto-social skills such as empathy, communication and attunement should be the main focus.

The mirroring of emotional states

In a randomised controlled trial about doulas in Texas, the prerequisite to participate in the study was personal experience of a normal labour and vaginal delivery with a good outcome (Kennel et al., 1991). The study results suggested that women are more likely to feel secure when protected by a midwife or other birth supporter who has had a positive experience of giving birth and can, thus, better understand their needs and connect with them. Those midwives who have not had a positive birth experience would benefit from mindfulness (mind-body) training, enabling them to work through any birth trauma and overcome fear. Body language and words from birth-related professionals, often reflecting their own trauma, emotional issues and attachment style, are powerful. Awareness of the effects on a mother's emotions and mental state, pregnancy and birth outcome should be encouraged by appropriate training.

It is now known that fear and anxiety enhance levels of adrenaline, inhibiting the release of oxytocin and making labour and birth longer and more difficult. Very often this modern knowledge is embedded in the midwife or other birth partner. The level of adrenaline released by a midwife in a birthing place, however, is also an important issue, since adrenaline is contagious and easily transmitted to the woman in labour. I recall the studies of brain-to-brain non-verbal communication (Schore, 2001b) or those on the role of the "mirror neuron system" (Rizzolatti & Craighero, 2004). This means that when we are in an emotional state, we can activate the same part of our brain as another person. Therefore, emotional states are contagious, including those associated with high levels of adrenaline, not only through the mirror neuron system but also energy exchanges.

Michel Odent represents the situation associated with an easy birth with only one person close to the woman in labour: an experienced and silent midwife, perceived as a mother figure, sitting and knitting in the corner of a small, warm room lit with a soft light (Odent, 2015). Odent suggests that the knitting midwife is helping the woman to keep her own level of adrenaline as low as possible and to let the oxytocin, the key hormone in the birthing and bonding process, flow. Interestingly, what we now call midwife used to be called *mammana* or *empirica* in some regions of southern Italy, which was a maternal figure who accompanied the woman throughout pregnancy, birth and the first postnatal months, just as still happens in many indigenous and aboriginal cultures. *Empirica* means "woman with experience." It is this consistency or familiarity, and human connection, of which sadly most Western modern birthing women are deprived, that is an essential element in a natural uncomplicated birth. Women nowadays may deliver with an on-call doctor or midwife they have never seen before.

Prenatal and perinatal holistic education should be an integral part of college training courses worldwide. Sarah Uzelac presents research investigating whether providing women with access to education and critical thinking skills in the area of perinatal care can positively alter the prevailing cultural belief that childbirth is a painful and frightening event requiring medical attention. The fascinating results of this research point to the need for more work in this area.

We should acknowledge that personality traits of self-development training – such as empathy, listening, engagement, non-verbal language and experience-based knowledge – may be more important than a scientific background for birth professionals. The woman-centred receptive side of midwifery (its true essence) needs to be protected and nurtured. The number of women who rely on their natural hormones and inner wisdom to give birth to babies and placentas is significantly decreasing. The domination of nature, of our mammalian competence and most human virtues is evident in every aspect of our lives and is seriously threatening humanity and Mother Nature.

Furthermore, we need to acknowledge our mammalian nature of giving birth and establishing a mother-baby bond benefiting from the psychobiological hormonal adaptation. Our society and obstetric practices often violate our evolved need for empathy and cooperation, which has been misinterpreted by our cultural conditioning that a woman does not have the power to give birth by herself. We need to acknowledge that enabling a mother to rely on her own mind-body resources, providing responsive and attuned care beginning in her own in-utero life, leads to healthy socioemotional development. These foundations lead to moral development and a cohesive peaceful society (Narvaez, 2014). One of the greatest revelations of my experience with Himba mothers and children, indigenous people of northern Namibia, was that we need to appreciate values from our indigenous cultures and create the conditions for them to be transmitted.

Sadly, many children in our society are raised with little or no empathy for others, and so the cycle of problems continues down the generations. Indigenous cultures teach us that our species has evolved to be strikingly empathic, compassionate and cooperative and has the capacity for "self-authorship". This evolved need is particularly important during pregnancy and childcare, and its fulfilment appears to have an impact on birth and child development outcomes. Studies found that having another woman offering consistent social support and mentoring throughout pregnancy correlated with a cascade of beneficial outcomes detectable for as long as 15 years after the birth. When compared with similar mothers not visited by a familiar figure, the children of visited mothers grew up emotionally more responsive, more resilient, acquired language sooner and were less likely to be abused by their mothers (Olds et al., 2007). Modern pregnancy, birth and parenting are missing the benefits of this most distinctive human need for consistent support, which is still paramount among the Himba and other indigenous cultures I visited. If we want to escape modern threats to humanity and blossom as a species, we must reconnect with our evolved needs and acknowledge our symbiotic (attuned) relationship with other human beings as well as with the natural world, including our mammalian nature.

When I told Badri, a Himba mother, that many children in our civilised world are born long before nine months, even at six, and many women decide to have a caesarean section (while mimicking the performance on my belly), she showed a quick visceral reaction and facial expression of puzzlement followed by the question, "Why would a woman decide to have her belly cut when there is a straightforward way?" as if I were talking about a different species. "Some women fear labour pain", I remarked. She must have had no idea of the kind of psychic pain I meant, a product of our modern way of life. How would she? At the final stage of labour, a Himba woman will sit on a rock and give birth, on her own or accompanied by one or two other women, who will be with her just to protect the birthing area, thus provide a sense of safety, and accompany mother and baby to the village, where they are accommodated in a shelter of mopane branches next to the sidewall of the main hut.

It is not all about technique: relying on the communication sensory-energy system

Intuition is the ability to know something immediately, without verbal explanation or conscious reasoning (Orlinsky & Howard, 1986). Badri intuitively grasped the implications of my information. Looking at ill-health statistics, we risk becoming a different kind of human being, as a consequence of environmental abuse, technological dominance, processed food, excessive stress generating anxiety, depression and other mental and physical conditions.

Another discovery I made during my experience with the Himba was that Himba women are masters in immediately connecting, despite language and cultural barriers. This could likely be linked to the context of their lives and society. They also probably sensed my profound interest in learning from them. Despite the translator's help, it was the desire to connect psychologically that helped us understand each other, beyond verbal language. There was a universal non-verbal language – gesture, facial expression, posture, rhythm of speech and laughing – which put our deepest human nature in touch and facilitated mind-reading. Later I found out that my insight was supported by Sarah Hrdy's intuition that what makes us human is not our ability to speak and ask questions, but the eagerness to "tell" someone else what is in our minds and to learn what is in theirs (Hrdy, 2011). The desire to connect psychologically with others and to read and share others' feelings and concerns had to evolve before language and provides the foundation for the evolution of cooperative behaviour. This is what is lacking in our midwifery today and what midwifery services fail to provide.

The spirit of openness, general respect and collaboration manifested by the Himba must have been the result of a social coherence that influenced each member of the community. A growing body of evidence suggests that an energetic field can form between individuals in a group through which communication can occur between all the group members (McCraty & Childre, 2010). In other word, there is a group "field" that connects all the members. This social coherence corresponds to a heart-based or physiological coherence that is reflected in a state of well-being. In this state, the group can achieve its objective more harmoniously and effectively. "Social coherence requires that group members be attuned and emotionally aligned and that the group's energy is regulated by care, not by threat or force from others" (Childre et al., 2016, p. 96).

Hyper-stimulation of the neocortex, that part of the brain involved in verbal language and intellect, is not a good ally in birth, as it appears to have an inhibitory effect on the physiological process of giving birth and bonding (Odent, 2015). Because we have become so hyper-intellectual, so dependent on spoken and written language, we have neglected our energy-sensing communication system. I believe that excessive stimulation of the neocortex also interferes with our evolved capacity to attune with our own needs and those of others. This occurs by hindering a midwife's intuitive capacity to understand and respect a mother's need for a quiet non-interfering environment, and thus create an energy field regulated by care.

Indigenous people, providing a window into the lives of our ancestors, have a vivid sense of the influence of the environment and their mind on conception, pregnancy and birth, which is what epigenetics acknowledges today. Our Western culture has emphasised the role of the left-brain hemisphere – with rational, linguistic, explicit reflection processes – as dominant. But a new paradigm shift acknowledges the right brain's implicit affective processes, expressing themselves through body language, operating at levels beneath conscious awareness as dominant in relationships and ill health (Schore, 2012). This is how a midwife or any other prenatal and perinatal practitioner can influence the experience of pregnancy, birth and bonding, and why it is important they become aware of these dynamics and care about them.

A mindfulness-based integrative programme could aid birth professionals as well as parents in understanding more in relation to preverbal communication (body movements, posture, gesture, facial expression, voice inflection and the sequence, rhythm and pitch of the spoken words) and its impact on maternal emotions and mind, and the value of connecting and communicating. This communication is supported by an infant/parent-centred care approach based on compassion, empathy and listening, all capacities fostered by the practice of mindful awareness.

Without the non-verbal, it would be hard to achieve the empathic, participatory and resonating relationship necessary to understand the other's experience (Stern, 2005b). A clinician or any other practitioner should be perceived by the parent (like any client/patient) as engaging in a natural meaningful dialogue growing out of their concerns; he or she should not be perceived as applying a stilted, formal technique (Valentine & Gabbard, 2014).

Most healthcare training courses focus on technique, but the focus should be on relationship and connection. The non-verbal channel of communication, not rational thinking and verbal communication, is much more important in human affairs than most people like to think (Buchanan, 2009). It is extremely naïve to take conscious verbal communication as the primary way that people respond to each other. While science and most training courses can describe aspects of emotions according to detailed models, there is a distance between such details and what a mother feels, and its impact on her baby's development. The complexity of human development – emotional, cognitive and social – emerges from the parents' meaningful experiences, in which others, culture and society play an important role. Later we see how my own subjective account of emotions, mental states and baby's engagement is free of the limitations of science. The narration of my perceptions and consciousness, and my baby's responses – a rich intimate embodied dialogue – cannot be replaced by science.

Deep listening, kindness and the sacred space

Deep listening is vital as it encourages self-confidence and emotional resonance, which facilitates parents' synchronic responsiveness with their baby, appreciation and enjoyment of the whole experience. "The feeling of being listened to or felt by a present attentive and engaging practitioner is what was so lacking in my own personal care, which was definitely where I can pinpoint the start of my birth trauma contributing to PTSD (Post Traumatic Stress Disorders)", says Cheryl. Emily remarks, "It took me 15 years to get the correct diagnosis of birth trauma and PTSD and my recovery and treatment was delayed, until I met a lovely psychiatrist who finally 'listened' without judgment".

July reports,

> As someone who had awful anxieties in my first pregnancy due to twice almost miscarrying my baby, to then having a traumatic birth which was ignored to then trying to cope with suffering PTSD while pregnant with my second baby, I only wish that there had been compassionate doctors around me. They might have seen the pain I was in and helped me to get support. I could have prevented many years of suffering for me and my family. So many families are affected by lack of proper understanding of perinatal mental health and perinatal processes. It is not good

that there is still stigma and lack of help, because the impact this has can be life-changing.

The feeling of being valued, rather than judged, corresponds to a physiological condition, which triggers healing. Liz tells us that the lack of understanding, especially around birth trauma, premature babies and baby loss, is striking. To the major human loss a human being can experience, this adds a lack of empathy and compassion for the birth experience with its huge impact on maternal health. Raising all healthcare practitioners' awareness of the importance of how these human virtues affect perinatal mental health and bonding/attachment is crucial. The way in which perinatal healthcare practitioners deal with a woman's pregnancy and birth experience can significantly have an impact on her well-being and affect her subsequent perinatal experiences if her emotional and mental suffering is not understood.

Alex reports,

> Following the loss of my first baby through miscarriage and the medics not removing my baby properly and then my having to have two general anesthetics in 5 weeks, I experienced a postpartum psychotic episode. It was horrific and I can remember it clearly to this day. It went on for a few short weeks but nonetheless it was a very real experience. Then through my other pregnancies I experienced antenatal anxiety. Although I didn't experience any further episodes of psychosis, I experienced some postnatal PTSD following the birth of my baby as a result of the midwife slicing my vagina whilst trying to look at my stitches and losing them. I was never treated for these episodes and was never supported through psychotherapy or human compassion and listening. I managed to pull through using the power of my mind and with as much sleep as possible. I know I have carried these issues into all my pregnancies and I'm sure this is part of the reason for my losing so many babies. The way I was treated by medics after my first loss many years ago was truly life-changing and horrific.

When synchronising with another person, thus feeling understood, the waves in each brain mirror those of the other, especially in the insula (which relates to the conscious feeling state). When a person is listening intently to another person's story, the listener's brain begins to anticipate the speaker's brain activity by a few seconds (Stephens et al., 2010). These researchers suggest that communication is an act performed by two or more brains and that during emotional moments, brains are more likely to become synchronous. This happens when we "resonate" with another person.

Throughout life, sympathetic others can become attachment figures (Mikulincer & Shaver, 2007). These may provide parents with an opportunity to enhance their skills and deepen their experience and the enjoyment from the relationship with their child. This is the case of contained multi-generational communities within which individuals know one another well; share the joys, burdens and sorrows of life; nurture one another in time of need; care for the well-being of each other's children and increasingly dependent elderly people; and feel rewarded by their essential contribution to the group that securely holds them. This is the most natural environment for parents to thrive and for children to grow up in (Gray, 2013). We are biologically wired for this kind of life, which has sadly become nearly impossible to find. The most tragic thing is that the absence of the village and its meaningful relationships is distorting many mothers' sense of self and the very foundations of attachment.

I recognise the value of preverbal responsiveness and attunement as paramount to the well-being of infants but also to parents' mental health. A mother's feeling of being listened to, seen, felt and valued by a health caregiver through an empathic relationship reflects her capacity to connect with and value her baby's needs and experience. Just as babies see themselves through the non-verbal and verbal exchanges of their caregivers (mirroring), so parents need to perceive themselves as compassionate caregivers through the communicative exchanges with their healthcare providers. Promoting mirroring is highly important, since by mirroring and validating, the parent helps the child to become more aware of his own needs and validate herself. But parents also need to be validated in this process. Connection is lost when the child's needs and feelings are rejected and thus invalidated, when for instance the parent is affected by mental challenges or excessive stress. Mirroring creates a sacred space between parent and child, a pause to slow down, which brings silent and still awareness to further awaken the spiritual aspect of self in the search of the core human experience.

Where it is given the time, with mirroring activities, the parent-infant relationship can bring a deep and fascinating state of being. I ponder that while verbal language has given human beings a huge advantage in the battle with their predator and competitors and helped in mastering their environment, it may have suppressed or weakened deeper processes, like those of the communicative sensory system that is fundamental to understanding the baby's cues. This may have affected the child's emotional, social and moral development. Understanding the baby's preverbal language and having this understanding facilitated by empathic others, through the practice of mindful living, offers every mother and father new ways to enrich their relationship with their child and offers the child lifelong benefits. It follows that we have to support these primal communications.

Being able to understand baby's non-verbal language, even before birth, may boost emotional communication and vitality, intimacy skills and emotional and social intelligence (Sansone, 2004). The experience of early mirroring enhances later empathy skills, setting the ground for a compassionate society and social services able to meet basic human needs.

Mirroring activities, involving movements, expressions, gestures, tone of voice and eye contact, fostered by parents' responsiveness, can enhance a sense of trust in others and lay the groundwork for lifelong empathy and cooperation skills. These are the foundations of human relationships and being at peace with the world, which benefits society at large. We can see the natural rhythmic unfolding of these mirroring activities among small bands of hunter-gatherers and the Himba of my study, still uncontaminated by the demands of our modern society.

Therefore, care providers need to be sensitively attuned to receive prospective and new parents' communications. Their right brain, involved in primary process communication (intuition and emotion), should be receptive to the music behind the words. In a world becoming increasingly multicultural and inhabited by refugee pregnant mothers and families struggling with linguistic barriers and isolation, practitioners' non-verbal skills and compassion are vital.

These high-quality exchanges require mindfulness and awareness training. When healthcare practitioners have trained in mindfulness, they become able to bypass verbal deficiencies and even cultural conditioning, by tuning in at the bodily affective level, which is more expressive and truthful than words. There is a sacred moment when parent and caregiver (or therapist) connect with each other as well as with their deeper selves, which can tremendously contribute to empowerment or healing. Mindful presence is a relational stance that is fundamental to evoking an experience and neurophysiological sense of safety in the client, which can have an impact on prenatal attachment, birth and parenting. Porges refers to the transformative power of feeling valued and safe (Porges, 2011). He deems that safety is critical in enabling human beings to optimise their potential. The neurophysiological processes associated with feeling safe are a prerequisite not only for social behaviour (e.g. connecting and bonding with the baby) but also for accessing both the higher brain structures that enable humans to be creative and generative, and the lower brain structures involved in regulating health, growth and restorations.

How can parents feel safe, thus value their birthing and parenting experience, if prenatal and perinatal healthcare practitioners do not empathically value it in the first instance? This may have to do, at least in some cases, with the caregiver's attachment style or experience of early trauma.

A new paradigm based on caring empathic interactions

Concerns about the quality of medical care provided by health services appear to be increasing. Deficits in care are frequently found to be associated with stress and with the apparent lack of recognition of psychological issues concerning doctors (Firth-Cozens, 2016). An article in *The Guardian* (2016) highlights that half of NHS (National Health Service in the UK) psychologists are depressed, feeling the strain of time limits and targets, with many suffering from the very problems for which they treat patients. Mental health is becoming a major issue among practitioners, threatened by the stress of long working hours and poor understanding of human needs. How can a distressed healthcare practitioner support a pregnant or birthing woman, or mother-infant bonding, if they need support themselves? The rate of burnout among doctors, midwives and other healthcare professionals is sobering and every training school programme needs to include stress-management, self-development training and mental health in their curriculum. A primary focus of all "others" relevant to mothers should be to provide a stress-free environment supporting health, allowing prenatal and postnatal bonding/attachment and all the mirroring activities to unfold.

A study conducted at Wake Forest Baptist Medical Centre documents results from a mindfulness stress-reduction training programme to help medical students reduce stress and prevent professional burnout, to enhance performance by improving working memory and empathy and by moderating performance anxiety, and to help familiarise future doctors with techniques recommended in many medical treatment plans for patients (McCann et al., 2013). The study used a practical approach to self-regulation training for third-year medical students that is a combination of applied relaxation and applied mindfulness (ARAM). Approximately 150 students have practiced this approach and overall feedback has been positive. Introducing students to self-regulation and self-care skills during medical school improved their personal health and professional satisfaction not only during school but also beyond. The study suggests that inadequate self-care and ineffective coping strategies are often established during medical training; they may persist after training and be self-destructive in long-term and undermine the quality of care for the patients.

With this in mind, a question is raised: how can practitioners concerned about their own issues be able to tune into expectant/new parents' and babies' needs, in the most crucial phase of their lives? This chapter addresses this much-neglected gap and proposes mindfulness-based relationship-focused training and prenatal and perinatal psychology for both professionals and parents to help babies thrive. This is a crucial topic that has seldom been looked at before. While supervision would be costly, mindfulness training combined with awareness of prenatal and perinatal processes could mitigate the impact of stress as well as value parenting and babyhood experiences. This would enhance the capacity for empathy, listening, connection and compassion, which caregivers may otherwise be unable to apply in their interactions with parents because of their early experiences and trauma, particular training or lack of analysis.

Other studies indicate that enhancing students self-regulation skills through self-care and communication approaches during their training may improve their personal and relational health. The practice of mindfulness has helped practitioners take different perspectives, improve self-regulation and be more open to cooperation, listening and attunement (Siegel, 2007). It changes the belief system and thus perceptual and behavioural patterns (Lipton, 2015). It transforms the way in which we perceive ourselves and the way we treat patients/clients. It is important that we experience mindfulness personally – from the inside – before we learn to pass the skills on to our expectant, birthing clients.

The work of Shapiro et al. (1998) also demonstrates that mindfulness education can improve empathy. Empathy is necessary for understanding and meeting human needs. A study with medical students found that those receiving a mindfulness-based stress reduction programme showed an increase in empathy over time. These findings suggest the possibility, to be tested in future research, that mindfulness may enhance professional as well as interpersonal connections, which in turn supports interpersonal well-being.

In conclusion, if women's regaining of their inner wisdom is the best path to a new maternity care, we must bear in mind that next to a woman's supportive husband/partner, a sensitive, understanding, present birth-related professional is the most critical figure in her pregnancy. Most of the unhappy stories I have heard from mothers-to-be and new mothers during my research and clinical work reflect a failure of compassion on the part of the medical and other healthcare personnel. The changing culture of medicine is becoming increasingly hyper-specialised, responsive to the imperatives of business and technology and less sensitive to the subjective reality of mother and baby. Lack of compassion may have medical consequences on pregnancy and birth outcomes. This is simply because mothers have evolved to receive empathic support (Hrdy, 2011). Receiving caring empathic interactions directly affects mothers' psychobiology and predisposes them to be empathic to themselves and others (Adler, 2002). This occurs by conveying emotional-physiological experiences to each other.

Mothers (and fathers), and not just those affected by mental conditions, need to receive a non-judgemental approach to both education and therapeutic work and great compassionate dedication from others. Our behaviour can promote tension or yielding in the other. There is a reciprocal influence, a back-and-forth flow of energy and openness between the "self" and "other." The way we behave towards others "creates states of mind in others" (Gilbert, 2005, p. 19). We can promote a state of mind that jeopardises the survival systems and safety ethic of others. Some people do this intentionally to promote submission to their dominance strategies; others do it unintentionally due to unresolved personal issues. Alternatively, we can facilitate a sense of safety in the other, so as to promote affiliative strategies, supporting relational attunement and engagement. This, in turn, supports parent-baby attunement and unleashes the potential for the mother-prenate relationship. The practice of mindful awareness promotes compassionate goals and non-judgemental and non-defensive behaviour. This is because the sense of presence and focus on this situation allows for understanding the process, in this case during prenatal and perinatal periods, and connection with the state of mind.

Through the practice of wisdom, we can gain self-authorship and create a life that is transformative in two ways. It is transformative for the self, because it nourishes the relationship between the self and all of life. Second, it can transform the world. The practice of mindfulness or primal wisdom engenders wise perception, which can create a culture of companionship promoting well-being. The practice of wisdom can teach us to open our heart and change mindsets we have established in our life course. By taking up purposeful self-authorship, learning and regularly practising self-calming techniques, e.g. sitting meditation and focusing on breathing, we can change our brains, reframe our behavioural patterns, expand our social selves and practise moral functioning, as contended by Darcia Narvaez (2014). An important message of this chapter and throughout this book is that by promoting common-self mindfulness, we promote healthy relationships and secure attachment between parents and children, and thus moral capacities and well-being. This should be a major concern of public health, humanity and society. Human beings are dynamic biosocial beings who, although most neurologically plastic during childhood, can self-author and transform themselves towards optimal development at any time of their life course through the practice of mindfulness or wisdom (Narvaez, 2014).

The practice of mindfulness and fostered wisdom offers a way to restore human virtues to their full potential and build mindful communities. Human beings – healthcare professionals, the parents, children, and every member of society – are perceived as an essential part of a cooperative, not competitive, natural world. Therefore, human relationships and moral responsibilities include the flourishing of all natural entities, thus our mammalian nature, which largely governs the mother-baby relationship.

Drawing on contemporary science, observation of other cultures and reflections on my pregnancy and developing baby, I urge all of us to understand human beings, in particular parents and their babies, as dynamic open systems susceptible to environmental influences. Intersubjectivity with others, reciprocity, co-regulates all our physiological and psychological systems, affecting our physical, mental, and social health and well-being. Responsive parenting practices, favoured by a mindful awareness state, optimise physiological systems, including emotions and self-regulation systems, and promote not only good health, but behaviours such as sociality and empathy. Joyful encounters (including healthcare practitioners) foster physiological systems in their underlying positive emotions and self-transcendence. This allows for community bonding and what Narvaez calls a "moral mood", both of which facilitate prosocial behaviour and empathic communal mood (Narvaez, 2014). These community bonding and mood promote nurturing practices.

When basic human needs are met throughout early life and adulthood, individuals and community develop the resources to thrive. This seems to be the case in small-band hunter-gatherer communities and the pastoralist Himba I visited, where under normal circumstances human needs are met as a matter of routine, especially the needs of infant and young children (Konner, 2005, 2010). When nurturing care meets needs, the evolved plasticity leads to outcomes typical of that species. When these needs are not met, atypical outcomes for that species are more likely. We receive myriad legacies from our ancestors. Recent findings in cell biology, neuroscience and epigenetics suggest that we are influenced by our ancestors' experiences, our mother's experiences when we were in utero, her nutrition, and our birth, bonding and attachment with our caregivers. These early and ancestral experiences can influence our genetic code and create implicit memories that in turn, influence our perceptions, experiences and choices today. Mothers' experiences, the sympathetic others she interacts with, whether they support her mental health and well-being or not, matter to everyone, to the whole of society.

We have learnt in previous chapters that epigenetics and research on developmental plasticity provide increasing awareness of how adult choices and practices influence the well-being of subsequent generations. What a person becomes is not only the result of genes, which play an important but small role, but how genes are expressed under cultural environmental influences during sensitive periods. Although much of who a person becomes is malleable and remains open to influences, early life establishes important foundations for future life. This is why prenatal and perinatal support (e.g. proper food; pregnancy, birth and breastfeeding hormones; and emotional and social support) leads to a body, brain, mind and soul that function more optimally and prepare a healthy womb environment and foundations for the baby development.

A mindfulness-based integrated prenatal and perinatal programme proposes a new paradigm of birth and parenting, which creates the conditions for a respected continuum of life and healthy society starting before conception and providing future generations with the capacity for companionship, interpersonal connection and compassion and empathy. This paradigm considers maternal mental health and developmental trauma as consequent on the failure of our society to meet our most fundamental needs. This empathy-inspired programme has not only a social and human impact but also a huge economic impact, since governments can save on the extremely high costs of premature births, the prenatal and perinatal depression and other conditions related to them and to unexpected caesarean births, difficult births or poor maternity and baby care, as well as the high costs of children's ill health.

8   Why maternal and paternal mental health and well-being matter

The World Health Organization (WHO) defines health in its 1948 constitution as "a state of complete physical, mental and social well-being and not merely the absence of disease or infirmity" (WHO, 1948). Therefore, this should also apply to the provision of comprehensive care during pregnancy for the optimal outcome for the mother and the child. But, sadly, addressing mental and emotional health has often been neglected in pregnancy care all around the world. This trend is rooted in the Cartesian dualism, individualism, materialism and "isms" in general. The seeds of dualistic thought are to be found in Descartes' famous dictum "I think, therefore I am": *Cogito, ergo sum*. However, I hold an emergent worldview based on relationships and connections between all things rather than based on the philosophy of dualism, division and separation. This view is encapsulated in a Sanskrit mantra, *So Hum*, which is well-known in India but less so in the West.

Prenatal and perinatal care needs this mantra, the mantra of non-dualistic and unfragmented relationships. Satish Kumar, among the most important educators of the twentieth century, translates *So Hum* as "You are, therefore I am": *Estis, ergo sum* (Kumar, 2002). This mantra should be the great fountain of wisdom underpinning a comprehensive pregnancy and mother-infant care, which acknowledges "You" as a human being and mental health and well-being as constituting an essential component of the care of parents during pregnancy. This is regardless of whether a mother has experienced any mental illness before pregnancy or in any previous pregnancy.

The evidence

Today we have abundant evidence of the impact of the mother's mental and social well-being on pregnancy, foetal development, birth and the transition to parenthood in terms of suggesting the best ways to support healthy prenatal and perinatal relationships and child development. Both perinatal and postnatal psychological distress have significant consequences on maternal well-being, mother-infant bonding and child development.

A review of 22 studies on prenatal attachment found that higher levels of mother-foetus attachment (MFA) were associated with higher levels of family support and greater psychological well-being. Factors such as depression, substance abuse and higher anxiety levels were associated with lower levels of MFA (Alhusen, 2008). Clinical accounts argue that parents' anxiety and stress may harm the vital intersubjective bonds, birth and development and even affect our capacity to empathise (Ammaniti & Gallese, 2014). Supporting mothers' emotional well-being during the prenatal and perinatal period is now recognised to be as important as the traditional focus on the physical health of the mother and child. A vast literature attests that mothers with more social support are more responsive to their babies' needs. In traditional societies, support from alloparents, which allowed our ancestors to evolve, not only improved a child's health, social maturation and mental development; it was essential for child survival (Coontz, 1992). Other studies have found correlations between a new mother's perception of low social support and postpartum depression (Miller, 2002; Hagen & Barret, 2007).

High levels of maternal stress, including antenatal depression, are a significant factor in the aetiology of postpartum depression, couple conflicts and the quality of mother-infant attachment (Austin et al., 2007). If a mother is persistently stressed while pregnant, her child is more likely to have emotional or cognitive problems, such as an increased risk of attention/deficit hyperactivity, anxiety and language delay (Van den Bergh et al., 2005; O'Donnell et al., 2009). Underpinning physiological mechanisms are likely linked to the woman's levels of cortisol, which has been found high in women with depression, anxiety and stress symptoms. Cortisol can be transferred to the foetus via the placenta, altering foetal development to prepare him or her for postnatal life in an adverse environment, which affects infant development (Glover & O'Connor, 2006; Talge et al., 2007). Talge and colleagues argue that it is still not known which forms of anxiety or stress are more detrimental, but research suggests that the relationship with the partner can be important in this respect. Antenatal psychological distress is known to have an impact on obstetric and neonatal outcomes, which often have significant consequences on perinatal bonding, attachment and child development. Dayan et al. (2006) found that the rate of spontaneous preterm birth was significantly higher among women with high-depression scores.

I should point out that stress is such as it is "perceived" by the mother at a certain level. Likewise, beyond a traumatising event, there is the survivor's interpretation of it at the foundation of the trauma experience. It is important to clarify that ordinary mild stress can be actually beneficial to the foetus's and child's development (DiPietro et al., 2006).

While many of us are aware of the adverse effects of toxic substances (smoke, alcohol, drugs etc.) and acute and chronic stress on foetal development, the protective function of the mother-baby relationship prior to birth is less well-known. The mother's emotional and mental states influence the relationship with her unborn baby, which is in turn a good predictor of the mother-infant relationship, as indicated by the videotaped mother-infant face interactions at about 12 weeks postpartum (Siddiqui & Hagglof, 2000). Both research and clinical work have so far underemphasised the quality of foetal-maternal interactions as prenatal psychobiological precursors to secure bonding and adaptive infant development, which have been examined in a study (Novak, 2004). Attuned interactions channel and enhance physical and visceral energy, and have a neurophysiological effect on infant well-being (Trevarthen & Delafield-Butt, 2013). Caregivers' early responsiveness and attunement prepare the growing brain for the capacities for self-regulation, creativity and social attunement, thus for empathy (Siegel, 2004). According to Schore's regulation theory: "Attachment is, in essence, the right-brain regulation of biological synchronicity between organisms" (Schore, 2003b, p. 41). As such, it represents the neurobiological history of the mother-child relationship, even though this fact is not always emphasised in discussion of attachment (Narvaez, 2014). Early experiences, including prenatal, create patterns that inform human development through neural pathways. As Siegel stated, "Human connections shape the neural connections from which the mind emerges" (Siegel, 1999).

A study of more than 700 mother-child relationships reached the conclusion that a low sense of attachment between an expectant mother and her preborn child could be associated with developmental delays (Branjerdporn et al., 2016). Early findings from this study suggest that mothers with a stronger bond to their preborn babies were more likely to have babies that were proficient in a range of skills. It follows that the quality of prenatal attachment is essential for development, for the interactions on which it is based provide a relational matrix on which the mind is created.

This evidence, resonating with the outcomes of my several years of observation and clinical work with parents and infants (Sansone, 2004, 2007), provides a foundation for looking more closely at assessing and improving parental well-being and maternal-foetal relationship, so as to give children a head-start before they are born. Furthermore, it informs future interventions, i.e. mindfulness practices, to support earliest human connections and promote infant development. Looking more deeply, this evidence indicates that the unborn baby is sensitive to maternal states, a sentient being capable of rudimentary embodied engagement with maternal communication, and that this engagement can be nurtured during intra-uterine life. The mother-unborn baby psychobiological narrative is a secure base, protecting both mother and infant, and therefore it needs to be supported by the father, the meaningful people surrounding the mother-to-be, including the healthcare providers and policy makers. The father in turn needs to be supported should mental issues alter his ability to provide a secure base to the mother and unborn baby and child.

If a mother's responsiveness and attuned bonding are an extension of the prenatal relationship, this may show that they are a process of shared attentiveness and engagement since life in-utero. This could be also a way of mapping the prenatal roots of intersubjectivity and explain the innate newborn's drive for relational engagement. However, if babies born to chronically depressed mothers show less drive for human interactions even with nondepressed adults (Field et al., 1988), it may well be that babies are sensitive to a prenatal dialogic narrative and that we can promote interrelatedness in the womb through a communal mindful relationship-focused approach.

A window of opportunities

Awareness that the preborn baby is already a psychological and social partner to her parents and, through them, to society as a whole must be brought to the fore. This awareness can change the way healthcare providers relate to expectant parents and the developing baby. It is time for the birth of a new awareness in society that the prenatal and perinatal stages are crucial in our lives, and that not only the mother, father and family matter, but the whole community as a vital source of well-being for our humanity. We need a perinatally informed culture of kindness and compassion.

It follows that the mother needs to be nurtured by an appropriate social network and emotional support to foster the feeling of "being felt and valued", of "being alive" that can nourish the vital embodied narrative with the baby, thus contributing to providing the best womb environment. We need to support this sacred early relationship because it has profound implications, with humanitarian, social and economic consequences. Nurturing is about meeting an individual's needs and innate expectations, which we evolved to do over millions of years. The brain changes and the self- and interpersonal awareness fostered by mindfulness practice are likely to promote awareness of the baby's evolved needs and expectations. As a society, our major concern should be with creating a sustainable programme to secure the foundations of maternal mental health and healthy child development. Every prenatal and perinatal healthcare professional, including psychotherapists, should adopt a mindful systemic/relational approach that considers the mother-baby-father triad at its core.

Significant opportunities to improve lifelong health and well-being for human beings begin prenatally. Many medical practitioners are not aware of the significant opportunities for emotional support during pregnancy and the postpartum period, which can increase positive outcomes for the birthing families and babies. All birth-related professionals, including physicians, psychologists, psychiatrists, neonatologists, mental health specialists, midwives, childbirth educators, pregnancy and parenting coaches and doulas should come together to share information and innovative strategies in order to improve the outcomes of our mothers and babies growing in the womb. World-renowned experts can provide observations, cutting-edge evidence of the baby's intelligence in the womb and insightful strategies inspired by primal wisdom for alleviating or preventing postnatal depression and other mental conditions.

Prenatal care and all professionals involved in it should adopt an integrated mindfulness-based approach that is also informed about trauma, enabling them to understand prenatal and perinatal processes and thus consider that what a pregnant woman thinks, feels and hopes, or her trauma, is embodied and influences pregnancy and birth outcomes and the baby's development.

Yana, 29 years old from Indonesia says this:

> I had a wonderful obstetrician at my recent birth a month ago and will thank him for the rest of my life for having a beautiful birth. Even though I had a caesarean birth, he helped me make a smooth transition and supported me to breastfeed immediately. This support made me happy and facilitated a strong bonding between my baby and me. My first son was stillborn at 26 weeks and 5 months later I was pregnant again and had a traumatic birth, an emergency caesarean section and birth complications, and I also experienced a rude attitude from nurses and midwives . . . all these incidents brought me to have PTSD and PPD (Postnatal Depression), which made bonding difficult. During my subsequent pregnancy (unplanned) I was afraid. Many friends supported and helped me through this. One of them recommended me to a psychologist, who helped me heal from my birth trauma, panic attacks and anxiety. Hopefully every mum who had a miscarriage, stillbirth, baby in NICU or other kind of traumatic birth experience receives appropriate compassionate help during pregnancy and beyond.

The consequences of a lack of continuity in care are evident in Yana's account. Therefore, we must create innovative ways to ensure continuity, starting by communicating with other members of the team to ensure mothers (and fathers) are getting the appropriate individual support.

Why paternal perinatal mental health matters

While the mother's impact on child development has been studied widely, the role of the father and his mental well-being in facilitating the conditions for mother-infant bonding to unfold has been neglected. Our patriarchal culture and social media put too much responsibility on the mother in child development, when the reality of the nuclear family already causes isolation and depression. In the absence of the village that supported mothers through shared childcare for millennia, the role of the father in our modern society has become far more important. A new paradigm that acknowledges the interrelational quality of human nature and the reciprocal influence of energy fields (quantum physics) on mental health and behaviour, which is central in primal wisdom, can help us overcome the Cartesian Western dualism that has considered the individual as a totally separate entity. This same dualism has led our culture to associate qualities such as "rational", "competitive", "unemotional" with men, at the expense of the so-called "female" wisdom qualities such as *intuition, compassion, listening, receptiveness, engagement, understanding,* which are essential in intimate relationships.

It is significant that, for cultural reasons – sexual role and social image – men are less prone to reveal their psychological difficulties (e.g. depressive symptomatology such as sadness, crying, a sense of failure, and impotence) and rather than asking for help they tend to somatise (develop physical symptoms) or turn to smoking, alcoholism, drug, sex or Internet addiction. Or they may manifest their discomfort through aggressive and abusive behaviour. This makes it more difficult to make an early assessment during pregnancy, since even when asked to fill in a *self-report* questionnaire, men are more reluctant to describe their psychological suffering but tend to state they feel anxious, stressed or report physical ailments. This can mask their depressive symptomatology.

Studies on perinatal disturbance have shown that in this crucial period, the mental states of fathers and mothers influence each other and can negatively affect their child's psychomotor development. This is different from the physiological influence (higher prolactin levels and lower testosterone levels) of some men in intimate association with pregnant women or new babies, who tend to be those more involved in caring for the baby during the first year of life (Bronte-Tinkew et al., 2007). I recall my husband putting some weight on around his waist during my pregnancy. I used to involve him in observing our baby's movements in response to my favourite classical music, reciting rhymes or using his voice and in stroking my belly. This intimate association with my pregnancy and regular communication with our daughter might have favoured his physiological influence as well as great involvement in caring for her during the years after her birth.

Studies have found a significant correlation between depression and anxiety symptoms in both fathers and mothers and their perceptions of stress (Goodman, 2004; Musser et al., 2013; Baldoni et al., 2009). If one of the partners is depressed, the entire *family system* is compromised. A fundamental aspect of parenting will be to offer a secure base to the offspring, e.g. an atmosphere of safety and trust in the relationship with the attachment figure (Baldoni, 2010). Franco Baldoni points out that another parental function very important for protection from traumatic experiences is to foster mentalisation. This function, a consequence of the quality of attachment, is fundamental for the development of the self and enables the child to regulate affects and their somatic correlates in stressful situations. While in the community the mother benefits from the entire web of social support, in the nuclear family the father's ability to provide a secure base for his partner, helping her cope with stress and suffering and allowing the mother-prenate/infant relationship develop undisturbed is crucial. This function is altered when fathers are too preoccupied, too anxious or depressed or show behavioural problems (aggressiveness, alcoholism and addiction disorders) (Baldoni, 2010).

Longitudinal studies on large samples have confirmed the relationship between paternal perinatal chronic depression and psychiatric disturbances in children at the age of seven (Ramchandani et al., 2008a, 2008b). On the one hand, a depressed father is less involved in the care of the infant and less motivated in supporting pregnancy and the mother-foetus bonding. On the other hand, a father who is not affected by perinatal disturbances and is more involved in the interactions with the infant can exert a protective function against maternal depression and compensate for the poor mother-infant interactions (Edhborg et al., 2003). This is why it is of utmost importance to assess the symptomatology from pregnancy, and when one parent is depressed, consider the possibility that the other may suffer (Schumacher et al., 2008). Franco Baldoni (2018) created the Perinatal Assessment of Paternal Affectivity (PAPA), a self-report questionnaire for the screening of affective symptoms in fathers during the perinatal period (anxiety, depression, hostility, relational and couple difficulties, somatic complaints, dangerous behaviours and addictions – smoke, alcohol, drugs, gambling, Internet, psychical or sexual compulsive and at risk behaviour). The PAPA doesn't allow for an accurate diagnosis but provides a simple and practical guide for detecting fathers at high risk of perinatal affective disorders.

The first two important protective factors (other than healthy nutrition) in pregnancy are the mother's relationship with the baby and that with her partner. These need to be investigated in any prenatal programme and therapy. If we want to prevent perinatal suffering and protect the mother-infant relationship, it is fundamental to acknowledge the importance of the father as early as pregnancy if not before, to support his role, identify his difficulties and promote his involvement in the journey to parenthood and his contribution. Healthcare professionals need to pay attention to the *quality of the couple relationship*. Perinatal depression is often accompanied by marital conflicts, which affect child development outcomes (Hanington et al., 2011). In these cases, it is necessary to offer the couple a space to discuss their affective and relational problems and help them improve their relationship (Schumacher et al., 2008). This is so important since by providing a couple relational model, parents are not only contributing to the child's well-being by reducing the adverse effects of stress but also shaping the child's capacity to build healthy relationships.

There are creative practices that fathers can use to enhance their perception of the baby in the womb, help bond with him/her and share the pregnancy experience. I used to involve my husband in observing our daughter's movements in response to the music, stroke my belly, interpret her movements, talk to her, imaginarily listen to her voice and story, and share my knowledge and wisdom about preborn babies' sentience. This shared experience helped him in the transition to parenthood, facilitated his understanding of the baby's signs and feelings and bonding post-birth, his involvement in baby care and co-parenting with me.

Richard Fletcher advocates that a father's mental health is vital to a well-functioning family and father-baby bonding helps a child for life. He warns health services they should provide screening and support for fathers as part of health care provision. Fletcher (2020) created a Focus On New Fathers (FONF) pilot program that will use a SMS4dads innovative digital platform to reach men expecting a baby/with a newborn to provide information and screen tool through the transition to fatherhood. The new program is being launched on Father's Day and will run in 2021. It provides, through text messages and the voice of the baby, information about the development of the baby during pregnancy and post-birth. Previous programs launched by Fletcher and his team have reported extremely positive responses from dads to the baby's voice and to the program overall. In a South Australian pilot study 92% of fathers said messages helped in their transition to becoming a father and to bond with their baby and co-parent with their partners. These practices can significantly mitigate the risk of perinatal depression and other psychological disorders.

The role of biological systems

We have intriguing evidence of the impact of the mother's and father's attitudes and feelings on their unborn babies. Based on the findings of many other researchers, as well as his own experience as a psychiatrist and psychoanalyst, Thomas Verny presents evidence that the mother's attitude towards her partner has a profound effect on the neuropsychological development of the child and on the birth experience (Verny, 1981). The mother's pattern of feelings, attachment and behaviour is the chief source of stimuli that shape a foetus's development. Therefore, it is plausible that the preborn baby memorises (visceral memory) not only the maternal voice, as we see later on, but also her emotions and mind states, through physiological mediation – emotions involve a neuroendocrine response – which would further explain how finely attuned human beings are, even before birth, to mental states and social interactions. This intertwining reveals the complexity of human hormones and physiological systems, and both their healthy and disrupted roles (due to various types of stress) in the lives of mothers and babies.

To understand the ways in which cells might remember and be affected by the experiences of the prenatal and perinatal time, we can use as an example the memory of the cells within the immune system which, once exposed to infection, are primed to recognise and attack similar future invaders. Verny and Weintraub (2003) write, "We do not need fully developed central nervous systems or brains to receive, store, and process information. Information substances from the mother, be they stress-related cortisol or feel-good endorphins, enter the baby's blood system affecting receptors at every stage of development, no matter how early in life. . . . Our earliest memories are not conscious, nor even unconscious in the stand-ard sense . . . we record experience and history of our lives in our cells" (pp. 159–160).

Both mother and foetus respond to stress. Prenatal development is designed to prepare the foetus to adapt to the environment she expects to live in outside the womb. Excessive stress may alter the foetus's adaptive response. Research suggests that this may occur even if the woman experiences excessive stress in the six months prior to gestation, which may increase the risk of preterm and very preterm birth (Khashan et al., 2009). The mother's loss of a child too close to the gestation of the subsequent child and her unresolved grief can adversely affect foetal development. In her book (2019), Luisa D'Elia Riviello describes the consequences of having been conceived a year after the death of her two-year-old sister. Her mother reports that the pregnancy with Luisa was complicated due to her mental challenges, which undermined Luisa's mental well-being as a child and adult. Her older sister was born a year before the child's loss and this had no significant adverse effects on her life. One and a half years after her birth, Luisa's parents separated, and she grew up missing her father's presence and all that comes with it. What transformed Luisa's suffering into healing and rebirth in her adult life was the combination of a man's deep love, psychotherapy with her mother with the aid of a psychiatric treatment, her mother's emotional and financial support, Buddhism and compassion for her parents and herself.

Because of the challenges that traumatic stress and unresolved grief may present for the mother, healing the consequences of traumatic stress is important to prepare the womb environment and for parenting. Sandman and Davis's (2012) research suggests that "When the predictive adaptive response occurs during prenatal development but does not match the postnatal environment, disease states may occur over the course of the life of the offspring" (p. 13).

We have looked at the evidence of the link between maternal stress, foetal behaviour (as recorded by means of 4D real-time ultrasound observations) and long-term consequences on the child development. According to Fred Previc, a former US government research scientist, the highly stressful, competitive environments characterising Western societies have affected the brain functioning by altering the brain's neurotransmitters (Previc, 2009). The neurotransmitters are biochemical, helping different parts of the brain to connect and work synchronically. When human beings are continuously stressed, the level of calming neurotransmitter serotonin falls, and the level of the motivational neurotransmitter dopamine tends to rise, inducing more self-driven behaviour. Previc believes that many of these effects are passed onto the preborn baby. When mothers are persistently under stress, their babies' brain biochemistry in the womb and in the period after birth can be affected (Glover et al., 2010). Nurturing practices such as mindfulness and social support may reverse this phenomenon by transforming our brains thanks to its plasticity.

The practice of mindful awareness and a combination of meditation techniques enhance interpersonal connection and the production of related feel-good hormones and change our attitudes by forming new neural networks. Positive interpersonal interactions have been correlated with good functioning of the vagus nerve, the tenth cranial nerve and the primary nerve of the parasympathetic nervous system, which is connected with our main organs and informs the brain about how they are working (Porges, 2011). The vagus nerve is implicated in the regulation of multiple biological systems. Interestingly, this correlation seems to be already present in prenatal development and to be influenced by maternal biological systems. Preborn babies of depressed women had elevated activity, lower vagal tone and more growth delays, and prematurity and low birthweight occur more often (Field et al., 2006). This study also found that newborns of depressed mothers are likely to show a similar biochemical/physiological substrate to that of their mothers, including elevated cortisol, lower levels of dopamine and serotonin and lower vagal tone. Elevated maternal cortisol during pregnancy seem to predict these neonatal outcomes.

The intrauterine environment can be altered if persistent stress in the mother changes her neurohormonal profile, blood flow and muscular tension. Cortisol appears to cross the placenta and thus affect the preborn baby and disturb the development of neural pathways in the preborn's brain (Glover & O'Connor, 2006). Two primary systems that mediate the influence of women's moods during pregnancy are the autonomic nervous system and the endocrine system (e.g. hypothalamic-pituitary-adrenal axis). For example, elevated/chronic sympathetic nervous system activation increases the release of catecholamines and vasoconstriction; increased catecholamine levels increase maternal vasoconstriction and blood pressure; vasoconstriction alters the utero-placental blood flow, reducing oxygen and calorie intake to the preborn, influencing his central nervous system development. Also, maternal cortisol crosses the placenta and influences foetal brain development and HPA-axis regulation (Bergner et al., 2008). Furthermore, when the mother is very anxious or stressed during pregnancy, there is reduced blood flow to the baby through the uterine artery, the main source of blood and nutrition for the baby, and this can lead to the baby not growing so well and also sets up a secondary stress response in the foetus (Teixeira et al., 1999).

As further evidence of how maternal psychophysiology influences prenatal development, a study has found that maternal hunger induces movements in the preborn that appear anxious (Piontelli, 2010). Piontelli suggests that chronic conditions such as maternal stress and inadequate nutrition establish chronic states that may become traits in the preborn baby. The rapidity of onset of a foetal response to a maternal event, mediated by foetal perception of changes in the intrauterine milieu, has been consistently observed (DiPietro et al., 2003). However, another study found that a combination of prenatal anxiety, non-specific stress and depressive symptoms were associated with more advanced motor and cognitive development in two-year-olds, while specific stress was associated with slower development (DiPietro et al., 2006). The authors speculate that because of the healthy sample, mild to moderate maternal mood dysregulation may not adversely affect the child. Instead, it may expose the baby to a variety of prenatal stimulation, which may benefit motor and cognitive development. These neurological and physiological studies establish a relationship between pre-natal experiences, behaviour and cognitive and emotional development. There is no determinism in human development.

A study on the preborn's responses to induced maternal relaxation argues that repeated and systemic exposure to periods of relaxation might gener-ate more persistent alterations to the mother's and the baby's functioning, with potential long-term consequences' for child development (DiPietro et al., 2008). The authors propose further investigation of active relaxation strategies and their associations with alterations to the intrauterine milieu related to blood flow and neurohormonal environment. There is signifi-cant research and clinical evidence of the formative influence of the moth-er's feelings and mind-body state on the psychological development of the unborn baby. The mother's psychological and physical states can affect her bond with her developing baby, as well as her baby's developing attachment to the mother. The mother unconsciously transfers her own fears, worries and emotional pain, or her bliss and elation, to the preborn and shapes the psychological "basic configuration" with which she is born. This "signa-ture" can be brought into consciousness and dealt with in psychotherapy, as clinical studies suggest (Janus, 2001).

Epigenetics

Considering epigenetics (how the environment and experiences affect the expression of genes) helps us better understand the importance of maternal experiences and well-being. The baby's gene expression may be altered by the pre-existing and perinatal environment. In numerous stud-ies over several decades, Michael Meany and colleagues have recorded the effects of maternal touch on gene expression (e.g. Weaver et al., 2002). Studies on rats show that maternal affection in the first week of life cor-relates with an altered expression of more than a thousand genes (Szyf et al., 2007). For example, rats with poor nurturance have a weaker feed-back system for controlling anxiety, resulting in more anxiety and height-ened stress responses to the unfamiliar throughout life. Maternal affection in the first ten days of life (the first six months in humans) determined methylation of the particular glucocorticoid receptor protein studied, whether the mother was an adopting mother or the biological mother, ruling out genetics. The methylation pattern matched that of the caregiv-ing mother. Moreover, the behaviour pattern was enhanced in the daugh-ter, proving the effects of poor bonding and poor brain functioning over generations (Weaver et al., 2005). In human beings, unhappy childhoods with poor nurturance have been found to be related to the methylation of mood areas of the brain, which are linked to schizophrenia and suicide (McGowan et al., 2008).

You might have inherited not just your grandmother's long nose, but also her predisposition towards depression caused by the neglect she suffered as a newborn. However, if your grandmother was adopted by nurturing parents, you might benefit from the boost she received thanks to their love and support. The mechanisms of behavioural epigenetics underlie not only deficits and weakness but strengths, resiliencies and wisdom. A number of studies show that we are born with an innate capacity for empathy for others and for nurtures, but past experiences are critically important for the development and expression of nurturing responses (Hrdy, 2011). In a study of infants and foster mothers, the best predictor of how securely attached an infant became to a given caregiver turned out to be the way the foster mother recalled her own childhood experiences and her state of mind about her past experiences (Dozier et al., 2001). Although genetics play a role in personality development, and of course these babies arrived in foster care with their heritable traits, attachment styles are known to be heritable in a different way. My nurturing practices during pregnancy, shaping my maternal consciousness, probably switched on the genome (blueprint of life) inherited from my nurturing parents, influencing the caregiving of my child and her kind empathic nature. Inadequate nurturing practices or traumatic experiences would have likely weakened that genome expression.

Traumatic experiences in our past, or in our recent ancestors' past, leave molecular scars that adhere to our DNA. Jews whose great-grandparents were forced to leave their Russian shtetls; Chinese whose parents survived massacres; adults of every ethnicity who grew up with mentally ill, alcoholic, or abusive parents – all carry with them more than just memories. However, traumatic experiences are also passed down through embodied implicit processes – heart resonance or coherence, sensory energy communication, muscular tension shaping the way of holding a baby, movements, facial expressions, emotional shutdowns, difficulties in connecting and feeling empathy.

Epigenetic changes in early life, including prenatal life, have cascading effects on developmental plasticity. In general, individuals more reactive to stress – that is with less ability to switch off "fight-or-flight" hormonal responses – are more likely to have a high resting heart rate and high blood pressure, experience increased appetite, and suffer from adverse effects on systems that regulate growth, reproduction, metabolism, immunity and emotion (Chrousos & Gold, 1992). Emotional dysregulation and poor attachment at six months predict poor social and cognitive performance (National Institute of Child Health and Human Development, Early Child Care Research Network, 2004). Growing up in a stressful household (and the resulting frequent and intense activation of stress hormones) leaves a susceptibility to physical ailments (heart disease, diabetes and obesity) and mental disorders (anxiety, depression and drug abuse) (Lupien et al., 2009; Meaney, 2010). High levels of glucocorticoid activated under stress tend to be specifically toxic to the neurons of the hippocampus (McEwen, 1999; Sapolsky, 1998). The hippocampus is involved in emotional regulation, a target of stress hormones and an especially plastic and vulnerable region of the brain.

In short, maternal experience (and her inherited caregiving) and related early caregiving have long-term epigenetic and developmental effects, some of which emerge only at a later stage, like adolescence, as late-forming psychopathology (Schore, 2003a, 2003b). Undoing or just mitigating these intergenerational cycles as early as possible by educating prospective and new parents and involving all prenatal and perinatal professionals and community is of the utmost importance. Brain plasticity allows self-care practices, such as mindfulness meditation, psychotherapy or other newer treatments in more severe cases, to heal parental brains and promote nurturing care to reverse the changes in genome regulation. A leading figure in the study of maternal influence, Frances Champagne, has learnt from her work that stress is a big suppressor of maternal behaviour (Champagne, 2008). We see it in animal studies, and it is true in human beings. She says that the best thing a mother can do is not worry all the time about whether she is doing the right thing. This prevents her from being present and connecting with her baby and being responsive. Keeping the stress level down is very important. So is tactile interaction, as the sensory input, the touching, is so important for the developing brain.

Encouraging a "mindful" approach can help promote maternal behaviour and also foster the reflective function with which she can make sense of the baby's sensory experiences and live motherhood in its wholeness. Mindfulness can slow the body and mind and increase feelings of being in control. It means the mother can put all her attention into what is actually happening between her and her baby in the present moment rather than being taken up by concerns and stress. This increases awareness of feelings, body sensations and movements and spiritual experiences, which is the opposite of being on "autopilot" (Astin, 1997; Vieten & Austin, 2008). Therefore, mindfulness can help mitigate the adverse effects of generational patterns.

The protective function of the earliest mother-baby relationship

Communication between mother and preborn occurs in several ways: physically (e.g. through hormones, blood flow and variation of abdominal muscular tone related to mental activity); behaviour (e.g. the baby's flow of movements, kicking, eye movements, facial expressions, the mother's voice and utterances or forms of vitality and touching the abdomen); sympathetically or intuitively (e.g. through love, a sense of relational presence in the womb, ambivalence, dreams, sensations, thoughts, imagination and maternal representations of the baby). These means of communication are interrelated. For example, any mental activity is a movement of energy or force – however virtual – thus inducing physiological changes and changes in forms of vitality (Stern, 2010). One of the more direct means of communicating maternal attitudes, feelings and mind states is the neurohormones the mother releases, which increase when she is under stress. These substances cross the placenta as easily as nutrients, alcohol and other drugs. In moderation, these hormones cause physiological reactions in the preborn, which stimulate his neural and physiological systems, but in excess they can adversely affect the developing baby (Verny, 1981; DiPietro et al., 2006). It is generally long-term stress (e.g. chronically anxious or depressed mothers) that may leave enduring negative effects, rather than isolated thoughts, feelings or incidents, which are aspects of life.

The mother's love, acceptance and positive attitude towards her pregnancy and preborn baby, as well as felt aliveness act as a strong protection, promoting the baby's healthy development. After nine months of gestational synchrony, human mothers and neonates under natural conditions move into an interactional synchrony of sound and movement within the first few hours after birth (Condon & Sander, 1974; Papousek & Papousek, 1992). Some call this *limbic regulation* (Lewis et al., 2000) or *psychobiological attunement* (Field, 1984), in which caregivers continue to act as external regulators of psychological and biological development (Eisenberg, 1995; Schore, 2001a, 2001b) just as the mother did during gestation. This *limbic resonance* or attunement with infants and children is key to empathic understanding and optimal emotional and social development (Decety & Chaminade, 2003; Decety & Meyer, 2008). It is also related to maternal well-being and therefore needs to be protected by all means.

For many years, perinatal mental health professionals believed that breastfeeding was actually a risk factor for postpartum depression. We now have evidence that indicates that exclusively breastfeeding mothers are at lower risk of depression. It is only in rare cases of psychoneurological dysfunction that breastfeeding may be a risk factor for mental conditions. Breastfeeding mothers report reduction in anxiety, negative moods and stress when compared to formula-feeding mothers (Groër, 2005). These qualitative findings are supported by physiological measures, indicative of a positive effect of breastfeeding on emotional well-being. For example, breastfeeding mothers have stronger cardiac vagal tone modulation, reduced blood pressure and reduced heart rate reactivity than formula-feeding mothers have, indicating a calm and non-anxious physiological state (Mezzacappa et al., 2005).

Indeed, breastfeeding is a regulator of psychobiological attunement and is generally protective of maternal and infant mental health. I found night breastfeeding a meditative, blissful and soothing experience. In the silence and dim light, I could open up my senses, only hear Gisele's rhythmic suckling, a lullaby-like tune for me, and pick up her bodily cues. Because of the long stretches of time spent with the baby, breastfeeding predisposes the mother to be more responsive. Maternal responsiveness is key to understanding long-term effects. When mothers consistently respond to their babies' cues, they set the stage for lifelong resilience in their offspring. Responsiveness is built into the extended breastfeeding relationship as well. Depressive symptomatology in the early postpartum period may increase the risk for infant-feeding outcomes, including decreased breastfeeding duration and likelihood to initiate breastfeeding, increased breastfeeding difficulties and decreased levels of breastfeeding self-efficacy (Dennis & McQueen, 2009). These findings support the need for early identification and support for women with mental challenges.

Emotions and mental states are perceived from forms of vitality – facial and body expressions, such as gestures and movements – and are mirrored by the perceiver (Stern, 2010). We also know that they are conveyed through energy fields and heart coherence (Childre et al., 2016). During gestation, emotions are perceived through other physiological routes, e.g. heart and breathing rhythms, hormones and muscular tension. Mental states are transmitted through face-to-face intersubjective exchange and regulated by emotions through dynamic interplay of movement and mirroring. As social mammals, human beings pick up cues that reveal the intended move-ment of others, through the mirror neurons (Gallese, 2008; Rizzolatti & Craighero, 2004). Attuned interactions are also based on these mirroring mechanisms. But mirroring requires time, a slow pace and a stress-free envi-ronment that favours presence of mind. The stresses of our modern life affect emotions and mental states and consequently interfere with the flow of exchanges during mirroring. From intrauterine life, attuned responsive-ness constructs the child's self and interpersonal world.

If the baby's evolved needs for attention, connection and care are not met, e.g. when parental mental health is impaired, his psychobiological development is undermined. A chronically depressed or anxious mother, whose mind is concerned about her own issues, is more at risk of with-drawing her love manifestations. She is less likely to engage and be respon-sive. Neither would the baby bond properly with a mother overburdened with anxiety or frustration. In his book *The Secret Life of the Unborn Baby* (1981), Thomas Verny described the case of a newborn girl who refused to bond with or nurse from her own mother, though she did not refuse other women. It turned out that the mother had wanted to have an abortion and bore the baby reluctantly at the father's insistence.

Chronically depressed mothers have difficulties in synchronising with the baby's positive emotions, while they are often synchronous with the nega-tive ones, with long-term effects on cognition and social emotion (Feld-man, 2007). By not being present, they have difficulties in picking up bodily cues and engaging with the baby's interactions. Babies of depressed, unre-sponsive or unpredictable mothers may have impaired self-organisational processes due to the lack of good feedback and dyadic meaning. The most common consequences of postnatal depression to the child – emotional and behavioural problems and cognitive delay – have been found by a number of studies (Murray et al., 1999). Unresolved maternal (and pater-nal) trauma predisposes to child abuse and neglect, which is the leading preventable cause of major mental ill health. In addition, child maltreat-ment has been shown to have lifelong adverse health, social and economic consequences for survivors, including behavioural problems (De Bellis et al., 2013; Fang et al., 2012); an increased risk of delinquency, criminality and violent behaviour; increased risk of chronic disease; lasting impact or disability from physical injury; reduced health and quality of life; and lower levels of economic well-being. Together these findings suggest that while maternal behaviour varies with changing circumstances, exposure to mater-nal depression in the early months post-birth may have enduring effects on child psychological adjustment. It is clear that primary prevention through an effective prenatal and perinatal programme to prevent harm before it occurs is of paramount importance.

Babies born of depressed mothers, while still loved, may have received low emotional and intellectual stimulation and aliveness, and their brains may not have benefited from the richness of neural networks that a baby born of a self-creative and content mother has available. The voice intona-tion and rhythm of a depressed mother reflects her state – it tends to lack vitality, although in some cases lows alternate with highs. We know that a mother's voice has an impact on her baby's developing brain (Dehaene-Lambertz et al., 2010). It is reasonable to assume that a predominantly sad facial expression and intonation, when for instance she is suffering from domestic isolation, affects the baby's range of expressions and motor tone through mirroring. A recent overview of the evidence found that babies born to depressed mothers had lower motor tone, were less active and more irritable. They also had fewer facial expressions in response to happy faces, disrupted sleep patterns, increased fussiness and non-soothability, and there was increased negative reactivity in two- and four-month-olds (Bergner et al., 2008). The authors highlight the importance of interven-tion that aims to improve maternal mood, address the mother's develop-ing relationship with her baby and positively influence the course of foetal development. Winnicott (1960) said there is no such a thing as a baby alone; this is more so during pregnancy. The protective function of a prenatal and postnatal nurturing relationship and the vital importance of supporting it by valuing the contribution of the father as well as the influence of the com-munity should never be underestimated.

Because most depressed mothers were already depressed or had emo-tional issues during pregnancy, it is extremely important to explore with the mother the relationship with her preborn baby and use a mindfulness relationship-based approach that encourages the mother to engage with her preborn baby. The practice of mindfulness encourages positive images of the baby and the exploration of any negative images that emerge and keep the mother "disengaged". If the mother is closed off from her body feelings and extremely disengaged, mindfulness practice may need to be combined with a psychotherapeutic work that considers the role of the body in mother-baby dynamics. Mindfulness also encourages the mother's body and sensory awareness, a sense of embodied presence and thus meaningfulinteractionswiththepreborn'smovements.Apreventiveorhealing programme should always take the mother-baby-father relationship – prenatal and postnatal – into strong consideration.

The importance of resonance

Asynchrony is an essential aspect of mother-child interaction and human development, provided synchrony is re-established after dysregulation, creating a flowing narrative. If a mistaken action or break in contact (misstep or rupture) is not followed by reparation, the child feels helpless and hopeless (Stern, 1985). The nervous system remains unregulated. Dyadic pattern of mutual sadness, hypervigilance, withdrawal or conflict may become stabilised and rigid and difficult to modify. This increases the risk of the child mistrusting the world (Sroufe et al., 2005). Children with poor early caregiving may have a greater sense of shame, leading to a propensity to depression (Alessandri & Lewis, 1996). Those who develop borderline personality disorder (BPD) report an inner "emptiness" suggesting that a critical period for nurturing the development of "self" was jeopardised (Carlsson, 1998). Constantly being misunderstood or ignored may lead to habitual shame, disconnection, dis-attunement and distrust.

Fredrickson (2013) suggests that attunement or positive synchrony equates with the experience of love in our body and we do not feel love when we are not in positive synchrony with others. Children who have never learnt the "intersubjective dance" with their mothers and others may never feel loved or be able to love. Mothers who are depressed after birth are less responsive to their babies, affecting the child's regulation of biological systems (Field, 1994), including the functioning of the hypothalamic-pituitary-adrenal (HPA) axis. Maternal depression is associated with disorganised sleep, decreased responsiveness to stimulation and a difficult temperament in infants. In childhood and adolescence, children are likely to have attentional, emotional and behavioural problems and, as adults, they may suffer from chronic illness (Field, 2011).

The modern lifestyle often does not meet the mother-child's evolved need for attunement. These days, often geographically separated from older generations, we turn to a book or the Internet for advice. Often advice is not only conflicting, but demoralising when our babies do not perform accordingly. Differing messages often make the women feel inadequate and the advice given is delivered "as a threat". A study found an association between use of infant parenting books that promote strict routines and maternal depression, self-efficacy and parenting confidence (Harries & Brown, 2017). One of the implications of the small families of the late twentieth century is that women rarely have the opportunity to care full-time for a small baby until they have their own. These days, girls are not raised to be mothers and they need to attend classes or read books to deal with parenting, while in traditional societies knowledge and wisdom are passed on and shared among members of the same community. There is no doubt that parents do need information, but there is now too much parenting information that is often conflicting, leading parents away from trusting their own feelings. There is an urgent need for inspiring shared experience, connection through human basic virtues and community engagement.

Nowadays there is an exaggerated need for tips and advice because women want to be in control of everything in their lives and feel frustrated if their baby does not behave as they expect. But this is a wrong approach, often contributing to making child-rearing difficult and a source of stress rather than reward and fulfilment. In the USA and the UK, child-rearing seems to have become about how well you get your baby to sleep, to feed and so on. But things with babies unfold smoothly when there is an empathic mother-baby-father relationship, in which the baby's evolved innate needs and expectations are listened to and thus met, as the mother discovers and relies on her own intuitive wisdom. In the same way, many women spend their entire pregnancy reading about different approaches to childbirth, receiving a variety of views and techniques, and many contradictions. Yet, the birth process and the baby's expectations have remained unchanged for millions of years. Natural, uncomplicated childbirth involves surrendering to elemental life-force energy, letting go attachments and allowing that "other power" to take charge. This means women letting their selves be loosened and transformed by the new ongoing experience and flow of life. This is aligned with primal wisdom abilities.

When adults receive meaningful emotional support, they are helped to work through their trauma and the related mental issues and to trust themselves. By practising nurturing practices such as mindfulness, their capacity for self-regulation, empathy and mentalising are fostered, and so is their capacity to provide responsive care. Mindful wise adults know how to respond to a baby promptly before things get out of hand. Their sense of presence and body awareness make them sensitive to movements, gestures and body signals, thus able to tune in. Their reflective function allows them to make sense of the baby's experience rather than getting anxious, being reactive or judgemental. Their *mindful movements* and gestures while responding to the baby coherently reflect their calm state, thus are graceful, rather than tense or jerky due to worry induced by unresolved inherited trauma. They reflect the flow of life, the feeling of being alive. And babies' optimal arousal reflects their caregivers' mindful state. Therefore, mindful parents can meet the child's nèeds before she becomes distressed, as indigenous mothers have done for millennia, supporting the development of a calm mindful personality. A caregiver who is sensitively responsive to the child fosters the child's emotional attunement with others and mentalising capabilities (Siegel, 1999). These children are the future of a cohesive compassionate society.

When the baby feels understood, his behaviour does not need to escalate into crying to voice his feelings, since his cues are picked up by an attentive parent through an empathic way of responding and reflective listening. In Grazyna Kochanska's model (2002), the development of the moral self depends on the quality of parent-child attachment, or the high-quality intersubjective environment shaped by shared positive affect. Inexperienced, distracted, mindless or irresponsible caregivers may be less skilled and less motivated to understand the child's needs; perhaps this is why community child-rearing ("cooperative breeding") evolved (Hrdy, 2011).

Indigenous and traditional cultures are far more communal than we are in their care of children. Child abuse and neglect are nearly impossible in hunter-gatherer bands or the pastoralist Himba of Northern Namibia I visited. If a mother or father gets irritable and acts harshly towards a child, others in the band will promptly step in and calm the parent while also gently taking the child. Because childcare is public, every community member, including young children, can witness all of the childcare in the band. Before becoming a parent, a young person has had plenty of experience holding and caring for other infants and children and witnessing many others doing so. No adult is left alone to care for a child unassisted. Our society has changed enormously. When modern mothers are under stress, they often have to deal with it on their own, which may put their well-being at risk. What can we do in our modern world to provide the kind of caring community that parents need for their well-being and children need for healthy development? The answer will come from the mindful parents' self-empowerment as well as a mindful society supporting them. It follows that it is paramount to promote nurturing practices as early as possible in pregnancy, ideally before conception, and establish a meaningful relationship between healthcare providers and parents and their children, which needs to be as close as possible to the traditional village.

Costs to society and economy

Currently, most local authorities in Britain and elsewhere tackle perinatal mental issues and child abuse and developmental problems by reacting after the event. What is missing is a commitment to prevent harm before it begins through primary prevention using meaningful effective communal action. Unfortunately, this focus on prevention is still missing in our Western culture, with consequences for the quality of parenting and childhood.

We now understand that it is vital to promote primary prevention through strategic approaches and practices, and thus prevent harm to preborn babies, infants and children. Grassroots campaigns and programmes should aim at ensuring national and local government support for all parents to prevent intergenerational patterns of mental health problems, abuse and neglect. The cost of failing to deal adequately with perinatal mental health and child maltreatment has been estimated at £23 billion each year in the UK (Mental Health Task Force, 2016), with other countries facing similar challenges. Imagine what else could be achieved with these funds if primary prevention was implemented. We should set goals to develop partnerships and alliances of organisations, individuals, practitioners, experts, academics and community, members of parliament and local authorities and share data and wisdom so as to implement them in everyone's practice.

However, I believe this implies a far deeper grassroots change. We need to recreate a way of life for which we are biologically wired, but which is nearly impossible to find in developed nations: communities in which individuals engage with and know one another well share the joys, burdens and sorrows of life; nurture one another in times of need; mind the well-being of each other's children and increasingly dependent elderly; and feel rewarded by the essential contribution to the group that securely holds them. This is the most natural environment for mothers to provide care and for children to grow up in, in which we have evolved for 99 per cent of human history. We know from epigenetics that from prenatal life, the environment shapes a child's health and personality predispositions towards empathy, compassion and moral development or selfishness, aggressiveness and violence. Today enormous pressure is put on parents as they try to make up for what entire communities used to provide. Social media platforms such as Facebook are illusionary substitutes for the village. Depression and anxiety skyrocket due to isolation and pressure, particularly during critical times of our lives when we need support more than ever and cannot find it. Research shows us that human connection is a biological necessity, and authentic, safe, fulfilling connections are essential for thriving (Porges, 2011).

I envisage that developing a mindfulness-based approach promoting healthy relationships with ourselves and with others, thus kindness, listening, compassion and empathy, and valuing human essence as a common goal can lead to amazing improvements in families' lives, society and the economy. This approach involves self-development, self-awareness, an awareness of prenatal and perinatal processes and lived experiences as foundations of well-being and interpersonal neuroscience. Furthermore, I see *self-love* in relational action, fostered by the practice of mindfulness, as the greatest gift we could possibly give to the mothers of tomorrow.

To envisage that future and believe in a possible new way, perinatal well-being, mental health and attachment, awareness of prenatal and perinatal processes and their continuum and child development must become a major concern for humanity, society and the economy. The benefits of this new paradigm will be immense. In the short term, local areas will benefit from lower costs due to fewer children being taken into care, and a reduction in court proceedings and costs resulting from educational disruption. There will also be lower costs from dealing with mental health problems and criminality, including terrorism. Ultimately, the benefits will be reflected in lower costs in health, criminal justice and welfare. As we have healthier contributors to society, this will also be reflected in lower taxes.

9 Acknowledging the intersubjective reality

It is clear that the mother's well-being and engagement with her unborn child are important sources of a child's healthy development. Science concurs that safe, responsive and nurturing early parent-child relationship promotes healthy brain and child development and protects against lifelong disease by reducing toxic stress and setting the foundations of socio-emotional health (Ordway et al., 2015). Most studies have been focusing on the correlation between the mother's stress and anxiety and the baby's behaviour in the womb and adverse outcomes. But how does the baby respond to the mother's life-enhancing emotions or prosocial virtues? Observations from my work with pregnant or new mothers and babies and my own experience of pregnancy reveal the preborn's responsiveness to manifestations of love, especially during the last trimester. I encourage mothers to lovingly touch the abdomen exactly where the baby's movement is coming from, so as to initiate a social game of reciprocity on which intersubjectivity is based. These sensory synchronic interactions are also about valuing and reinforcing the baby's responses.

Usually the baby tends to respond rhythmically with a kick, arm-stretching or ovoid movement when the mother touches her abdomen. With repetition of these interactions, the baby can even learn to anticipate the mother's touching by "asking" for more through his motions. It may be hard to believe, but a conscious attuned pregnant mother can report such communicative events. My baby's specific movement patterns (end of the sixth-month gestation) straight after a phone conversation with my husband abroad for work also indicates her responsiveness to my emotional nuances. I often noticed her anticipatory motor pattern, thus her possible perception of my intention, probably through subtle biochemical changes, for example a few minutes before I approached food, began listening to my favourite piano music or lay in the sun. Indeed, the preborn is sensitive to the mother's mental state. Theory of mind may have its roots in prenatal life, in these earliest sensorimotor experiences.

The mother's aware perception of these intimate communicative exchanges – the foundation of prenatal bonding – requires a mindful state incompatible with preoccupations, chronic stress or emotional issues. In recent decades, this reflective and intersubjective mother-baby space has been curtailed mainly by a work-centred and materialistic culture, with adverse consequences for parents' and children's well-being. One of the most revealing discoveries during my visit to the Himba was the mothers' vivid sense of a human presence in the womb during their pregnancy. I recall Badri reporting, "When I felt the baby move in the womb I knew he wanted to talk to me". She was ascribing an intention to her unborn baby. Indigenous mothers are known for anticipating their babies' need for a wee by picking up their bodily cues.

Recent studies describe possible prenatal mirroring mechanisms on the basis of coordinated intentional motor patterns, thus sophisticated development of the motor system at 22 weeks of gestation (Zoia et al., 2007). These movements, traditionally described as reflexes rather than intentional actions, are not uncoordinated, but are directed at specific targets. We can think of a rudimentary MNS (mirror neuron system) operating in the foetus during the prenatal period. In this regard, Carter Castiello et al. (2010) explored whether the propensity to social interaction is already present before birth. Therefore, elementary mirroring mechanisms may be shaped by mother-preborn intersubjectivity (shared experience). A two-dimensional (2D) ultrasonographic study showed a congruent mouth-motor response by the foetus to maternal acoustic stimulation. In particular, when the mother sang the syllable "la" in a nursery rhyme, foetuses significantly increased mouth openings. This finding suggests that foetal matched responses may be rudimentary signs of early mirroring behaviours that become functional in the postnatal period (Ferrari et al., 2016). Such responses may play a role in the development and emotional attunement with their mothers long before birth. It is interesting that all those infant's movements of lips, tongue and mouth, described as already so communicative by Dr Vivien Sabel (2012), are consistently practised in the womb, showing that the body parts involved in speech later on are already used by the unborn baby to explore his or her environment and own body. These movements serve for sensorimotor practice, which feeds brain and development of a rudimentary self. The preborn in the third trimester can hear very well and thus produce congruent mouth-motor responses to acoustic stimulation, in particular maternal sounds. I always encourage expectant parents to read books, rhymes or poems out loud to the baby, as this can help with bonding and intersubjectivity.

A study conducted by Prof Vincent Reid, a psychologist from Lancaster University, found that the foetus in the third trimester actively seeks out information from the environment (Reid et al., 2017). The study showed that when a face-like image was projected through the uterus, the babies turned their heads to look at it. When the face looked upside down, and so harder to recognise as a face, the foetus did not react. This could happen because the way light falls in the womb primes him to recognise these "face-like" shapes. It may be due to prenatal visual experiences. This also shows that an unborn baby's senses are already well developed and parents should interact with the baby while still in the womb. There are many ways of interacting and setting the roots for bonding and empathy. We know that straight after birth babies prefer to look at faces than any other stimuli. A human baby seems to be hard-wired to interact with human beings and establish meaningful human connection. However, this innate predisposition needs to be nurtured in the womb so as to unleash its potential.

Another study shows preborn babies at around 24 weeks of gestation looking upset and touching their faces more often if their mothers had been anxious, helpless or under pressure. Researchers at Durham and Lancaster universities (Reissland, 2015) believe they are picking up on their mother's anxieties, and then trying to soothe them away with the power of touch. As adults we do this by holding our head in our hands. The study may indicate how unborn babies pick up on stress and respond to stress and negative emotions such as high anxiety. Human beings are astoundingly attuned to subtle emotional shifts from intrauterine life. Slight changes in muscular tension, energy, heart and breathing rhythms signal to the baby how happy, comfortable, relaxed or frightened the mother is. After birth, the maternal state and emotion are picked up by the slightest changes in the tension of the brow, wrinkles around the eyes, curvature of the lips and the angle of the neck (Ekman et al., 1980, 2007). The muscles of the mother's face and those involved in her holding and gestures give the baby clues about how calm, excited or worried, or how connected she feels, whether her heart is racing or quiet. Dr Stephen Porges considers that connection and love are a human biological necessity (Porges, 2011). When the message the baby receives is "you're safe with me", both mother and baby relax, in the womb as well as in the world outside the womb. But the mother needs to feel safe herself. Then the relaxed baby can look into the mother's face and eyes. These body cues and exchanges shape our capacity for empathy and future relationships.

The unborn baby as an active social partner

During my 33-week scan, my baby looked content, almost like attentively perceiving my favourite musical piece and showing attunement with my emotional response to the music. This is consistent with Zimmer's thought that when the preborn baby hears music, he responds to the mother's emotional response to it, thus to its biochemical mediators (Zimmer et al., 1982). These observations suggest a possible prenatal impact on mirroring, which implies that the roots of empathy may reside in intrauterine life. This could even suggest that our capacity to empathise with others is mediated by embodied prenatal and perinatal mechanisms, that is by the activation of the sensorimotor circuits underpinning our own emotional and sensory experiences (Gallese, 2003; Ammaniti & Gallese, 2014). The other is present in the self-experience from the beginning of life. Prenatal and perinatal experiences form the blueprint of our predispositions. Intersubjectivity is at the core of our experience of self and other, and its quality is shaped by the mother's psychosomatic resources and well-being. Our culture promotes individualism, but at a deeper level, we barely exist as individual organisms. At conception, we interact with myriad cells. In the womb, we interact with the complexity of our mother's mind, body and soul. Bessel van der Kolk (2014) states that our brains are designed to help us function as members of a tribe. Perhaps this is true from life before birth. Much of our energy is expended on connecting with others. Without connection, a baby would not survive. One of the signs of mental suffering is difficulty in creating functioning and satisfying relationships.

Bonding long before birth is vital to growth. A mother's mindful love of her baby before she meets him out of the womb has a significant impact on his development. Clinical accounts suggest that the anxieties of mothers and fathers may harm these vital intersubjective bonds and undermine a child's developing self-confidence (Ammaniti & Gallese, 2014).

Through companionship care, from conception the environment signals "all the way down" to cells that the child is welcome, setting the roots for the capacity for love and empathy. Environmental signals form a cellular memory beginning at conception and an energy state that is transferred to subsequent generations (Emerson, 1996; Lake, 1979; Meaney, 2010). Through mindfulness abilities – presence, reverence and synchrony, loving attitudes and behaviour – as early as conception and gestation, parents provide the optimal developmental niche, as the child can build emotional systems that form her values; she learns the value of companionship, empathy and compassion (Narvaez, 2014). Therefore, parents can contribute to building a cohesive peaceful society.

However, this embodied formative process is far from concerning just mother, father, baby and family. The baby, as early as intrauterine life, is an active social partner not only to the mother and father, but through them, to the community and wider society. The parent-baby system is open to environmental influences from conception, and anyone can exert an influence on it, including healthcare providers and policy makers. After birth and beyond, through early mindful relationships with others, thus in the most natural environment for children to grow up in, the child expands his learning of the value of cooperation, community and mutual respect, on which a cohesive healthy society is based.

It is not surprising that negative interactions can have adverse effects. Research and clinical work, some of which I have cited, show how high levels of stress, depression and anxiety have deleterious effects on intersubjectivity, development, attachment, empathy and emotional, cognitive and social development. This, in turn, speaks to the importance of the use of early prenatal nurturing practices and compassion to support the mother's mental health, the mother-baby prenatal relationship, and foetal development. In this way, we can prevent birth and postnatal trauma or depression and other conditions, and their harmful effects on infant and child development.

A strong nurturing mother-baby bond, supported by a mindful community, can protect the baby and child against the impact of stress or traumatic shock. The womb is the child's first home and his perceptions of it as warm and caring or hostile create personality predispositions (Piontelli, 1992). As he enters the outside world, this will be largely a continuum of his first home and birth experience. If he felt the womb to be a rejecting and hostile place, the child will be predisposed to distrust others, to find it hard to relate to others and to have poor self-confidence. Yet, I point out that predispositions can be strengthened or weakened by subsequent experiences, thanks to brain plasticity – its capacity to be moulded by experience – which stays with us throughout our lives.

In the first few months of her life, my daughter Gisele already manifested a tendency to trust others, to be interested in others, engage with them and feel empathy – all qualities fundamental to being human and major assets to a cohesive society. Her creative imagination and her love of reading and early writing have mirrored the creative epistolary, narrative and musical relationship I formed with her during her prenatal and perinatal life. Every baby and child is potentially gifted, but for her potential to unfold she needs to be nurtured nutritionally, emotionally and creatively.

A mother's (and father's) quality of love and vitality affects the baby physiologically, by nourishing the baby's neural connections as early as prenatal life. This helps the baby regulate his emotions, physiological systems and social engagement by influencing his vagal nerve functioning (Porges, 2011). Therefore, a mother's love shapes the baby's predispositions and sets the roots of his social, moral and human behaviour. Indeed, we can say that what a mother can be and do for her developing baby and teach him – with her mindful nutrition, creativity, narrative dialogue and nurturing practices – has a huge impact in shaping the baby's brain and capacity for empathy and healthy relationships. In a study by the Washington University School of Medicine in St Louis, the brain images revealed that a mother's love influences the baby's brain morphologically (Luby et al., 2012). The learning and memory centre of the brain that is also associated with stress responses is called hippocampus. The hippocampus in children who were nurtured well was found to be 10 per cent larger than those children who were not nurtured. In her book *Why Love Matters*, Sue Gerhardt explains how loving a baby benefits his growth since gestation (2014).

Motherhood and love are intrinsically linked to human well-being, and a lack of respect for maternal love is at the root of widespread mental issues and dissatisfaction with modern life. Receiving support from meaningful people, in particular her husband or partner, and thus the promotion of their mental well-being, are of high concern for the mother and society. We can consider the mother the holder of science as the survival of our species relies on motherhood, which lies at the core of all human functions – biological, social, cultural, spiritual, economic, educational and artistic – and every other aspect of human existence. It follows that the health of the mother significantly matters to society and economy, as the future of a cohesive and productive society rests on healthily and happily developed and resilient children. Therefore, maternal (and interrelated paternal) well-being should be supported by all healthcare professionals they interact with, every member of the community and policy maker.

A remnant of the old mind-body split paradigm?

I am now posing a question: if we have such abundant evidence of how maternal emotions and mental states affect foetal and child development outcome, why are conventional medicine and healthcare services still so often unaware that emotions, thoughts, consciousness and subconsciousness are connected with the mother's physiology and thus her baby's development? Why are prenatal and perinatal healthcare professionals and services often unintentionally mindless – though well-meaning – towards a pregnant and new mother, for instance by using inappropriate words and nuances or being indifferent to the delicate implicit dynamics? For instance, mothers' accounts reveal that labour and birth outcome can be disturbed by apparently minor events. A midwife's loud repetitive words such as "push, keep pushing" to get her baby out quickly can be intrusive and affect a labouring woman's feelings and physiology. There is overwhelming evidence that directed pushing induces stress in both mother and baby and results in increased morbidity for both, and among other things is associated with altering the mother's body fluid pH, resulting in inefficient uterine contractions, maternal fatigue and metabolic alterations and interfering with the baby's gradual descent and rotation, causing the baby more stress and increasing the risk of hypoxia and heart-rate abnormalities (Brancato et al., 2008). The obstetrician is usually called in to rescue the baby and pull him out. It is extremely important that the birth environment acknowledges the importance of feelings and helps a woman feel confident and safe to let her hormones do their job and support her mental health. We should remember that safety is a biological necessity (Porges, 2011), especially during critical life events.

The tendency to ignore the role of emotions in health is *an* old thought-habit, a remnant of the old paradigm that focuses on the physical level of health (Frazzetto, 2013). Most healthcare practitioners are still uneducated about the impact of parental attitudes and mental ill health on their baby's development. Foetal development is still considered to be mechanically controlled by genes because of the notion of genetic determinism healthcare practitioners learn as medical students (Lipton, 2015). The major concern of many obstetricians and most of us is about nutrition, exercise, taking vitamins and elimination of alcohol and drugs. The words "healthy lifestyle" are for most of us associated with these. While these are all health-enhancing strategies, most of us miss the attention to daily emotional self-care. But maternal emotions, like everyone's emotions, are a key element in self-care, even to take up a form of exercise, yoga or nutritional plan. Emotion is what connects a mother to her baby, a mother to her baby's father and a father to his baby. It is what creates a flow not just within the mother's body but also between them and thus creates emotional resonance or empathy.

Emotional resonance is in fact what allows us to feel what others feel, what makes relationships cohesive. Affective attuned responses to infant cues help the infant organise his emotions and physiological experiences, leading to reflective functioning (Greenspan & Shanker, 2004). Paediatricians' main concern is often still about body weight, food intake, and not how bonding and these attuned infant-caregiver interactions are involved in eating behaviour and growth. It is enough to visit some neonatal intensive care units (NICU) to become aware of this reality: the preemie is often still considered unable to suffer, to be marked by his trauma. But the ground-breaking approach of some neonatologists understands the vital need of preemies to be put on their mothers' chest, breastfeed and talked to (even though connected with tubes and still very small) in order to thrive.

The old paradigm considering mind and body as independent is still predominant in our culture and affects training courses and thus practitioners' attitudes towards mothers, often regardless of their possible influence on maternal mental health and baby's development. Practitioners often do not realise that perinatal mental conditions (e.g. depression) are by far the commonest major medical complication in pregnancy and often the leading cause of maternal death in the UK (Oates, 2003). They may not be aware that the prenatal and perinatal period is the most efficient time for detecting or preventing depression in women. This lack of awareness is one of the neglected areas in maternity services.

This misunderstanding goes back to the Cartesian mind-body split, which is an arbitrary division that current research has shown to be invalid (Frazzetto, 2013). As a result, women have learnt to distrust their bodies and feelings and to trust, sometimes unconditionally, other authorities instead of their own inner resources and wisdom. But the main preoccupation of doctors, midwives and all those involved in prenatal and perinatal care should be to acknowledge and respect parents' emotions and needs and reduce their anxiety. This will not be possible as long as prenatal education and care are medicalised and merely aimed at making women aware of all the risks associated with pregnancy and birth. Therefore, healthcare in pregnancy and postpartum should be promoted in a humanistic fashion. Pregnancy and birth should be considered not as mere physiological or pathological events but a celebration of life and humanness.

Every practitioner dealing with expectant couples, all of us, must never forget priceless human values such as kindness, listening, smiling and the use of appropriate words and body language during interactions with mothers and their families, so as to support their emotional and mental health.

Body language and words from birth-related professionals, often reflecting their own trauma and emotional issues, or work schedules, are powerful. Awareness of their effects on maternal emotion and mental state, on pregnancy and birth outcome, should be widely promoted. This is even more important for deaf pregnant women and new mothers who, due to impaired hearing, rely far more on bodily cues – visual, tactile, gestural and motor information. Support is one of the biggest issues for new mothers today. Many do not have family who live close by. The modern urban lifestyle and social media limit the availability of real human connection and support, and refugee pregnant women and new parents struggle with language problems and the demands of adjusting to a new culture. This is a community and societal issue that is calling for change.

A dialogue between science and intersubjective mother-baby experience

A mother's subjective experience should be seriously considered by science to embrace a wisdom-based way of knowing, including engagement with emotional presence. If it has not been valued, this is because science has been associated with competition, control and rationality – all qualities characterising a male-dominated, materialist and even aggressive twentieth-century culture. But a mother represents the essence of what science should be: observing, understanding human nature, intuitive caring, connecting, unifying, cooperating and communicating.

A dialogue between scientific research and subjective experience – relational attunement, imagination and emotional presence – has always been difficult, if not impossible. This relates to a culture created by the seventeenth-century philosopher Descartes, who declared body and mind to be distinct, separate entities, almost entirely unrelated to each other (Ryle, 1949). The view that scientific objectivity requires complete detachment is a recent development that still dominates scientific discourse today. But there are new neuroscientists who consider soul, mind and emotions to be interrelated and to play an important role in health. Scientists are expected to be uninvolved and distance themselves from what they study, to measure events as static objects, pulled out of the movement and flow of life (Narvaez, 2014). Ancient Greeks argued about this view (e.g. Heraclitus emphasising change and Parmenides emphasising the eternal). The focus on objectivity implies disengagement from emotional presence, a position of control over the Other (e.g. medical control over the birth process and mother-infant dyad). Relational attunement, wisdom, emotional engagement and imagination are essential sources of well-being for pregnancy and prenatal and perinatal development and need to be included in our Western medical frame of mind. There are new neuroscientists who consider the soul, mind and emotions to be interrelated and to play an important role in health and well-being. Allan Schore proposes a new paradigm that acknowledges maternal emotions and mind as relevant to science (Schore, 2012).

Traditional ecological knowledge characterising indigenous cultures derives from "millennia of lived experience . . . rich in models for the philosophy and practice of reciprocal, mutualistic relationships with the earth" (Kimmerer, 2013, p. 57). Unlike indigenous science, Western science treats the natural world as an object (the known) and the scientist as the subject (the knower). This view may reflect the tendency of modern women and medicine to ignore the resources of caring mammalian nature. This orientation neglects relational attunement and interrelations, which are not always measurable by scientific methods, yet are vital for sustainability. It narrows awareness and frames the world materialistically. Such an emphasis on intellectual, non-personal knowing, which dominates science as well as our education system (including school and parenting education), has damaged the ability to perceive, sense, know and understand what is valuable and meaningful in the world. Such views are contrary to the way of thinking in other societies and throughout history, when human beings were more humble about their place in the world and more embedded in their environment. Science is only one way, often very helpful, of knowing, and one "mode of existence" (Latour, 2013). But science today tends to have a sense of superiority to other forms of knowing or understanding the world, resulting in detachment from imagination.

Indigenous cultures and all wisdom traditions consider an emotionally detached approach to life, relying on a mind that can rationalise anything very dangerous. Rationalism, emphasising the left-brain-dominant intellect over other forms of being and knowing, cannot capture the essence of reality – its values, meanings and purpose. Smith beautifully explains, "The worthful aspects of reality – its values, meaning, and purpose – slip through the devices of science in the way that the sea slips through the nets of fishermen" (1991, p. 356). This scientific view dominates the Western medically orientated healthcare system, obstetric practices and parenting culture, with detrimental effects on child development and well-being. The modern lifestyle, which generates stress and mental suffering, further favours emotional detachment and disconnection and curtails parent-child emotional availability and thus interactions, reinforcing the dominant science-based paradigm.

For science to facilitate well-being and sustainability, it needs wisdom, humanity and connection with the landscape. Scientific knowledge in traditional indigenous societies is personal and experiential, based on practical knowledge. In contrast with the detached intellectualism of Western science, indigenous science builds a deep and understanding interrelationship with the landscape (Cajete, 2000). Their culture is ecologically and community-centred, which fosters sustainable lifestyles. Connection to land, Gaia (topophilia or love of the land), spirituality and ancestry, kinship and cultural continuity are commonly identified by indigenous people as important health-protecting factors. The types of modern science that are closer to this ancient science are the descriptive sciences (e.g. anthropology and biology), being interested in the interrelations of elements. Ecological sciences have moved towards the indigenous perspective, whose worldview, knowledge and practices inspire sustainable life. They have moved away from a human-centred perspective and towards a "unity of mind and nature" (Bateson, 1972; Berkes, 1999). My view is that this new mindset and sustainable way of life has to embed pregnancy, birth and parenting and the healthcare system, by reconnecting with mammalian nature, thus with the natural as well as social landscape, and becoming aware of and interested in the interrelations of elements. Parenting needs to move towards eco-parenting and connection to the land; spirituality and meaningful kinship networks have to be considered as important health-protecting factors.

Scientific research is reductionist, in that it can only reduce reality into parts that can be mathematically and separately measured and quantified. This is possible in physical relationships but not in biological and social relationships. Neuroscientist Candace Pert acknowledges two levels of emotions. Emotions exist in the body as informational chemicals, the neuropeptides and receptors, which can be measured, and they also exist in another realm, the one we experience as feeling, inspiration and love – beyond the physical (Pert, 1997). Emotions flow freely between the two levels and thus connect the physical and non-physical, just as is acknowledged in primal wisdom.

Pregnancy is a complex reality and scientific research can only have access to very limited aspects of it. Psychoanalyst Ludwig Janus and obstetrician and Prof Lucio Zichella consider that when these limited aspects become the major focus of scientists, obstetricians and midwives, the understanding of the whole complex situation of pregnancy is deformed and this can enormously impair the competence of doctors and midwives and put maternal health at risk (Zichella & Janus, 2012). Too often, scientific methods hinder wisdom-based ways of knowing and alter the perception of the more complete reality of a pregnancy.

If we want to contribute to the well-being of parents, thus of their children and humanity, scientific research on which healthcare is based, especially in the prenatal and perinatal realm, needs to give more space to maternal experience – emotions, thoughts, beliefs, expectations and consciousness – since much wisdom resides in this personal dimension. Mindful healthcare practitioners will create an environment where mothers (and fathers) can express their joy and concerns without any fear of being judged. Listening with an open heart will take over from mere rational assessment. My experience of pregnancy pre-empted and consolidated my scientific and clinical learning, since some of what I had learnt about neuroscience, prenatal and perinatal development and mindfulness, I experienced first-hand.

Personal experience presents the complexity of real-life situations, of which scientific research can only measure one single aspect or correlation between two or three. This is something that is likely to occur and is only a piece of a more complex puzzle; it is certainly not representative of the whole situation. To comprehend the whole reality of pregnancy, we cannot ignore the interaction between different levels of reality – the intelligent psychosomatic network, including its interdependence with the natural environment. Therefore, laboratory results need to be considered more cautiously and responsibly because their generalisation can hinder the comprehension of the reality of pregnancy and mental ill heath in mothers. Therefore, a true comprehension of pregnancy, prenatal and postnatal development is not possible without a dialogue between the mother's emotional/psychological experience and scientific findings, which can only access very limited aspects of it. It follows that mindfulness-based education can open healthcare providers to this human dimension by enhancing their interpersonal connection and empathy. A mindfulness training can enable them to individualise care according to the unique needs of parents and their infants and children. By learning to listen deeply to the mother's unique experience, we challenge generalising beliefs and ideas, and frequently useless diagnosis, if these do not serve the best interests of human lives.

A new trend of scientists is acknowledging the limits of science and the valuable contribution of personal experience (Siegel, 2007; Gallese, 2005; Schore, 2011; Frazzetto, 2013). We are discovering the complexity of human development. It is time to minimise reductionism and oversimplification, otherwise we miss savouring the essence of human life, with adverse consequences for our mental health. There is an increasing awareness of the need for science to embrace subjective experience and intersubjective engagement as the essence of human development. The lyrical tone of this book provides a sense of the depth of the unborn baby's life as well as maternal experience. The scientific data on prenatal development, which have unlocked many secrets of the unborn baby's life, is modest compared with the complexity and wonder of a mother-baby relationship and their intersubjective experience. Certain aspects of maternal emotions and their impact on prenatal experiences are simply not amenable to scientific investigation. Often a mental condition is silent and there is no "physical test" to assess its impact on the quality of life, the mother-baby relationship and bonding and the family dynamics. It is only by listening to the pregnant mother's and father's stories with compassion that we can pick up the signs and their need for support. Healthcare should always be accompanied by human virtues that are not only healing but have a mirroring effect on the parents' child-rearing abilities and on those of future generations.

Moreover, personal experience can resonate more lastingly than a measured phenomenon. If we consider the discovery of the mirror neurons (Rizzolatti & Craighero, 2004), eminent paediatrician Donald Winnicott had originally described the mother-infant mirroring process at the basis of attachment by observing mothers and infants (Winnicott, 1971). What research did was to identify a possible neurological substrate of a much more complex phenomenon. While neuroscientists can bring valuable contributions to our understanding of foetal and newborn brain development, they cannot measure or explain the ongoing mother-baby narrative in mathematical terms. Neither can they explain, for example, why a large number of healthy women have repeated miscarriages in the first few days, weeks or months of their pregnancies, still births, preterm births or negative birth and maternal outcomes. While in some unhealthy mothers one cause of this may be genetic faults, nutritional deficiencies or pollutants, in other cases it may be the embryo's or foetus's sensitivity to maternal ambivalent emotions or unwanted pregnancy (Mohllajee et al., 2007). We cannot explain in scientific terms how a woman has become pregnant shortly after buying herself a dog after three years of failed attempts to conceive. The healing power of emotions, connection and love of a dog is immeasurable.

A number of studies have suggested that the degree of intentionality about pregnancy may be important in understanding its health impact (Pulley et al., 2002). Pregnancy intention, particularly unwanted and ambivalent, may be an indicator of increased risk for some poor outcomes and should be considered in interventions aimed at improving the health of mother and child. The desire to become pregnant or happiness at being pregnant is an important factor in healthy pregnancy. Pregnancy intention is a complex concept, including emotional and psychological factors that may not be captured by current intervention strategies (Sable, 1999).

Acknowledging the complexity: the art of the journey

Intersubjectivity, or the sharing of another's experience, has been a topic of great interest and activity. Only recently has there been a scientific and academic interest in intersubjectivity before birth, which has yet to reach the mainstream (Ammaniti & Gallese, 2014). The topic of subjectivity is one that modern neuroscience has avoided, focusing mainly on cognitive, behavioural and linguistic aspects rather than implicit processes. It is generally agreed that there are no direct, objective ways to measure the subjectivity of other human beings. Only their words and actions give us clues about their inner experiences. Indeed, it is possible that the very nature of the human mind will not be fathomable until neuroscience comes to terms with this potential contribution of the internal representations, some of which are affectively experienced states (Panksepp, 1998).

Preborn and infant development depends on an intricate balance of factors that are hard to isolate. On the one hand, we have our parents' genetic contributions and their histories – including early traumas. On the other hand, we have our own genes – the product of our parents' genes and experiences – neurotransmitters circulating in our bodies, all the stimulation from the uterine environment, including our mother's feelings, thoughts and everyday activities, which mould our neuron circuits, emotions and sensorimotor system, our behaviours, core self and our soul. And there are other factors that our limited mind cannot figure out. Then comes the mother's social environment, her culture, all subtly transmitted to the baby. The most powerful force for healthy human development, and the only one of which a mother can be sure, is her mindful love. Sadly, we live in a society that encourages competition, achievement and success rather than attachment and love, although there is a shift towards a valuation of human essential virtues. What matters most in pregnancy is the art of the journey, the creation of a trusting relationship with the baby day after day, because even if he does not know the world outside, he does sense whether he is loved or rejected and learns about trust and empathy.

The fusion I have described during my baby's gestation between scientific knowledge, professional and personal experience, and also art and memoir on what makes us human, translated into an ongoing bodily narrative between my baby and me, formed the ground for mental development. It gradually shaped my baby's predispositions, manifesting themselves through her love of art, playing piano and composing music, writing, reading, designing, and her empathic and sociable nature. Writing a book, composing a rhyme, singing, listening to music, meditating and other kinds of intellectual and creative endeavour are pleasurable and meaningful activities, which support maternal mental health and have physiological effects on her and consequently on the developing baby. During my pregnancy, I wrote an epistolary dialogue with my baby, a rhyme I regularly recited to her; shared a musical experience with her; practised mindfulness; contemplated in Nature; and came to see the influences of all these activities on her personality. I did gain gratification from chiselling out my intimate dialogue with my baby, my emotions and insights, making sense of random thoughts and images.

In the twenty-first century, governed by science and technology, we can all learn to integrate neuroscience, wisdom, psychology, poetry, philosophy as well as our own observations and insights as human beings. To understand the roots of our human nature and preserve our health, we need this integrative view of life: to be at once scientific and lyrical.

While providing a version of what scientific and professional knowledge has revealed about the foetus's life, I later describe what this meant for me as I walked through the path of pregnancy and motherhood. Sometimes this knowledge did shed light on my journey, but most times it was my maternal wisdom, insights and developing relationship with my baby. These gave meanings and philosophical explanations to the wholeness of experience. Science cannot, at least not exclusively, explain and give meanings to mother-baby-father communications and intersubjective energy-fields. The mother-baby relationship is primal, not rational, even if we try to convey it on a piece of paper, as I am doing here. It involves the deep primal-brain systems – brain stem and limbic systems – which interestingly are the first to develop in an embryo. In evolutionary terms, the earliest brain and body parts are the most important. Studies on embryos' brains indicate that the emotional system or the brainstem/hypothalamus self-regulatory system monitors cortical development (Trevarthen, 2003). Emotional systems influence cognitive, behavioural and even language development from early prenatal life, contrary to what cognitive neuroscience typically describes. It follows that our earliest emotional and sensorimotor experiences are embedded from very early intrauterine life and monitor subsequent elaborated mental development as intentional or goal-directed in more advanced forms (Delafield-Butt & Gangopadhyay, 2013). This ground-breaking work also seals the gap between mental and physical agency into an integrated embodied mind.

A new neuro-philosophical perspective to seal the gap

This new neuro-philosophical perspective brings neurological issues to bear on the old questions concerning the nature of human mind. This is in line with Panksepp's belief that this new integrative discipline may shed light on the highest capacities of the human brain. If we understand important brain processes at a deep neurobiological level, we will better understand the fundamentally affective nature of the human mind (Panksepp, 1998).

However, we must acknowledge that emotions are not entirely amenable to the scrutiny of science. This is often the attitude of healthcare practitioners. Our own experiences, embedded with our own values and our own meaning for our lives, tend to prevail over any more universal laws, such as those of science. The German philosopher Martin Heidegger, the author of *Being and Time* (1972), one of the most influential philosophical works of the twentieth century, made a huge contribution to the understanding of emotions. He makes the distinction between two main ways of looking at the world: a theoretical understanding of reality, which is how we observe and theorise about things – the way a scientist would – and how we engage with the world, how we connect through our interactions with objects or people in various circumstances. The latter way also refers to the intersubjective mother-baby field.

According to Heidegger, our personal experience of the world overshadows our scientific knowledge of it. It is how we initially get to know the world in our earliest life, our related beliefs or internal representations, which shape our mind and our health. We can say that our *subjective* experience of our emotional life prevails over our theoretical knowledge of it. Heidegger believed that science cannot fully grasp the *lived experience* of an emotion. It follows that a mother-baby-father experience has the greatest power and has to be taken into strong consideration. In fact, it is not a stressful event itself that most affects a prenate's or infant's development, but the mother's emotional response to it and her interpretation of it.

Prenatal and developmental psychology, midwifery and medicine need to integrate the psychological, neurological and philosophical aspects because this is the only way to understand the complex psychosocial and biological reality of pregnancy, birth and childhood more completely and so more responsibly. Buddhist philosophy and psychology, which have been found to offer similar answers to those provided to neuroscience by the latest research, can help us to see the interdependence of different aspects of our reality, including pregnancy and birth, and child development. Pregnancy also brings about a spiritual dimension in many women's lives, which we know has an impact on physiology and well-being, thus on pregnancy, childbirth and bonding outcomes (Lipton, 2015). The profound experiences of pregnancy and parenting, lived with an embodied awareness of the continuum of prenatal and postnatal development, can raise and help solve important philosophical issues, for instance about self-knowledge, creativity, imagination, truth, love and empathy, which can be all connected with Buddhism as well as to the latest findings in neuroscience. This is also relevant to midwives, obstetricians, psychologists, neonatologists and all professionals working with expectant/new parents and babies, in order to understand the whole reality of a human being.

Spirituality is about a deeper search for meaning in our lives and makes our life purposeful. In concert with Bruce Lipton's ground-breaking attempts to combine spiritual and scientific perspectives (Lipton, 2015), we should never see spirituality as antagonistic to science, but rather as a complementary way of looking at reality. It is a fundamental dimension of human existence, and it is vital in pregnancy to maintain health and produce a fully human being. Spiritual emptiness is a major cause of stress and a result of modern technology and materialism. According to the Australian Prof David Tacey (2003), today we can speak of a client-led or grassroots recovery of the spiritual dimension in healing and health, although we are trying hard to find a personal language for our yearning, our search for meaning. In my view, spirituality is an essential component of the mind and has to be integrated with the practice of psychology, medicine and all professions with a concern about ill health and can even coexist harmoniously with a scientific mindset. This is the mindset that healthcare professionals need to achieve in order to provide the best quality of care.

There is a complex dimension behind the visible, which is the mother-baby relationship, an energy field. This is a sacred intimate space which has to be protected by attuned compassion, understanding, kindness and listening so as to unleash its full potential. Ancient and traditional wisdom teach us that this communal attuned support promotes the well-being of the mother, the infant, the family and society. Neglect, abuse and lack of respect towards motherhood (and fatherhood) and this profound early relationship undermine the preborn's life-support system and his development, threatening the well-being of humanity.

Prenatal and perinatal healthcare professionals (obstetricians, midwives, nurses, psychologists, psychotherapists etc.) should train to become able to support the well-being of both parents throughout pregnancy and beyond and to recognise the early symptomatology, often somatic, of a mental disturbance, while empowering their human and health resources. Mindfulness-based training can enable them to observe and recognise bodily cues, listen attentively, connect, understand and have compassion. In this way, they can also offer a mirror that promotes the same relational abilities within the couple, as well as with the unborn and new baby. Couples can also benefit from a mindfulness-based course themselves, combined with therapy if needed, by enhancing the same self-regulation and relational abilities.

Perinatal staff should train to inform both parents properly about how to recognise perinatal disturbances in themselves as well as the other, as a family *biopsychosocial open system*. Becoming aware of the risks and potential impact on their child's development and well-being long before birth can help parents seek help at any stage, preferably during pregnancy. This prenatal and perinatal education can benefit from a neuro-philosophical perspective and the integration with *self/couple-development* and continuing mindfulness practice. Through mind-body and sensory engagement, this nurturing practice can foster the reflective, stress-reducing, self-regulatory and relational abilities required for fulfilling parenting and secure attachment in both parents and child.

The sacred early bonding is where the very roots of empathy and humanity reside, and thus needs to be protected by every possible means. The brain changes, self and interpersonal awareness fostered by mindfulness practice promote awareness and understanding of the baby's evolved needs and expectations and at the same time the couple's mutual understanding and resonance. We have supporting evidence of the benefits of mindfulness on mental, social and physical well-being and the alleviation of anxiety and depression (Kabat-Zinn, 2003a; Goleman & Davidson, 2017). A systematic review suggests that mindfulness-based interventions can be beneficial for outcomes such as anxiety, depression, perceived stress and levels of mindfulness during the perinatal period (Dhillon et al., 2017). Mindfulness-based stress reduction (MBSR) has been used in antenatal classes for both parents, with the aim of preventing the negative impact that acute stress and fear have on maternal and neonatal outcomes (Duncan & Bardacke, 2010).

The benefits of mindfulness extend to the wisdom-related abilities required by parenting. Mindfulness practice fosters reflective function, intra/interpersonal attunement, receptiveness, connection with the present moment, resonance (right-brain to right-brain communication), attentiveness and compassion, all abilities promoting attachment and fulfilling parenting (Siegel, 2007). Studies of secure attachment and mindful awareness practices have overlapping findings (Sroufe et al., 2005). In fact, both processes affect the prefrontal cortex and amygdala activity (emotional regulation) of the brain. This book aims to inform future preventive strategies to support the prenatal relationship and intersubjectivity, prevent psychological distress in the early postnatal period and birth complications and promote infant and child well-being.

Showing that prenatal nurturing practices such as mindfulness and mindfulness-based therapies can break the cycle of an intergenerational transmission of the effects of depression has epigenetic implications. It also unleashes the potential of mother (and father)-preborn relationship and empowered parenting. This is also an urgent call for healthcare profession-als and science to acknowledge the prenatal intersubjective relationship and adopt a compassionate approach towards mothers, fathers and sentient babies in the womb.

10 A mindfulness relationship-based model to support maternal mental health and the mother-baby relationship in pregnancy and beyond birth

It is clear that the modern science of epigenetics, interpersonal neuroscience, attachment and mindfulness resonate with the primal wisdom that has allowed us to evolve into human beings. Very often, research findings confirm what humans have intuitively known for millennia. Training the mind to see interrelationships is the wisdom-based way of knowing. It helps us become compassionate rather than judgemental. For instance, when a child has a tantrum, rather than mirroring his or her stress and punishing him, we understand what is behind his behaviour. We look into the story his body is telling, the dynamic relationships with his parents, the family energy the child absorbs, whether he receives proper attention and so on. We listen and witness.

Compassion has cerebral networks that are traditionally associated with positive emotions such as maternal love and affiliation. When altruistic love encounters suffering, it manifests as compassion. We can face our own suffering or another's with courage, motherly love, benevolence and determination to find a way to help. We can feel benevolence towards all others in all situations and limitless kindness that we can extend to all beings. If healthcare professionals were trained to see connections, listen deeply and be compassionate, their clients or patients' health outcomes can improve considerably. Perhaps we can begin to implement the ancient wisdom view and support scientific evidence through a prenatal interdisciplinary model based on health advancement and reflecting a scientific and cultural paradigm shift; indeed, it begins long before birth.

The wisdom and evidence gathered in this book support a prenatal and perinatal mindfulness relationship-based (PMRB) approach as a comprehensive model of care that offers a promising opportunity to deliver a collaborative service that supports conception, pregnancy and early parenting, as well as infant development and health outcomes. This may occur through a sustainable and cost-effective strategy that legitimises the study of age-old collective and wisdom-based practices, such as mindfulness meditation, breathing techniques, yoga and other methods that cause shifts in the autonomic/visceral state and emotional experiences. Such a strategy is supported by polyvagal theory, which indicates physiological mind-brain-viscera communication as the royal road to affect-regulation and invites a radical shift in therapeutic approaches to a number of psychopathological states, such as anxiety, depression and trauma-related dysfunctions (Porges, 2011). These new approaches would invite pregnant mothers to cultivate interpersonal rhythms with their prenate and infants, to nurture their age-old capacity to use their voices, facial expressions and touch to regulate their babies' sensorimotor, visceral and emotional experiences and develop a profound connection that prepares parent and infant for bonding after birth.

The purpose of this model of care is to support improvements in the mother's self-regulation and co-regulation with the prenate and infant, her mental health from conception through pregnancy, leading to the development of an attuned maternal-preborn/infant relationship, and the infant's physical, emotional and social development. We have created a sophisticated technological society and healthcare system that have forgotten the basic never-changing human needs of mothers, their babies and families, which have been the foundations of health and well-being for thousands of years. We can use modern infrastructures and sensibility while recreating the old village, the community that used to support the child, mother and family – and still does in some traditional and indigenous cultures – with companionship, shared childcare and parenting (alloparenting), empathy, compassion and other human virtues. We have looked at research indicating that social support, family functioning and relationship satisfaction significantly buffer any stress the mother and developing prenate and infant experience. This is the norm in indigenous and traditional societies. Body-mind interventions that are inspired by polyvagal theory thus either promote the activation of the social vagus or dampen sympathetic tone, improve relationships and family functioning by reducing the negative impact of perceived stress on the emotional well-being of expectant and new parents.

While the PMRB model is designed to support parenting age-old inner resources and abilities, the prenatal programme content also aims to help mothers and fathers (and other caregivers) understand the importance of the early period of their infant's life, including prior to birth, the mother's as well as the prenate's and infant's nutritional, emotional and relational needs, and how to nurture them. This raised awareness occurs through reflection as well as sensory, breathing and body awareness, and awareness of baby's interactional abilities (even if rudimentary). It is fostered by the practice of mindfulness and leads to improved sensory emotional co-regulation and maternal reflective functioning, which forms the basis of bonding and attachment. Trauma-informed care and how positively to transform the consequences of trauma into care is a fundamental aspect of mindfulness awareness.

Understanding the prenate as able to engage with interactions and communicate indicates awareness that the prenate is a sentient being, responding to and affected by maternal attitudes, emotions, thoughts, stress, soul and consciousness. This understanding can bring wisdom and depth to healthcare practitioners, interventions and parents and revolutionise the old paradigm of perinatal healthcare. It can change the way healthcare practitioners and the entire community relate to pregnant parents and unborn babies and offer a more humane interactional approach. With this knowledge or frame of reference, the focus of the present model shifts from the thought about "expecting the baby" to "the baby is already here and I am connected to my baby". This feeling of connection is the baby's lifeline, just like the placenta and umbilical cord.

This mindfulness relationship-based approach implies a mind-body, or biopsychosocial, and ecological theoretical framework of attachment having its foundations in the prenatal period, replacing a psychological one that neglects the body and its contribution. It resonates with the indigenous sustainable way of living. The Australian Aboriginal and Torres Strait Islander people view health as "not just the physical wellbeing of the individual but the social, emotional and cultural wellbeing of the whole community, in which each individual is able to achieve the full potential as a human being, thereby bringing about the total well-being of their community" (Houston, 1989). Connection to land, spirituality and ancestry, kinship networks and cultural continuity are commonly identified by Aboriginal people as important health-protecting factors (Zubrick et al., 2014). This is in line with the science of quantum physics identifying the biological substrate of spirituality, connectedness and belonging to a community.

The new paradigm proposed in this book and leading to the development of the PMRB programme draws on the latest discoveries in the fields of interpersonal neuroscience, epigenetics, attachment theory, sensory approaches, mindfulness, primal wisdom, quantum physics, eco-mindfulness, anthropology, prenatal and perinatal psychology, infant mental health and eco-parenting. It is hoped that the insights gained through my work with expectant/new parents and their infants, as well as findings of the research project further supporting this programme, will advance changes to the current perinatal mental health paradigm. The inclusion of interdisciplinary mindfulness relationship-based approaches in pregnancy and the postnatal period is expected to heal and prevent trauma, perinatal stress, depression, anxiety and psychosomatic symptoms and bonding difficulties, which pose a risk to child development and the welfare of society. Therefore, prenatal and perinatal mental ill health is a major public health issue that must be taken seriously.

The reason for focusing on this crucial period of human development is the growing body of evidence in support of primal wisdom, which shows that experiences during this period can have lifelong consequences for health and well-being, and why healthcare during pregnancy and even before should be a community priority. As noted in the report of the World Health Organization's Commission on Social Determinants of Health

(2008), "Many challenges in adult society have their roots in the early years of life, including major public health problems such as obesity, heart disease, and mental health problems. Experiences in early childhood are also related to criminality, problems in literacy and numeracy, and economic participation". There are currently three key concepts that are supported by this growing body of evidence and will help raise awareness of early support.

- Developmental plasticity and the developmental origins of health and disease (DOHaD) hypothesis (Barker, 2004), as well as the latest data on susceptibility to transmission of disease. The DOHaD hypothesis is that health/disease is likely to have originated during prenatal development as the result of environmental influences: altered nutrition, stress, maternal and paternal mental disorders, drugs, infections or exposure to environmental chemicals.
- Change in the social environment and the "mismatch" hypothesis (evidence is now accumulating that some of the physical and mental problems that are now prevalent arise from a mismatch between human evolutionary capacities and modern environments (Kearns et al., 2007; Lieberman, 2013). The PMRB programme aims to ameliorate the adverse effects of this mismatch by integrating primal wisdom and the related human qualities developed through evolution with modern sensibility.
- Ecological (natural environment) impacts on development and health, and the social determinants of health and disease.

Evidence relating to these concepts raises our awareness of how children develop and highlights the critical role of the very earliest stages of development – the first 1,000 days from conception, and the importance of nurturing practices during this period to prevent or mitigate later problems.

The importance of maternal and paternal mental health

Pregnancy and the postpartum period can be times of joy and positive expectations but also of challenges and stress for the mother, her infant, her partner and family. Perinatal and infant mental health refers to the emotional and psychological well-being of mothers, their infants, partners and families, from conception through pregnancy to the first three years postpartum (Queensland Health, 2014). These first 1,001 days can be a window of opportunities for parents to contribute to their babies' healthy development, as well as a time of high risk for the onset or relapse of mental issues, with consequences on maternal functioning depending on the severity. This time is critical for the future development of the infant across all developmental domains (Centre of the Developing Child at Harvard University, 2009).

The importance of maternal mental health during pregnancy and in the postnatal period for the well-being of individuals and societies has been recognised in the literature (Bauer et al., 2014; Mental Health Task Force (MHTF), 2016). Evidence suggests that depression affects up to 20 per cent of women during pregnancy and the postpartum period, which indicates women's need for support during pregnancy (Rich-Edwards et al., 2006). Perinatal mental health problems have a considerable impact on economics. In the UK, depression, anxiety and psychosis have a long-term cost to society and economy of about £8.1 billion for each one-year cohort of births (MHTF, 2016). The cost of untreated perinatal mental illness and its adverse consequences on children, such as maltreatment and neglect, have been estimated at £23 billion each year in the UK. In other countries, the reality is not different. The MHTF report indicates that treating perinatal mental health problems effectively during pregnancy could save many of the serious long-term human and economic costs. It has been demonstrated that health advancement programmes in the prenatal and perinatal period can be both more achievable and more cost-effective than cure (Bauer et al., 2014). The World Health Organization (2018) launched a Nurturing Care Framework for Early Childhood Development, which recognises the mental health of pregnant women and mothers as a key to the health, growth and development of very young children. As a result of the importance of maternal mental health during pregnancy and in the postnatal period, a sound understanding of maternal mental health and the factors associated with it is essential.

For too long, the importance of the father's mental health and its links with maternal and child mental health has been ignored and their experiences either sidelined or treated in isolation from that of mothers. I showed in Chapter 8 how a depressed father is likely to be less involved in the care of the infant and during pregnancy less motivated in supporting pregnancy and the mother-prenate relationship. I looked at evidence for the associations between depression in fathers in the prenatal and postnatal period and behavioural/emotional problems in their children. Studies from 1980 to 2007 (Schumacher, 2008) found that birth-related paternal depression was closely associated with maternal depressive symptoms and higher risks for children's emotional and behavioural problems. Couple conflict can also explain emotional problems in very young children. Relationship dissatisfaction was found to be the strongest predictor of maternal emotional distress (Røsand et al., 2012). Relationship satisfaction appeared to buffer the effects of stressors such as moving, somatic disease, family outcome, irregular working hours, dissatisfaction at work, work demands, and maternal sick leave.

These findings highlight the need for support for couples before, during and after pregnancy to prevent stress during pregnancy and post-birth and improve outcomes for children. The importance of a good partner relationship that consists of both emotional and practical support should be highlighted to all expectant couples and in all programmes. Prenatal programmes should aim to strengthen positive wisdom resources within the couple's relationship, strengthening the foundations for the family's future development. The PMRB programme is inclusive of both expectant mother and father. However, even if the father is not a participant in the nine-week programme, the PMRB facilitator has the mother's relationship with her partner in mind. By enhancing women's mindful awareness and prosocial abilities (e.g. compassion, communication, empathy, acceptance and love), the course is expected to positively influence the relationship with the partner. Because of the group sharing experience and compassionate PMRB facilitator, by not feeling judged, women can talk openly and can be empowered with tools to better deal with issues with the partner. Experiencing an improved relationship with the partner can make some types of stress more tolerable. Further, by providing a positive relational model, parents not only contribute to their child's well-being but also influence the child's capacity to build healthy relationships.

Maternal mental health and its links with foetal and infant developmental outcomes: the missing link between associations

There is both theoretical and empirical literature suggesting that poor maternal mental health during pregnancy, in particular depression, anxiety and stress, has an impact on foetal and child neurodevelopment outcomes, highlighting the need for a better understanding of antenatal factors that influence maternal mental health and child development (Glover et al., 2010; Stein et al., 2014). There is evidence that maternal mental, emotional and social well-being correlates directly to the quality of mother-infant interactions and the infant's mental, emotional and social well-being and development (Mason et al., 2011; Murray et al., 1996). Maternal postnatal depression has been linked not only with developmental challenges in young children but also with affective disorders in adolescent offspring in a 13-year longitudinal study (Halligan et al., 2007). Developing postnatal depression also appears to increase the mothers' susceptibility to relapse and consequently to the development of depressive disorders in offspring. These findings underline the need to investigate antenatal factors predicting depression post-birth and reduce the risk of developing it through efficacious support during pregnancy that responds to mothers' evolved need for social support, thus human connection. As our indigenous cousins teach us, when this basic need is met, maternal consciousness and mammalian and wisdom abilities can naturally unfold.

While the adverse consequences of poor maternal mental health on infant outcomes can be explained, among other reasons, by the high rate (70 per cent) of women with postnatal depression having relationship difficulties with their infants (Milgrom et al., 2006), there are likely to be underpinning mechanisms during pregnancy linked to the woman's levels of cortisol, which have been found to be high in women with depression, anxiety and stress symptoms (Glover, 2014; Van den Bergh et al., 2005). Cortisol can be transferred to the foetal environment by crossing the placenta, disturbing foetal developmental processes, which affects the infant and consequently the mother-infant relationship and maternal care. This link is often omitted in developmental psychology, leading to undervaluing an important window of opportunity in the prenatal period. Therefore, there is a need to develop comprehensive support programmes to reduce maternal stress in pregnancy and the risk of its impact on foetal and child development, and to enhance the first human relationship.

A consistently observed adverse outcome of antenatal chronic stress in a review of 14 prospective studies is attention deficit hyperactivity disorder (ADHD) symptoms, observed in children four and 15 years of age (O'Connor et al., 2002; Van den Bergh et al., 2005). Some critical gestational stages have been reported to increase foetal vulnerability to the long-term effects of antenatal anxiety and stress and consequent alteration of her hormonal profile. Physician and author Gabor Maté tells us about the link between his mother's pregnancy with him during the Second World War and his frequent crying as an infant and later ADHD.

I assume another underpinning mechanism of antenatal stress may be poor quality of maternal interactions and receptive attention, transmitted to the baby in many subtle ways, e.g. increased muscular tension, tone of voice, fast breathing and heart rate. Recall that if we view a video of a mother and father having a loud argument while the mother is undergoing a sonogram, we can clearly see the foetus arching his body and jumping as the argument starts, showing his capacity to respond to maternal stress. Imagine the impact of chronic stress on the baby's behavioural and emotional patterns and way of dealing with stress as a child. It is not occasional discord that affects a baby's development but continued perceived stress, which also makes it more difficult for the mother to have nurturing positive feelings towards her baby. Differences in genetic make-up may make some babies more vulnerable to unfavourable prenatal situations than others and put them at greater risk of being born with problems and vulnerable to postnatal stress. It is the matching of genes and experiences that shapes the childhood outcomes, which can never be predicted but only minimised or maximised as a risk.

Depression, anxiety and stress during pregnancy have been also associated with foetal weight, in particular intrauterine growth retardation, and premature or complicated birth (Dayan et al., 2006; Maina et al., 2008). The intrauterine environment can be altered if stress in the mother changes her neurohormonal profile, blood flow and muscular tension. Furthermore, when the mother is very anxious or stressed during pregnancy, there is reduced blood flow to the baby through the uterine artery, the main source of blood and nutrition for the baby, and this could explain why the baby doesn't grow well and also sets up a secondary stress response in the foetus (Teixeira et al., 1999). A systematic review investigated the long-term risks associated with caesarean delivery for mother, infant and subsequent pregnancies (Keag et al., 2018). There is evidence that the stress experienced by the foetus or neonate during some obstetric interventions can have long-term effects on the function of the HPA axis in later life through increased cortisol levels (Gitau et al., 2001). The study highlights that unlike normal vaginal or even caesarean delivery, a difficult forceps delivery raises the newborn's cortisol levels. Receiving the first contact with an artificial device instead of warm human touch can be a traumatic experience for the baby during his transition into the world. The increase in cortisol level activates the amygdala fear circuits in the brain. Regular stroking and maternal voice (e.g. lullaby singing) can normalise brain function and weight gain, counteracting the traumatic birth experience or missing out on the sensory experiences of late gestation in premature infants (Standley, 1998).

Supportive trauma-informed programmes in pregnancy aimed to reduce anxiety, depression and stress symptoms, and therefore the risk of premature and birth complication, are therefore needed. Mode of deliveries have also been associated with the practice of breastfeeding (Saeed et al., 2011), with a higher rate of bottle-feeding mothers who had caesarean deliveries compared with those who had normal vaginal deliveries. The benefits of breastfeeding for infant and maternal heath, as well as for society and the economy, are well documented (Bachrach et al., 2003). A cohort study of 1,745 women found that postnatal depression had a significant adverse impact on breastfeeding duration (Henderson et al., 2003), highlighting that the impact of maternal mental issues on breastfeeding is poorly understood. Antenatal factors have been associated with breastfeeding duration, which suggests recommendations for prenatal intervention focused on maternal breastfeeding self-efficacy (O'Campo et al., 1992). However, we need to keep in mind that it is the combination of breastfeeding and mindfulness care that leads to the best child outcomes, as our wise indigenous cousins teach us. When serious circumstances impair breastfeeding (e.g. medical conditions or unresolved trauma), receiving emotional support is crucial in promoting the most powerful force in infant development, which is maternal caregiving.

A case study I followed up during my research project at a birth unit in London revealed how a mother's experience of emotional neglect in early life may have led to her intolerance of physical contact with her baby and how this manifested through her body narrative and breastfeeding difficulties (Sansone, 2007, 2018a). This case study addresses the important questions about the impact of deep emotional issues rooted in the mother's early childhood on her pregnancy, breastfeeding, bonding with her baby and the baby's development. A mind-body, mother-baby relationship-focused approach from healthcare practitioners, implementing mindfulness abilities, provides mothers with a vital avenue of self-knowledge and transformation. It can also mitigate the intergenerational transmission of developmental trauma and prevent bonding and breastfeeding difficulties.

It is also well-established that maternal mental problems are key determinants of difficulties in the mother-prenate relationship (Alhusen, 2008); bonding formation (Ammaniti & Gallese, 2014; Glover et al., 2010); parental sensitivity and responsiveness (Zeanah & Zeanah, 2009); and mother-infant emotional availability (Barfoot et al., 2017). Nevertheless, little is known about the relationship between maternal mindfulness and the mother-prenate relationship, or the influence of antenatal factors, such as mindfulness and mother-prenate relationship, on mother-infant emotional availability, engagement and attunement post-birth. We need a radical shift in healthcare approaches to pregnancy and parental and infant psychological dysfunctions, and to address this gap in the literature and clinical practice.

The cited studies highlight the need to investigate and understand antenatal factors that might be associated with infant outcomes in order to support outcomes for mothers and infants through humane support during pregnancy that reduces depression, anxiety and stress and potentially other psychophysiological disorders. Before psychological issues manifest, for example triggered by the birth experience, there are implicit physiological/emotion dysregulations leading to dysfunctions. These larval states of illness are sources of discomfort or pain, the so-called uncommunicable disease, and often go unnoticed by the so-called experts. The PMRB programme can promote stress-coping skills, nurturing affects and a positive attitude to pregnancy, which can be self-regulatory, and antidotes to the development of psychophysiological conditions.

Because of links between maternal mental health and foetal and infant development outcomes, treating maternal mental issues alone does not improve infant/child development outcomes. Therefore, focusing on both the mother's and father's well-being, and the parent-prenate/infant relationship through daily interactions is crucial. Research (Berlin et al., 2008) has found that early interventions that focus on promoting secure parent-infant relationships, mental health and well-being and safe and supportive social connections for families are more likely to result in improved outcomes for these families. Growing evidence suggests that day programmes support maternal mental health and the attachment relationship, leading to improved infant development outcomes (Meschino et al., 2016). The PMRB programme is one step ahead in proposing that the best outcomes for mother and infant are correlated with support in pregnancy (and even before conception) focusing on the mother's and father's well-being as well as their relationship with the prenate, through meaningful interactions. These prenatal connections are considered a biological necessity and prepare parent and infant for adaptive relational engagement.

Interactions and relaxation as antidotes to stress

A small to moderate level of non-chronic antenatal stress may be helpful for the child's development, and perhaps the association between prenatal stress or arousal and child outcomes is best represented by a u-shaped curve. The mother's conscious perception of the links between her emotional/muscular tension or mood and her prenate's movements and quality of aliveness can help her develop an attuned relationship, which is the foundation of attachment. This is a key aspect of the PMRB model, aimed at strengthening stress-coping strategies. Through her responses to maternal emotional nuances, breathing and postural changes, the baby may learn about a variety of stimuli and responses, and the presence of an "other" with whom she interacts.

> I recall one night during my pregnancy lying awake with tension in my chest. Something about my husband had upset me. The baby persistently kicked – she may have dreamt of my fears, sensed my cortisol, my heart pounding or the tense womb, the change of energy. She produced movements different from the flowing ones she used to make while I was listening to my favourite piano music, softly talking or singing to her, or touching her through my abdomen. My awareness of the connection between us made me access my inner wisdom resources passed on through evolution and rediscovered through the practice of mindfulness. I could then calm my baby by becoming aware of my breath, and through that come into the present moment, when everyday activities can take on a joyful, miraculous quality. My nervous system influenced and was influenced by the interactions with the baby. We were co-regulating each other in a work of art, a dance designed by Nature. This intimate deep connection was our leading force in labour, birth and postnatal bonding, in the maintenance of the continuum. If we are mindful, or fully present in the here and now, anxiety disappears and a sense of timelessness takes hold, allowing our highest human qualities, such as kindness and compassion, to emerge.

When a woman experiences an emotional swing, it is reassuring for the baby if she rests her hand on her belly and strokes it until she feels that calm envelops both of them again. She can also softly talk to her baby while breathing deeply and sensing the energy reaching the baby. It is important to reconcile with her partner as well, so that any emotional tension left melts away. Her emotion (anger, grief and anxiety) is being transformed and physiological balance re-established. I used to listen to classical piano music and felt my baby's abrupt kicks switching into flowing movements during the *Adagio for Organ and Strings* by Albinoni, *Fur Elise* by Beethoven or a rhyme I had composed for her. Her behaviour was clearly reflecting my emotional flow. This ancient maternal wisdom and self-art therapy is supported by scientific findings indicating links between maternal emotional state and foetal behaviour. Indigenous people have been aware of these links for millennia and use contemplative practices and dances to positively influence the mother-baby dyad (Sansone, 2018b).

A study (DiPietro et al., 2008) on foetal responses to induced maternal relaxation suggests that repeated exposure to periods of relaxation might generate more persistent alterations to maternal and foetal functioning, with potential long-term consequences for child development. Foetal responses to induced maternal relaxation during the thirty-second week of pregnancy were recorded in 100 maternal-foetal pairs using a digitised data collection system. The 18-minute guided imaginary relaxation generated significant reductions in maternal psychological tension, heart rate, skin conductance, respiration period, cortisol levels and an increased respiratory sinus arrhythmia. Significant alterations in foetal neurobehaviour were observed, including decreased foetal heart rate (FHR), increased FHR variability, suppression of foetal motor activity (FM) and increased FM-FHR coupling. The study revealed significant associations between maternal autonomic measures and foetal cardiac patterns, lower umbilical and uterine artery resistance and increased FHR variability, and declining salivary cortisol and FM activity. It also reveals the close relationship between imagination and physiological effects. The authors also observed that it is possible that guided maternal relaxation may generate a biphasic response including a rapid sensory-mediated component and a secondary response mediated by neurohormonal or vasodilatory processes.

These observations are consistent with my observations of my unborn daughter regularly responding to music with ovoid movements not straight after the onset of the piano musical piece but after a few seconds. It is possible that this secondary response mediated by my neurohormonal changes induced by the music relaxation was preceded by other subtle rapid changes in the baby, e.g. in FHR. If mindfulness meditation induces relaxation among other effects, we can hypothesise that it can induce positive physiological and behavioural responses in the prenate. Maternal experiences generate a cascade of physiological and neurochemical consequences that may alter the intrauterine milieu either directly or indirectly, and thereby generate a foetal response (DiPietro et al., 2008).

It is important to remark that findings only help us understand links and possible influences of maternal stress and psychological disturbances on foetal development. No study can capture the complex interplay of factors affecting development outcomes. Besides, the brain is a social organ susceptible to change and mitigation of adverse effects through good continued practice at any stage of our lives. However, understanding links can help parents as well as healthcare professionals to raise awareness of the importance of parents' consciousness and well-being from before conception through pregnancy to create a healthy womb environment to welcome the baby and exert positive epigenetic influences on development. The implication of the existing research is that programmes during pregnancy to improve parental mental well-being and primal wisdom resources can reduce the risk of socio-emotional and cognitive problems in the child and later adult.

A meta-analysis of several studies highlighted that mothers' attitudes towards the baby during pregnancy may have implications for child's development (Foley & Hughes, 2018). In particular, mothers who "connect" with their baby during pregnancy are more likely to interact in a positive way with their infant after birth. Interaction is important for helping infants learn and develop. We know that positive social interactions and affects can improve oxytocin levels (pleasure/love hormone), which in all mammals improve uterine contractions and cervical dilation during birth, improve mother-infant bonding and promote breastfeeding. Higher levels of oxytocin have been shown to evoke feelings of contentment, reductions in anxiety, and feelings of calmness and safety. Even receiving empathy and compassion during pregnancy (e.g. from the partner or healthcare practitioner) can have a positive impact on the mother and baby's overall health, assist with a positive birth experience and reduce the risk of postpartum depression. The higher levels of oxytocin a mother has, the more loving and caring she will tend to be towards her baby.

Reconceptualising the mother-foetus attachment (MFA) relationship

According to attachment theory, an infant needs to develop a relationship and have experiences with at least one primary caregiver to support healthy physical, social and emotional development and, in particular, to learn to regulate feelings (Bowlby, 1973). A sensitive and responsive caregiver will provide the infant with a "safe base" from which to explore. Attachment theory has provided an understanding of the contribution of the parent-child relationship to child development.

This important theory has only relatively recently been applied in pregnancy, consequent to an increasing awareness of the prenatal roots of human development and infant mental health. Mother-foetus attachment (MFA) has been viewed as an emotional tie, an affectionate relationship between a pregnant woman and her foetus, which begins in utero and continues after birth (Condon, 1993). Rubin (1976) suggests that the immediate bond between mother and her neonate is an extension of mother-foetus experiences. MFA has been described as "the extent to which women engage in behaviours that represent an affiliation and interaction with the unborn child" (Cranley, 1981, p. 282).

The conceptual understanding of the MFA phenomenon is still being debated, however. Van der Bergh and Simons (2009) and Laxton-Kane and Slade (2002) suggest that the term "attachment", as defined by Bowlby (1959), cannot refer to prenatal experiences and requires a different conceptual framework due to a lack of reciprocity between the mother and her foetus. While the prenate's capacities for perception, sensorial learning and memory are known, there is no consensus about whether the prenate is a sentient being capable of reciprocal interactions, e.g. responding to maternal touch, vocalisation, rhyme, music, mediation or induced imaginary relaxation.

Studies on MFA synthetised in a systematic review have primarily investigated the factors that influence the mother-foetus relationship and highlighted the importance of intervention to support this relationship (Alhusen, 2008). Nonetheless, these studies on prenatal attachment have focused on the expectant mother's representation of the baby, rather than on a bidirectional process outside her mental image. Therefore, most MFA scales refer to the foetus as an internalised image in the mother's mind, a product of her own creation rather than the actual being developing in her womb capable of engaging in an embodied relationship (Van der Bergh & Simons, 2009). This has influenced healthcare professionals' attitude towards pregnant women, their way of relating to them not as the carriers of a developing sentient being sensitive to maternal states, determining whether she receives humane compassionate care or not.

Research, education and clinical practice need to focus on the mother's actual feelings, perceptions and actions in an embodied relationship interacting with her baby, instead of just thoughts of the baby's arrival, which often brings anxiety or idealisation of the baby. This is in line with the primal wisdom and mindfulness worldview emphasising the importance of connecting with the present moment and the richness it brings.

This new concept of prenatal attachment based on shifting attention from when the baby arrives to the baby is already here and I am connected to my baby reflects into Prenatal Bonding Analysis, a method created by Dr Jenö Raffai (1998). A collection of case studies reveals that Prenatal Bonding Analysis provides the possibility of creating an intense bonding between mother and foetus, witnessing the development of the foetus in the womb and realising early development of personality predispositions. At the same time, any prenatal trauma or dysfunction can be recognised, including the capacity for healing (Schroth, 2010). Schroth argues that the method can be at the same time an instrument of prenatal and perinatal research, empowerment of bonding between mother and foetus and a great help for preparing for easy birth. After birth, the baby is likely to be more settled and have access to her or his full potential. This method has also proved to mitigate the transgenerational impact of prenatal violence. In one detailed case study, the influence of the transgenerational history over four generations manifests in the perception of the baby in the womb on a symbolic level. The effect of this history may have been a risk factor in the actual pregnancy contributing to premature birth or even miscarriage. Through the prenatal bonding and contribution of the father, the trauma or challenging emotion can be elaborated and managed.

To understand the complex process of mother-prenate relationship, there needs to be an understanding of the prenate's capacity to engage in reciprocal interactions. There is a need for research that recognises this earliest capacity and the contribution of mother-baby reciprocal interactions during pregnancy to the later mother-infant relationship. A new conceptual framework may also inform later studies for the development of a new mother-foetus relationship, rather than attachment, scale. A communal awareness of foetal consciousness can humanise prenatal and perinatal care.

The prenatal relationship: impact on foetal development and its relevance to epigenetics

Neuroscience provides evidence that a foetus's physical and emotional development is affected by epigenetic factors (Yehuda et al., 2016). Epigenetics refer to the changes in gene expression fostered by environmental influences, including maternal stress, developmental trauma or positive emotions (Alegria-Torres et al., 2011). Other factors such as nutritional habits, physical activity, yoga, meditation, mindfulness practice, spiritual practices, working habits and substance abuse can trigger changes in gene expression. It has been shown that, through modification of gene expression as a result of exposure to stress hormones circulating in the blood, significant pain or trauma experienced by the parents in their early life is passed down to the next generation and even the generation after that, leaving a memory in our physical being. Cellular memories may be transferred and stored during prenatal life as impressions (DiPietro, 2010; Wade, 1998). This is an astonishing discovery because if Darwin believed that it would take many generations for evolution to shift, epigenetics is proving that changes can happen in one generation through foetal exposure to certain environmental conditions, including the mother's perceptions and emotional experiences.

A study of 32 Jewish men and women who survived the Holocaust showed that genetic changes induced by trauma appeared to have been passed on to their children (Yehuda et al., 2016). The genes of these children showed changes that those of Jewish families living outside of Europe during the war did not. They also had increased likelihood of stress disorders in comparison to the control group. These mechanisms may interfere with the development of a prenatal attachment relationship. Depression during pregnancy was found to be negatively related to MFA scores (McFarland et al., 2011), suggesting that the links between postpartum depression and poor mother-to-infant attachment may be mediated by antenatal factors.

Gabor Maté recalls having been conceived during the Second World War and born during the Germans' invasion in Hungary. When his mother called the doctor concerned that baby Gabor was crying all the time, the doctor said that all Jew babies were crying frequently. Maté also links his and his son's ADHD to the excessive stress experienced by his mother during her pregnancy. He was a workaholic father for a long period as a consequence of his mother's lack of emotional support during the war and transmitted the same emotional disconnection to his children by working all the time. Maté explains that children's disorders are their way of coping with stress, as they picked up on the parents' stress since pregnancy. Stress prevents parents from picking up non-verbal cues from their children, thus from being responsive, connecting and developing a secure attachment. So, it can be highly beneficial that parents engage in mindfulness practices equipping them with stress-coping and attachment-formation strategies as early as possible before birth.

The origins of psychological disorders have also been traced to conception, embryonic, foetal and birth experiences. Study participants have accurately recalled events and affective states from conception through birth that have affected their lives (Chamberlain, 2003; Emerson, 1996; Tashaev, 2007), giving rise to the hypotheses that prenatal memories may be retained unconsciously in the body and personality predispositions may begin to be established during these initial stages of life. However, epigenetics and neuroplasticity are also affected by positive environmental influences. While trauma and symptomatic effects (e.g. depression) affect offspring through the malleable process of gene expression (as well as relationship), epigenetic effects of early stress can be mitigated or reversed by providing nurturing support as early as pregnancy to influence the next generation. Therefore, prosocial capacities such as love and compassion may emerge easily from nurturing caregiving and their seed sowed since the earliest stages of human development. The quality of the mother-prenate relationship is therefore essential for development due to foetal susceptibility to environmental influences and neuroplasticity. Maternal imagination can widen her perception and awareness of her baby, enhance emotional engagement and availability, and thus have epigenetic effects. Paternal imagination and emotional support can significantly contribute to this process.

Despite the contention that prenatal and perinatal experiences have an impact on the mother-foetus relationship, most MFA scales and models still refer to the foetus as an internalised representation in the mother's mind, a mental image to which the mother is attaching. My research is focused on the contributing role of the mother's body during pregnancy and post-birth, her embodied mind, in the relationship with her baby, and infant outcomes. It is intended to inspire clinical and non-clinical practice.

Foetal consciousness and engagement

To understand the origins of human connection, which is at the centre of the PMRB model, we need first to understand the prenate as a sentient being. We know now that unborn babies are far from being passive dwellers in the mother's body but perceive pain, maternal stress or joy; react to sensory stimuli such as touch, smells and sounds; and manifest a wide range of facial expressions in response to them. Studies on premature babies have focused on the importance of maternal physiological rhythms such as breathing – having a strong emotional connotation – as a stimulation of the foetus's neurobehavioural development (Thoman & Graham, 1986). Long before birth, the prenate memorises sounds and the maternal voice. The PMRB model implies that more attention needs to be paid to the development of prenatal support focused on maternal physiological cues, such as breathing and vocalisation.

Some researchers have investigated the presence of consciousness in the womb. Emerson (1996) deemed prenates as conscious beings with experiences and behaviours *in utero* that will affect their future life. Chamberlain (1994/2011) posited that babies learn, dream and remember, are sensitive and aware and are social and communicative. He asserted that the prenate is a sentient being who can communicate with his or her mother, and whose well-being and birth experience are affected by this relationship. Newborns' recognition of their mother's voice among others and stories read during pregnancy, based on their acoustic experience, has been widely evidenced, indicating prenatal learning. It has been shown that unborn babies who had been recited a short child's rhyme aloud in the last trimester responded with a decrease in heart rate whereas the control babies did not (DeCasper et al., 1994). They showed a preference for the story read by the mother during late gestation compared to a novel story.

A newborn recognises the mother's unique melody or voice and is soothed by it and drawn to it when there is a range of voices present (Hepper & Shahidullah, 1994; Kisilevsky et al., 2003). This requires that the sounds heard *in utero* were perceived and registered in memory and later recalled. It also requires some level of attentiveness and awareness. A mother noticed that as soon as her newborn sleeping on her chest after delivery heard her father's voice, she opened her eyes and smiled. The father had talked and played with the baby throughout pregnancy and always told her that he loved her so much. He used to say "Good morning" when he went to work, "Good afternoon" when he arrived, while stroking the mother's belly. Amazingly, the baby started to move at the same time (anticipatory conditioning).

By listening to the mother's voice, the prenate is introduced to its emotional content, her form of vitality and his first experience of safety. Human language, in particular maternal prosody, is rich in dynamic features of vitality, and without these forms of vitality, babies, and presumably prenates, are much less engaged (Stern, 2010). Maternal melody is a source of musical stimulation and rich in empathic messages. It is precursor of attachment and verbal language. In fact, the neonate's recognition of it secures attachment to a familiar person. The melodic patterns of vocalisations and facial expressions influence physiological states and can elicit a sense of calmness and safety (neuroception of safety) in the listener (Porges, 2011). On the basis of these findings concerning foetal sentience, we can assume that maternal prosody may regulate the social engagement system and enhance the physiological state in both mother and baby during pregnancy, with the positive effects of improved emotional engagement and socio-emotional behaviour after birth and beyond. One of my next studies will use physiological measures (e.g. infant and mother's vagal tone, eye contact, vocalisation and skin-to-skin contact) to investigate the social engagement system post-birth.

Unborn babies seem to be predisposed to respond selectively to specific maternal vocalisations. A study found that when mothers sang the syllable "la" in a nursery rhyme, prenates significantly increased mouth openings (Ferrari et al., 2016). Other stimuli provided by the mother did not produce other significant changes in the baby's behaviour. The authors suggest that this selective sensitivity to specific maternal vocalisations ("la") may suggest that foetal matched responses are rudimentary signs of early mirroring behaviours, responsiveness or early motor resonance that become functional in the postnatal period, helping the infant to establish behavioural and emotional attunement with the mother. Such early imitative responses might facilitate positive social affect between the mother and the infant. In the light of Porges's polyvagal theory, these infants' matched responses to maternal prosody may have a regulatory effect on the social engagement system.

This evidence and my observations of indigenous mothers who have used similar sounds (vocalisation and singing) during pregnancy for millennia inspired the inclusion of a rhyme containing "la" sung by the mother in the PMRB programme, with the aim of facilitating emotional engagement and a connection with the prenate. These mother-prenate psychophysiological synchronisations seem to be the design of Nature's wisdom, a primal resourceful wisdom that has guided mothers and infants for millennia. Unfortunately, expert dominance and modern obstetric practices generally neglect and disturb this delicate implicit co-regulatory narrative between mother and baby, which in normal conditions leads to natural birth, attuned bonding and secure attachment.

Newborns have been found to exhibit changes in their movements when they were played a tune that was heard during pregnancy (Hepper, 1991). Prenates increased their movements on hearing the tune; newborns decreased their movements. This is consistent with observations of my unborn baby's increased flowing movement on listening to my favourite musical pieces and decreased movements after birth, though sometimes these movements increased, according to the musical piece. A baby who was a few weeks old, Gisele showed a distinct orientation reflex towards the source of music she had been exposed to during pregnancy, a typical response to familiar stimuli. She looked very peaceful, almost with an expression of reminiscence. She was soothed by a rhyme I composed during pregnancy and used to regularly recite to her. Neuronal traces had formed implicit memory, a blueprint, which underpinned Gisele's predispositions, such as her capacity to play a piano tune at four years and compose music, her sense of rhythm and aesthetics, imagination, empathy, gentle and caring nature, interest in people and capacity to attune to human relationships.

Mothers I have worked with have often reported noticing their babies' recognition of the music they had regularly listened during pregnancy by either relaxing or moving in rhythm with it, depending on the musical piece. Indigenous mothers used to sing the same song to the baby from before conception through pregnancy and beyond to create a familiar element that elicits continuum and safety.

A sensorimotor intentionality view presents brain ancient structures – the brainstem and midbrain – developing during the earliest weeks of gestation and involved in regulation of visceral organs and transmission of sensory and motor information, as underpinning conscious experience (Panksepp & Northoff, 2009). This new theory of consciousness suggests that the function of conscious experience is to integrate sensory information to guide motor action and identifies the brainstem and midbrain as responsible for this goal-directed control from earliest embryonic development (Delafield-Butt & Gangopadhyay, 2013). This view identifies the integrative neural substrate of conscious experience at the interface of a bodily self-awareness (visceral and proprioceptive senses) and environmental awareness (exteroceptive senses). Therefore, the cerebral cortex should not be regarded as in charge of goal-directed control of bodily movements, but as a further development in cognitive and reflective understanding of the world, based on early primary subcortical consciousness experiences (Vandekerckhove & Panksepp, 2011).

This phenomenological neuro-philosophical perspective conceives that since prenatal life, mental experience is necessarily grounded in this pre-reflective sensorimotor intentionality and embodied self that is responsive to a relational world. This new body of research identifies this unfolding of mind-body unity – not mind-body duality, from the earliest prenatal development. It highlights a continuum from primary consciousness to more complex levels of consciousness developing with experience and time. Understanding the embodiment of human mind and self from prenatal life may contribute to the development of prenatal interventions promoting a mother-prenate relationship based on sensorimotor exchanges and physiological co-regulation, rather than a mother's mental representation of the baby. The latter is more likely to disconnect from body awareness and embodied engagement.

From sensorimotor attunement to mental beginnings

Foetal propensity to interact before birth has been explored, as newborns appear to be wired to engage in social interactions (Carter Castiello et al., 2010; DiPietro, 2010). Castiello and colleagues reported that, in the fourteenth week of pregnancy, twin foetuses displayed movements specifically aimed at the co-twin with kinematic characteristics different from movements orientated towards the uterine wall or towards their own body. In particular, twins exhibited a higher degree of accuracy in their movements performed towards the eye or mouth regions of their twin sibling than for self-directed movements.

The infant's innate ability to initiate interactions with an adult, and then to expand this communication through bodily exchanges, such as eye contact, vocalisation, smiling and other integrated bodily functions rhythmically and cooperatively, is well established (Trevarthen, 1999). The imprinted neuropsychological mechanisms of fine attunement and musicality characterising prenatal experiences may explain why the baby is born with a pre-formed system in his brain that can create a musical or rhythmic body and communication. Caregiver's human interactions and body communications, such as skin-to-skin touch, are regulators of the baby's nervous system, and when they meet the baby's needs they contribute to good functioning of the social vagus and dependent visceral organs (Porges, 2011). This suggests that an infant's drive for social engagement, intersubjectivity and sharing experience may not emerge after birth (phylogenetic), but commences in utero through a psychobiological interpersonal relationship with her and others close to her (ontogenetic). This drive may serve to regulate the baby's physiology and affect the social engagement system, so it needs to be nurtured pre- and post-birth through maternal emotional and relational engagement.

A study's findings indicate that Kangaroo Care training, or skin-to-skin contact, appears to positively influence both neurodevelopmental trajectories and infant functioning, more specifically to stimulate the infants' left frontal area of the brain implicated in higher-order cognitive and emotional regulatory skills (Hardin et al., 2002). Extended tactile stimulation would also influence the physiology of mothers and their full-term infants by increasing peripheral basal oxytocin – the "cuddle" or "love hormone" in mothers and suppress cortisol reactivity – the "stress" hormone – in infants and their mothers. Oxytocin is the hormone associated with caregiving and affectionate behaviour, while cortisol is implicated in the stress response system. Oxytocin has also important implications for postnatal depression. It is reasonable to assume that supporting maternal mindfulness and mother-foetus positive interactive experiences may stimulate neurodevelopmental trajectories and promote maternal warmth and sensitivity predicting greater regulatory abilities and secure attachment.

From the very first weeks of embryonic development, movements serve important biological as well as psychological functions, allowing tissue growth and neural connectivity and providing experiences for learning. As a consequence of the prenate's vital activity, touch is the very first sense to develop, from which the baby receives information about his body and his environment. Touch is the primary source of stimulation, is perceived very early and enhances prenatal learning (Brazelton, 1995). When a pregnant mother gently and mindfully strokes her abdomen, she forms an emotional lifeline with her sensitive baby. In the last trimester, when the growing baby stretches the abdominal wall, he is very sensitive to parental touch, which is parents' common way of connecting with their baby. Affectionate touch is vital for an infant and child to thrive. It is so throughout our life. Further studies demonstrate that the infant's sensorimotor engagement with the world is characterised by exploration and repetition of a desired sensory effect, intended to explore new actions and their consequences and learn to control movement to achieve desired effects in what Baldwin (1895) first identifies as "circular reactions". Very attuned mothers have reported their unborn babies' ability to signal their need for sensory stimulation by producing specific kicking patterns towards the abdominal wall in response to touch, suggesting anticipation and operant conditioning.

I recall my baby's gentle kicking in the womb subsequent to my repeated gentle strokes, which I perceived as her request for reassuring tactile stimulation, a neuroception of safety in Porges's terms – a pattern she formed through habituation. I perceived similar anticipatory movements shortly before putting my favourite music on. She may have sensed my intention or other subtle psychophysiological cues. These observations and studies and many others (Tomasello & Carpenter, 2007; Trevarthen & Delafield-Butt, 2013) contribute to a growing body of literature and shed light on the importance for learning and development of pre-conceptual, goal-directedness and relational engagement. These implicit processes will become our powerful neurophysiological heritage, shape our body language and being and affect our relationships throughout our life.

These exploratory perception-action cycles and their sensory effects – active from before birth – not only enable the emergence of meaningful content, but are also the ground for the baby's developing knowledge of how the environment responds to his or her demands for interaction (Piaget, 1954). This cycle of embodied sensorimotor actions shapes the cognitive processes that deal with increasingly complex information, as perceptual, motor, memory and planning systems mature. Therefore, "knowledge of the world is necessarily embodied, structured by an awareness of how experience unfolds within the actions of a primary and pre-reflective sensorimotor intentionality" (Delafield-Butt & Gangopadhyay, 2013, p. 406). Mental experience is therefore grounded in this sensorimotor intentionality and mother-prenate emotional sensorimotor engagements, which may regulate the baby's nervous system eliciting the social engagement system. These primary experiences shape the baby's interoception, which, as according to Porges, serves as the neurophysiological substrate of the higher processes.

It is in the light of this evidence, my work with pregnant mothers and my own pregnancy, motherhood and mindfulness experience, that I developed the Pre- and Perinatal Mindfulness Relationship-Based (PMRB) programme, using mother-prenate sensorimotor and neurophysiological co-regulation mediated by maternal (and other family members') touch, melodic voice, breathing, movement and music. These creative media occurring within the practice of mindfulness as a way of being promote maternal sensitivity and reflectivity, as a foundation of connection and secure attachment. All the mother's varied creative mind-body expressions and activities and emotional nuances contribute to the baby's psychophysiological development (DiPietro et al., 2006).

The prenate is particularly sensitive to a mind-related communication, particularly fostered by the practice of relationship-focused mindfulness and needs emotional connection as much as he needs nutrients passing through the placenta. He needs reassuring messages from the mother's pregnant and birthing body and her environment to continue to thrive. He needs a mindful caregiver able to infuse him with an experience of trust and love. By communicating with her baby, the mother is conveying a visceral sense of safety to the baby and nurturing his or her mind and consciousness.

A few months old, my daughter Gisele showed remarkable memory, learning and prosocial abilities, which had been sown in her richly nurtured womb environment. She seemed to manifest a preference for *Prelude in E Minor (Op 28 No 4)* and *Nocturne in F Minor (Op 55 No 1)* by Frederic Chopin and *Fur Elise* by Beethoven (which I greatly enjoyed) by producing coordinated movements. Unborn babies have been found to be able to discriminate between low-pitched piano notes (testing cardiac deceleration) (Lecanuet et al., 2000). The authors of the cited study argue that this ability to discriminate between notes and possibly musical pieces may play a role in the earliest developmental stages of speech perception. This could explain Gisele's linguistic skill at a very young age. One of the mindfulness exercises I teach pregnant mothers in their advanced stage is to hold the baby's body (through their belly) and touch each part of it. The gentle tactile stimulation may enhance interoception, neuroception of safety, attentiveness and awareness by sending messages from the body to the brain and creating connections. It contributes to forming a core embodied self.

Nevertheless, mind-body programmes supporting mothers' understanding of foetal sentience and mother-foetus communication and attunement, physiological co-regulation and emotional availability following birth are needed.

Mother-infant emotional availability and the neuroception of safety

The concept of emotional availability (Biringer, 2000) refers to the parents' sensitivity and receptiveness to their infant's body cues and verbal communication.

Good emotional availability in the first year indicates well-attuned pre-verbal interactions between infant and parent; that is a well-functioning mother-infant relationship (Vliegen et al., 2009). These parental abilities and preverbal communications are key factors in the parent-infant relationship, shape the child's ability to regulate emotions and are essential contributors to infant development (Van Zeijl et al., 2006). Before developing verbal language, infants express their feelings and needs through bodily signals (e.g. movement, gestures, facial expressions and vocal tone), which are perceived and interpreted by a sensitive and receptive parent to meet the infant's needs (Sansone, 2004). In an environment free of the stress of our fast-paced modern life, like the community of indigenous cultures, these mother-baby balancing co-regulatory mechanisms are maintained by default. These parental abilities can be fostered by cultivating mindfulness and mother-baby relationship during pregnancy.

Attuned interactions, the foundations of secure attachment, channel and enhance physical and visceral energy, thus have a neurophysiological effect and impact on infant well-being. Parental responsiveness and related parent-infant attunement can be conceived as a nature's regulatory system, ensuring that the infant regulates the type and intensity of incoming sensations and maintains an optimal neurological state to learn (Whittingham et al., 2016). I suggest some rudimentary mechanisms of this regulatory process may occur during prenatal life according to a Nature or wisdom-based design and be preparatory for life outside the womb. Therefore, supporting parental responsiveness from pregnancy may be useful to help infants achieve calm-alert neurological systems to support learning and well-being. Being responsive to an unborn baby implies maternal embodied awareness and inner attunement, as well as an understanding of the baby's emotional and relational needs.

A responsive mother is able to perceive with an open heart, observe, make sense of the signals her baby is sending through his movements and behaviour and respond through sensory/arousal modulation (e.g. touching, talking, singing and dancing) and reflection. This mindful awareness practice focused on compassion promotes sensitivity and reflective function, establishing the foundations of human virtues and secure attachment long before birth.

Can the earliest human connection nurture a sense of safety, of "feeling felt" in the unborn baby? Can this primal sense be infused with the mother's own sense of safety? When we come to "feel felt" by another person, who is therefore *emotionally available* for us, our brain likely establishes a state of what Porges has called a "neuroception" of safety (Porges, 1998). Porges's polyvagal theory proposes that our nervous system evaluates whether a situation is threatening or safe and activates the brainstem's vagal and autonomic nervous systems to respond with either open receptivity in "safety" or with "threat". When a pregnant or birthing woman does not feel safe, this affects her nervous system and consequently her baby.

When there is attunement between two people, creating a sense of safety, Porges (1998) proposes that activation of the myelinated vagus nerve occurs with the softening of facial muscles, relaxation in vocal tone, and opening of the perceptual system to receive input from outside. I assume this state of psychophysiological attunement can be nurtured between mother and pre-nate (and between mother and father!) to prepare for postnatal bonding. Porges proposes that *myelination* creates more rapid neural signals transfer, thus more learning, and with the neuroception of safety, the vagus nerve supports the individual becoming open, receptive and approaching others. Myelination is the process of forming a myelin sheath around a nerve to allow nerve impulses to move more quickly. This process of neuroception of safety involves both the mother's and the infant's social engagement system and is bidirectional. Porges proposes a *social engagement system* that "pro-vides a system for voluntary engagement with the environment with spe-cial features associated with the prosocial behaviours of communication" (1998, p. 850). The activation of this vagal system may involve the release of the pleasure/love hormone oxytocin and its distribution throughout the body with sensations of positive states associated with physical touching and proximity. In a mother-baby dyad, this corresponds to emotional availability and mutual engagement, indicators of responsiveness and attunement.

Daniel Siegel (2007) proposes that we can extend these interpersonal mechanisms into the view of internal attunement, a self-engagement system that activates a form of interpersonal communication that is embedded in Porges's interpersonal notion of "love without fear" (Porges, 1998, p. 847). Siegel associates love without fear to the state of mind in mindful aware-ness. Siegel suggests that internal attunement may activate the same neural circuitry involving the myelinated vagus in a state of safety as we create a lov-ing relationship of self-engagement with our own direct experience. There-fore, maternal self-attunement interweaves with attunement with the baby, also because the baby perceives this loving relationship through physiologi-cal cues. This maternal attuned relationship with herself as well as with her baby is associated with a sense of neuroceptive safety, or neural integration, which allows for clear sensing, fundamental to be responsive (Siegel, 2007). This sense of safety is essential in a birthing woman and bonding formation.

When secondary influences, such as trauma and mental suffering, or envi-ronmental influences such as some obstetric practices, impair this engage-ment with the self and moment-to-moment lived experience (with curiosity, openness, acceptance and love – without fear), then internal engagement does not occur. In this case, the pregnant or postnatal mother is unlikely to engage with her unborn baby and infant. The practice of mindfulness, in particular self-compassion and self-empathy, can alleviate suffering and create a stabilising sense of being connected to both moment-to-moment experience and to her authentic sense of self. In this state of safety, atten-tion becomes open and receptive. This open state or open heart is founda-tion of love and connection.

Siegel proposes (2007) that the sense of safety fostered by internal attune-ment then initiates receptive awareness. Receptive attention is then open to whatever arises in the field or ongoing experience of pregnancy, developing baby, birth and parenting. This is the reflective state of awareness that is at the heart of mindfulness and sensitive conscious parenting. The reflective qualities of receptivity, self-other observation and reflexivity are each part of mindful awareness as well as secure attachment and are established with intention and practice. The PMRB programme promotes these abilities through self-attunement and mother-prenate engagement. It resonates with the wisdom qualities that have been practised by default for millennia and still are so by indigenous cultures.

Depressed mothers, though loving their baby, tend to have less receptive attention necessary to connect with the baby's ongoing experience. Furthermore, they have been found to be less likely to engage in eye contact and tactile interactions (Cohn et al., 1986; Field, 1984). These psychophysiological media positively influence the social engagement system. Depressive symptoms have been found to reduce parent sensitivity during interaction and capacity to respond to the child's bodily signals and thus meet their child's developmental needs (Barfoot et al., 2017). Mothers suffering from depression have also been found to be more intrusive and hostile towards their infants (Cohn & Tronick, 1989) and the content of their language more negative (Murray et al., 1993) and conveying fewer affective signals typical of child-directed speech called "motherese" (Stern, 1985). Mothers facing this kind of mental challenge are the most in need of cultivating mindful awareness, combined with individual psychotherapy if needed. However, mild worries are part of ordinary life and false steps in mother-infant communication are part of the dance, as long as they are followed by repair. It is when a mother is overwhelmed by challenging emotions or consequences of trauma that her sensitivity or ability to pick up the baby's cues and meet his needs can be jeopardised.

With increased evidence for the need for support to improve maternal mental health by reducing the risk of depression, gaining an improved understanding of antenatal predictors of emotional availability (sensitivity, mutual involvement and attunement) post-birth may highlight support strategies to promote better mother-infant relationship, potentially leading to better outcomes for infants.

Interoception or embodied awareness

Interoception has become a major research topic for mental health, and in particular for mind-body interventions. Interoception or embodied awareness has been defined as "the process by which the nervous system senses, interprets, and integrates signals originating from within the body" (Mehling et al., 2018, p. 1). The interoceptive focus of mindfulness practice enhances the capacity to look "inward", which allows one to sense their inner world and pick up and interpret bodily cues (Siegel, 2007). A pregnant mother's ability to focus inwards has been described by Winnicott as a universal psychological change in pregnancy and as necessary to connect with her baby (1965). Parent capacity to interocept and interpret has been associated with the capacity to respond to the infant's bodily signals and meet the infant's developmental needs (Negayama et al., 2015). However, the importance of a pregnant woman's interoceptive awareness to perceive and interpret the unborn baby's cues and what is going on in her body has not been acknowledged or investigated. The role of the maternal body and sensory awareness and its links with mental health during pregnancy, the mother-prenate relationship and the mother-infant relationship have received little attention, yet it could be a key antenatal factor in the quality of these domains, which is a focus of my research and clinical work. We know that embodied awareness and interpersonal attunement are both promoted by the practice of mindfulness. Identifying associations between maternal interoception, mindfulness and the mother-baby relationship pre- and post-birth may inform antenatal support strategies for mothers and their families during pregnancy and the child's earliest relationship and development.

The PMRB programme aims to support parental sensitivity, responsiveness, and parent-infant attunement through interoception (body awareness and inward focus) and sensorimotor engagement fostered by a sense of safety and open receptivity. It utilises a deep understanding of the roots of psychomotor development and implicit messages contained in people's posture, movements or inhibition of movement as a consequence of stress or trauma. From prenatal life, the baby responds to adverse or favourable conditions, transmitted via maternal physiology, through movement, muscular tone, vocal tone and breathing. This is why the pregnant mother's interoception and inward focus are vital for self-regulation and co-regulation with the baby. Because the PMRB programme is focused on the embodiment of maternal mind and mother-prenate relationship, it seals the gap between these two domains generated by Western approaches to interventions in pregnancy, either focused on the mind (psychological approaches) or on the body (medical/pharmacological approaches).

The intergenerational impact of adult attachment style

One factor influencing maternal mental health is the pattern of attachment a pregnant woman developed during her earliest experiences with her primary caregivers. These relationships lead to the establishment of internal working models or representations of oneself and one's attachment figures (Bowlby, 1973). These attachment patterns guide future relationships, including romantic relationships and future parental caregiving. However, what we know today is consistent with the life of indigenous and traditional societies: the most powerful predictor of a child's socio-emotional development is not only a secure attachment to his mother but involves the quality of the entire attachment network (Van IJzendoorn et al., 1992).

Mothers with more social support have been found to be more responsive to babies and correlations between alloparenting support, maternal sensitivity and child well-being have been identified (Coontz, 1992). Within the modern nuclear family, the support from the father and his mental health is very influential. Low social support in the prenatal and perinatal period is likely to lead to postpartum depression (Miller, 2002). When infants are exposed to entire social worlds and multiple interactions with adults and children, thus more mature reflective minds, they later begin to think of themselves as organisms with a mind and develop empathy (Fonagy et al., 2002). Novel rearing conditions may have developed when children depended on a wider range of caretakers (Hrdy, 2011). Therefore, mothers evolved to receive the same empathic support from the community as they did as children.

In the village, infants grow up feeling secure, an extended family and the cultural context remain predictable, a mode of birth and childcare customs are transmitted and everyone conforms to the same customs; in contrast to the fast rate of cultural changes in our society, which puts huge pressure on children and adults. Not surprisingly, nowadays the most severe threat to social relationships and mental health seems to be uncertainty. The isolation and pace at which we are moving in our lives are overwhelming, scorching and leaving us with a sense of deep dissatisfaction, predisposing children to trauma. By providing pregnant mothers with social compassionate support, we can mitigate the risks of developmental trauma and promote secure attachments. Through the practice of mindfulness, we can strengthen stress-coping strategies, resilience, ethical grounding and integrity in uncertain and morally challenging times.

Parents' unprocessed early childhood adversity is likely to be transmitted to offspring and affect their health and well-being through epigenetic biological mechanisms and maternal attachment patterns or caregiving behaviour during pregnancy and in the postnatal period, which influences foetal and infant development outcomes. Children of mothers who have been exposed to adverse childhood experiences (ACEs) have been found to be at increased risk of a multitude of poor health and development outcomes, including parent-infant relationship difficulties (McDonnell & Valentino, 2016). The impact of exposure to psychosocial risk (e.g. prenatal depression, anxiety and stress) and related adult attachment patterns on child development have been identified in a number of studies (Monk et al., 2012).

More securely attached parents are likely to be more responsive, sensitive and involved, compared to adults with insecure attachment styles, which results in more positive outcomes for their children (Edelstein et al., 2004). We learnt in Chapter 5 that mindfulness practice promotes secure attachment.

A longitudinal study revealed that women with higher avoidant attachment styles and greater depressive symptoms were more likely to have children with early developmental problems than those women with less avoidant attachment styles and less depressive symptoms (Alhusen et al., 2013). When a parent is upset and absent, she or he can hardly get into a baby's needs, thus respond and attune. Furthermore, women with stronger mother-prenate relationship during pregnancy had more secure attachment styles and children with better developmental outcomes than those women reporting lower mother-prenate attachment and less secure attachment styles. This indicates that attachment style may be a mediator of maternal mental health as well as attunement. Alhusen and colleagues suggest that poor prenatal attachment may be indicative of the mother's attachment style that hinders her capacity to engage in intimate relationships with others, including her unborn baby, and through the child's earliest life.

These findings may be an indicator that pregnancy is a most sensitive period, through which psychosocial risks are expressed in complex physiological and behavioural responses that influence foetal and infant development. Despite these associations, research and support programmes examining antenatal and postnatal factors that lead to the intergenerational transmission of risks are severely lacking. Providing such understanding can facilitate the development of support programmes in pregnancy and preconception that aim to tap into greater fields of possibilities, insights, wisdom abilities and creativity and break transmission of risks across generations. Both the preconception, prenatal and perinatal period provide windows of opportunities for support to improve maternal mental health, attachment patterns and infant developmental outcomes. Nevertheless, this support should be focused on fostering the parental inner wisdom and mammalian abilities that have guided mothers and sustained their mental health for millennia, and not on expert dominance and merely technological modern advances.

Western approaches to mental health are still typically embedded with seventeenth-century Cartesian dualism in addressing mental and physical disorders and emphasising the value of the intellect/rational over wisdom qualities, such as intuition, insight, embodiment, compassion and mindful awareness. Within the last few decades, there has been an increased interest in the use of mindfulness in addressing illness. Yet the very essence of mindfulness is a humane way of life and aiming to foster self-knowledge and self-development, individual psychophysiological regulation and wellbeing, creating a cohesive and healthy society. However, we can only access aspects of ourselves through the practice of mindfulness in relationships and cooperation. Mindfulness is the most ancient practice cultivated by humans to cope with life challenges and nourish depth and spirituality, which are an essential aspect of health and create a conscious humanity. This broad focus of mindfulness resonates with the maternal ancient wisdom of pregnancy, birth and parenting that guided women through evolution, and where healing of human suffering resides.

11 Visioning the future

Contemplative science provides an understanding of how inseparable minds, bodies and brains are and the many ways they can be moulded through practice towards health, affecting future generations. Mindfulness practice and meditation can greatly shape health and well-being. By cultivating mindfulness and related wisdom virtues in their daily lives, parents can positively have an impact on their children. The development of capacities in children such as kindness, caring and compassion, along with receptive attention, self-regulation, empathy and a capacity for human connection, is largely ignored by many parents, as well as the education and healthcare systems. From the moment we are born until the day we die, mindfulness and compassion, which are interwoven, affect our lives for the better.

Neuroplasticity teaches us that the repeated experiences children have shape brain circuitry and personality, including human virtues. In indigenous and traditional small-scale societies, human virtues develop by default thanks to cultural stability, shared childcare and intergenerational transmission of knowledge. At present, how our children develop human capacities has been mainly left to chance, both by parents and in our education system, although many families of course instil these values in their children. What if the roots of these capacities are set during pregnancy, even around the time of conception, through the mother's being present in her own body and inward receptive attention towards her unborn baby?

By focusing on the very first human relationship in the womb, caring and respecting this sacred space, perhaps the baby can develop a kind, caring and compassionate nature through underlying neurological mechanisms of co-regulation with his pregnant mother. The prenatal and perinatal period offers an important window of opportunity for development in the brain's circuitry, and by cultivating wisdom abilities, we can strengthen those circuits.

The science of cultivating attention is supported by abundant evidence and indicates that the benefits of cultivating attention during pregnancy can be huge not only for the pregnant mother and the father but also for the baby. There is no human connection without receptive attention, without "noticing". Our increasingly technological society and school system do little to strengthen attention and human virtues in children. Actually, our society and healthcare system suffer from an attention deficit. The digital devices children grow up with offer constant distractions, and boosting attention skills and human virtues is an urgent public health need. It has to begin from the beginning of life – in the womb – through contemplative attention during the most sacred period of human development.

I envision mindfulness-based programmes in pregnancy and community building, promoting parents' well-being and consciousness of the crucial period of their children's development and windows of opportunities as being part of the standard offerings for all expectant parents. By cultivating receptive attention, kindness, listening and compassion as a community, including healthcare practitioners and policy makers, as well as parents, not only can we prevent or mitigate the impact of parents' trauma and mental dysfunctions on children, but we can also enhance parental wisdom resources. In a technological digital society that contributes to the attention deficits in adults as well as children, we need to cultivate wholesome states and virtues, perhaps even using a little bit of technology such as video games as a tool, but only as a first introductory step, for example to listen to while driving. Changes will only be permanent with continued practice, ideally without the game, as it is the practice that engages our body, brain, genes and soul, thus our whole being.

I envision a time when our culture cares for the mind and mental health of pregnant women in the same way as it cares for the body, with practices to nourish the mind becoming part of our daily routine. This mental cultivation would be reflected in healthcare practitioners and policy makers caring for the mental health of pregnant mothers and their partners through mindful attention, listening and compassion, as these significantly benefit pregnancy, the mother-unborn/infant relationship and infant development and ultimately society itself and Mother Nature. Listening is a key tool to help establish a healing relationship between practitioners and their clients/patients. The recent crisis in maternal mental health, witnessing mortality and morbidity of pregnant and birthing women/parents in developed countries, is related to the lack of clear and open space where listening skills can be lifesaving. Most cases reveal how pregnant and birthing parents do not feel listened to or believed, which leads to a culture of denial of fundamental emotional human needs and a delay in care. Listening to one's self as well as the other is a key element of mindfulness-based approaches. It allows human communication to tune in and turn into healing music (Jensen & Nelson, 2017).

A sense of oneness

This communal flourishing includes less division between "I" and "you", and between "us" and "them". His Holiness the Dalai Lama gave a talk to religious representatives of diverse religious traditions of Buddhism,

Christianity and Islam among others, from 40 countries. His first words after greeting them at the meeting were, "Each one of us wishes for a happy life yet we keep making life difficult by putting a great emphasis on 'us' and 'them'". He noted that even religious affairs are dragged into this egocentric concept designed by man when in fact all religions are universal in their promotion of love and compassion.

I sometimes find the division between religions, even among those of the Christian faith, anti-religious and incoherent, so in the wrong direction to goodness, God. Mindfulness is what links all religions. It is how we practise the religious teaching in our lives, and with our children, that makes a difference. We should teach our children to respect the diversity of religions, of cultures and nations and of people's views and opinions. There is so much I share with Buddhism, and I do not see any antagonism with the Catholic Church in which I was brought up. I like to embrace my tradition and wisdom with my scientific knowledge and my Eastern teaching. By no means do I see them in conflict.

The Dalai Lama's core message is that in this difficult time, all religious traditions of the world have the moral obligation to bring world peace by channelling inner peace first. He advocates Buddhist philosophy by converging it with modern science through human intelligence for a practical approach. Buddhist teaching in fact has much in common with the latest neuropsychology of child development, as it bases ethical behaviour on a real appreciation of human nature, which is interdependent and intersubjective.

What if birthing a humanity successfully happens, one that will be hard-wired to live in peace and respect for all life in all its forms and with a sense of oneness among all human beings and elements of Nature? What if, by transforming our minds we can improve not only our own health and well-being, but also that of pregnant mothers and fathers by better supporting them and their developing babies through humanised care and policy making? Mindfulness practice can produce a greater sense of our interdependence not only within our organism (cells, organs, systems, mind, body and soul), but also on one another, and on every life on the planet and the cosmos, ensuring life's sustainability. When this sense of interdependence and awareness of the unborn baby as a sentient being are nurtured on a grand scale, they inevitably affect the way in which practitioners relate to pregnant mothers and their babies and families, leading to changes for the better in our communities, our societies and our nations.

This nurture of human virtues has epigenetic effects and thus mitigates or breaks cycles of transmission of the adverse consequences of trauma and mental illness as well as social ills such as poverty, intergroup hatred and mindlessness about our planet's well-being. The findings presented in this book further our understanding of how genomics and stress interact and suggest that further investigations of the genomics of stress response can uncover mechanisms that lead to depression and other mental dysfunctions, therefore to societal and ecological problems. These findings show the importance of the history of stressful childhood events of traumas in the response to stressful events, which determines a child's and adult's resilience. When parental wisdom is allowed to unfold thanks to an appropriate environmental provision, compassion and attunement are possible and infants and children can thrive. Mothers do not need instructions on how to observe, mirror and respond to their babies when they feel supported, fearless and safe.

I view mindfulness-based programmes during pregnancy and in the perinatal period as one solution to an urgent public health need, reducing selfishness, fear, hatred, greed, us/them thinking, the threats of eco-calamities and promoting more kindness, affiliation and calm. While I have taken up the science adventure of a PhD to explore some uncharted prenatal and perinatal avenues, I am aware that the scientific data, though important, are by no means sufficient for the change many of us envisage. New ideas and innovative paradigms lead to shifts in thinking and science. Science is close to culture and restricts our view of what is possible, especially when it comes to human science. Modern psychology has had to embrace Eastern systems as they offer paths towards possibilities of transforming a person's very being (Sansone, 2007). Today many empirical studies confirm the ancient wisdom that guided individual and community well-being, including motherhood, for millennia, and the effects of mindfulness practices that shape the brain both structurally and functionally. In the same way, studies provide evidence that continued mind training can reshape the brain and alter human traits and behaviour.

So, why this book now? I envision that the more youth practise mindfulness and related wisdom abilities and the more they are inspired by a compassionate community, including healthcare providers and politicians, the more we can positively shape future generations for the better. Epigenetics tells us how children's genetic expression is moulded by environmental influences for better or worse, according to the quality of experiences, whether fostering love and compassion, or threats, fear and hatred. The most favourable time is when the brain is more plastic and experience-dependent, from pregnancy to the first postnatal years, though change is possible at any stage of human life through continued practice. At a time when major global challenges are affecting everyone and everything on the planet, we have the chance to make a difference in human evolution by implementing a paradigm shift. This is synthesised in the 8 May document released by WHO, UNICEF and other partners:

> We now understand that the period from pregnancy to age 3 is the most critical, when the brain grows faster than at any other time; 80% of a baby's brain is formed by this age. For healthy brain development in these years, children need a safe, secure, and loving environment, with the right nutrition and stimulation from their parents or caregivers.

> This is a window of opportunity to lay a foundation of health and well-being whose benefits last a lifetime – and carry into the next generation.
> (World Health Organization, 2018, p. 7)

It is clear from both science and primal wisdom that healthy child development lays the foundations for lifelong health and emotional security and is key to shaping a thriving human family, community and society and planet. Investing in the youth of the country can save many societal problems and reduce the costs of mental dysfunctions, criminality and disrespect for the Earth, because an educated and conscious youth will be continuously open to growth and transformation and create a new generation of enlightened citizens. It has to begin with a comprehensive training for frontline maternal and child healthcare delivery staff, which includes the practice of human virtues and integrates science, philosophy and spirituality deep into the inner being in preparation for serving humanity. This will help improve maternal and neonatal/child outcomes and prevent health issues.

I have shown the evidence that it is possible to cultivate positive human qualities and physiological regulation transforming our being in depth, and that any of us can walk the deep path leading to compassionate caregiving practice, as well as flourishing parenting and childhood. We don't need to be in a crisis to take up mindfulness practice. Human qualities are like seeds: we can sow the seeds of love, kindness and compassion or of anger and fear, and transmit them to children. The future of our Earth and its Mother Nature relies on wisdom caregiving qualities, thus from training the mind and heart.

Compassion and self-compassion – a game changer

From the moment you are born until the day you die, compassion will affect your life for the better. Compassion is an intelligent response to emotional pain, rooted in wise courageous action, since it implies turning towards others' suffering, embracing it, rather than turning away, being overwhelmed and frightened or denying it. It is more than empathy. While empathy, the emotional resonance with another's pain, when it is intense and repeated many times, can lead to emotional distress, anxiety and even avoidance, compassion is associated with positive emotions such as maternal love and affiliation. When altruistic love encounters suffering, it manifests as compassion in the trained mind and is determined to find a way to help. We can feel benevolence towards all others, including ourselves, in all situations, and extend this kindness to all beings. Compassion allows for deep reflective listening and its healing power is especially helpful for those working with expectant and new parents to have the felt sense of being supported, so that they can compassionately support their own babies and other family members. Compassion enhances one's experience of being alive, immune system function, heart variability and the physiological functions. It enhances treatment and outcomes and can prevent and mitigate mental dysfunctions.

Self-compassion is an intelligent response towards our own difficult emotions and pain, and it opens our window of tolerance. It can be an antidote to self-judgement, shame, poor self-esteem, depression and anxiety. It creates a sense of self-care and safety. People with high self-compassion who have experienced trauma are less likely to feel threatened by and therefore avoid painful emotions, thoughts and memories and thus develop post-traumatic stress disorders (Neff & McGehee, 2010; Thompson & Waltz, 2008). Self-compassion may be an important buffer for those who have experienced early childhood trauma and reduces the risk of it developing into more complex mental disorders. Compassion and self-compassion bring a stronger sense of meaningfulness and purposefulness into life. Without self-compassion, we can either be overwhelmed by pain, disconnect from ourselves, sow the seeds of anger, or we can go into denial or flight, lose our sense of tenderness and humanity, undermining the relationship and care for expectant parents and their prenate/infants. Parents' lack of self-compassion can prevent them from connecting with their baby. Compassion and self-compassion change the relationship between brain regions, teach us how to manage the stress response and therefore are essential for resilience (Neff & Seppälä, 2016; Stevens & Woodruff, 2018). Because of this neurological transformative power, they can be a game-changer.

A child nourished with compassion and self-compassion from conception will learn to love his or her upset, angry, crying and loving mother, in all her being, and to appreciate the full range of human emotions in others and within himself. He won't deny suffering but will learn how to suffer. Honouring and respecting childhood from conception requires compassion and self-compassion on the part of the caregivers, including the entire community. Mindfulness, or loving awareness, and compassion, when interwoven, are fundamental human capacities to be present and open to experience with care, either the care of the new parent or the care of the prenate/child. This quality of care changes everything. Youth, the future parents, practitioners, society and the healthcare system need it today more than ever.

Thich Nhat Hanh teaches that we do not have to spend years on a mountain to benefit from mindfulness wisdom (1991). Instead, he says, just become aware of your breath and senses, and through that come into the present moment, where everyday activities, including the care of the prenate or child for parents, or of the parent from practitioners or the community, can take on a joyful, miraculous quality. If we are mindful, or fully present in the here and now, anxiety disappears and a sense of timelessness takes hold, allowing our highest qualities, such as kindness and compassion, to emerge.

It begins from the beginning

It is clear that the roots of social peace and a thriving humanity are set at the beginning of life within our very first relationship in the womb with a compassionate Mother and will shape the blueprint for how each human being treats the world and Mother Nature. Imagine a world where human beings all held deep within them the roots of a secure early beginning. This is why I developed a prenatal programme based on the universal ancient practice of both mindfulness and awareness of the unborn baby as a sentient being capable of learning from a compassionate focused relationship. The programme gathers all the latest converging findings from interweaving disciplines: epigenetics, interpersonal neuroscience, quantum physics, mindfulness, sensory processing, attachment, anthropology, evolutionary psychology, prenatal and perinatal psychology and Buddhist psychology. Therefore, what sets the strategy for human flourishing is the integration of primal wisdom, which has guided human well-being for millennia, and modern science. We have learnt throughout this book the evidence showing what wisdom traditions have long taught, that the key to well-being and true fulfilment greatly depends on the state of our minds and the quality of our consciousness. These can be trained from early life, as early as far before birth, to prevent or reduce the risk of trauma and its adverse consequences on health.

Human science often confirms what mothers and communities have intuitively known and practised for 99.9 per cent of human history. This is why science needs to be integrated with primal wisdom in professional training and practitioners' practice. Science cannot do justice to the depth, complexity and richness of the prenatal and perinatal realm. It took me one year to assemble the theoretical framework of this book into a PhD research design. Science can help us find associations, pieces of a complex, though important, puzzle. Therefore, science needs to be humanised and its implementation by professionals in their practice has to be mediated by a mindfulness relationship-based approach towards the potential generators of children's well-being and thriving. The future of humanity as well as our planet depends on how we care for pregnant and birthing mothers, fathers and their families. I envision the future of mental health based on prenatal and perinatal psychology as forming part of its foundation.

The PMRB programme

> For the unborn baby to reveal him/herself,
> mothers need to be ready to abandon
> their idea about him/her, listen and connect.
>
> Antonella Sansone

Amishi Jha's group at the University of Miami now offers mindfulness training to high-stress groups such as football players, firefighters and teachers.

The Garrison Institute outside New York City offers a mindfulness-based programme to help trauma workers in Africa and in the Middle East deal with secondary trauma, e.g. fighting the Ebola epidemic or helping traumatised refugees. The Prison Mindfulness Institute now teaches mindfulness inmates in 80 prisons across America. More companies and healthcare institutions should offer mindfulness approaches and contemplative methods to employees interacting with pregnant mothers and new parents as part of their training and development programmes. Why wait until modern parenting challenges are triggered by the birth of the child or later? Why not prevent or mitigate them during pregnancy or even before conception? This question led me to develop the Pre- and Perinatal Mindfulness Relationship-Based (PMRB) programme.

The PMRB programme is an adaptation of the one-year Youth Mindfulness certified teaching course and has much in common with mindfulness-based stress reduction (MBSR, Kabat-Zinn, 1990), with a particular focus on mother-prenate connection. The PMRB programme is held for two hours once a week for nine weeks. In addition, there is a three-hour reunion session 2–3 weeks and 10–12 weeks after all the women have given birth. The recommended class size ranges from 10 to 15 expectant women. The mindfulness facilitator has completed a certified one-year teaching course comprising four five-day mindfulness retreats and has an interdisciplinary knowledge of prenatal and perinatal psychology. Although the PMRB programme is explicitly designed for expectant mothers, participants' partners (baby's father, friend, mother's parent or any support person) are welcome.

The teaching of mindfulness is integrated with the following techniques and knowledge:

- Breathing technique and meditation, mind-body pain and stress-coping strategies for childbirth and awareness skills for coping with daily life stress, self-compassion – noticing new sensations, baby's movements, with receptive attention to the present moment, to enhance body awareness and allow for connection with the baby, reducing mind wandering which makes one vulnerable to anxiety and depression.
- Mother-prenate sensorimotor modulation techniques using maternal touch, vocalisation, foetal movements, and voice of the baby providing information about her/his development and needs.
- Perinatal education, including foetal development and psychobiological needs, psychobiological processes of pregnancy, childbirth, postpartum adjustment, breastfeeding and breastfeeding self-efficacy and psychobiological needs of the infant.
- Walking meditation to cultivate connection with Nature.

In the PMRB programme, formal mindfulness meditation instruction is given and practised in each class for 20 minutes, following a topical discussion. A key element of the PMRB programme is the focus on the mother-baby relationship during pregnancy from a new body-mind perspective based on the mother's embodied awareness and acceptance of the unborn baby as a conscious being, capable of engaging in bidirectional interactions. The key factor reflects a new concept of prenatal attachment based on shifting attention from "when the baby arrives to the baby is already here and I am connected with this baby".

Participants will be asked to commit to practising mindfulness meditation at home using guided meditation on YouTube for 20 minutes a day, ideally five days a week, throughout the course. Further, as part of the programme, participants are invited to write at home a diary of their perceptions of the baby's movements and cues, and a dialogue with the baby during the programme to enhance interoception (embodied awareness and inward focus), a sense of presence, sensitivity and reflective functioning, connection with the baby and relaxation. The emotional and health benefits of expressive writing have been documented (Baikie & Wilhelm, 2005). It seems that the very act of telling a story and articulating the emotions forms connections between different areas of the brain. But before we can narrate the story, we have to pay attention to the emotions and their embodiment. It is our attention that influences our neuroplasticity, the capacity of the neural networks to be formed and transformed by our attention.

Mindfulness practice is centred on training attention to what is going on in the present moment. Mothering benefits from training the mind to attention, as babies need sensitive and mindful attention to thrive. Imagining the baby voicing his feelings and experience by writing and reading letters to him on the basis of the acquired awareness can be a tool to cultivate empathy for the unborn baby and infant. Conveying feelings of love and gratitude to the baby has physiological effects and nourishes prenatal bonding. For millennia, indigenous mothers have practised mindful attention by singing a song to call for the soul of the child before conception, then celebrating the conception through dances and ceremonies and singing the same song to the child throughout pregnancy, birth and beyond to establish a reassuring continuum (Sansone, 2018b).

The importance of continued practice and maintaining engagement is explained during the first session. Selected reading and resource lists will be provided for those who are interested in expanding their knowledge.

An essential element of the course is to encourage a sense of community, sharing and belonginess among the expectant mothers and every element of Nature to reduce the potential impact of social isolation on mental health for the new parents in the post-partum period.

Coda

Supporting the maternal-prenate/infant relationship and maternal mind state through good practices facilitates maternal compassionate love and emotional availability and has potential advantages for the mother's and father's well-being and infant development. Early human connection is a biological necessity and without it, humans' being cannot flourish. Support during pregnancy should aim to improve the mother's mood, decrease anxious preoccupation with her infant, increase attunement to her infant's needs and inputs, modify negative perception of the baby, increase pleasurable interactions and develop confidence in parenting abilities (Paris et al., 2009). The relationship with the father should be highly considered in any support group.

The influence of the mother's embodied awareness on her relationship with the prenate and infant has been considered for the first time in this book and is being investigated further in my PhD. Further, the PMRB programme outcomes may temper the influence of trauma, mental disorders and insecure attachment on maternal mental health, prenatal relationship, and mother-infant relationship and infant development, thus having epigenetic effects. The programme may have implications for reducing the risk of postnatal depression, anxiety and stress, and the adverse consequences on mother-infant relationship by supporting mother-foetus relationship. Due to the documented effects of maternal mental health challenges on foetal development, mother-infant relationship and infant development, exploring associations between mindfulness, maternal mental health, mother-foetus relationship and maternal emotional availability may provide important information with clinical implications not only for future research, but also for perinatal mental health practitioners working with pregnant women from a community as well as clinical population.

Understanding the unborn baby as an active agent responsive to maternal stress and mind state and capable of sensorimotor interactions highlights the implications for maternal-foetal relationship-based interventions, and the need for healthcare providers to change the way they relate to pregnant mothers and their developing unborn babies. It is anticipated that this book and findings from the research project can inform later studies to examine implications for intervention and prevention in pregnant mothers with mental disturbances, therefore mitigating their potential adverse consequences on mother/father-infant relationship and infant development and well-being.

In the face of ecological, economic, social and political challenges, the world stands in need of a cultural shift. We need individuals and communities that are educated in prosocial qualities and behaviours such as trust, cooperation, kindness, compassion, truth-seeking, receptive attention and emotional availability and that embody these qualities, so as to support pregnancy, parents' health and well-being, foetal development and future generations in becoming agents of positive change in the world. Mindfulness and relationship practice play key roles in prosocial development across the lifespan of individuals within communities. These individuals are the practitioners or policy makers having an impact on those becoming parents, the parents or schoolteachers affecting future generations and so on. We are all interdependent and the future of our planet depends on our collective human abilities, which derives from every child's nurturing experiences. Integrating scientific, contemplative and artistic knowledge and wisdom can help us address how the development of prosocial qualities, health and well-being can be promoted at different stages of life – from prenatal life, infancy and childhood to adolescence, and from early adulthood to old age – and in different cultural-historical contexts, through mindfulness and related wisdom practices, community-building and social programmes. When these programmes involve pregnant mothers and their partners, we can have the most powerful impact on future generations because the period from pregnancy to age three is the most critical, when the brain grows faster and is highly experience-dependent.

This broader perspective on health embraces self-development to become intentionally wise as well as cooperation with the social and natural world. We need to remember that the way we behave towards others creates states of mind in others, which affect next generations. If a pregnant and birthing mother feels loved, nurtured and safe in her environment, the baby feels loved, wanted and safe, and this shapes his development and well-being. This mind state allows a mother to care for her well-being while creatively communicating with and caring for her baby. It will coherently manifest post-birth through her engagement/nurturing system – voice intonation, facial expression, eye contact, quality of holding her baby and posture. Honouring children begins in the womb.

Sharing compassionate goals, practising mindfulness, reflecting wisely, being non-judgemental and non-defensive but open to listening, connecting and understanding have an impact on the next generations. The health and well-being of women and couples simply create health and well-being in our society, and supporting it must be our community's priority. Humanity and the natural world are at high risk, as reflected by our society, but we can protect the next generation of human beings by reforming how we care for women and couples during the crucial pre-conception, prenatal and perinatal time. Then the new generation will learn the pleasure of social and intimate relationships, whereas when care is inadequate, relationships may be painful and avoided. Wisdom practice and all practices fostering wisdom beget wise perception, which is necessary to create a culture of compassion and cooperation also embracing appreciation of the value of Nature, including mothers' mammalian caring nature. This culture affects the quality of parenting and therefore next generations.

The following are some wisdom steps based on contemplative traditions and leading to human well-being:

- The health and well-being of women, men and couples create the health and well-being of next generations, thus of our society.
- Early life, including the prenatal period, sets up trajectories for health, emotional, social and moral capacities, rooted in neurobiological and socio-emotional development.

- Human creativity and imagination greatly reside in how children are raised and the culture humans create.
- Multiple perspectives and interdisciplinary approaches promote wholesome mental qualities related to prosociality – empathy, compassion, altruism and ethics (peace).
- Projects that nurture empathy, compassion, kindness and well-being in children, from conception through mindful parenting and improving romantic relationships, and across the human lifespan must be supported.
- Primal wisdom practices offer a way to restore human nature to its potential and needs to be integrated with scientific evidence in all professional training and practice with a concern for pregnancy, birth, fertility assistance, parenting and infant and child health.
- The natural world, including human beings, needs to be viewed as more cooperative than competitive, leading also to an appreciation of maternal mammalian caring nature and the body as sources of well-being rather than being neglected in the name of intellectualism and rationalism.
- Acknowledging the health and well-being benefits for both mother and prenatal/child of universal mammalian practices, such as nurturing mother-foetus communication, extended breastfeeding and co-sleeping, is likely to promote their implementation, leading to a healthier humanity and Mother Nature that takes care of us.

Parents who are resistant to ancient mammalian childcare practices such as breastfeeding and co-sleeping, which have been our human heritage for 99.9 per cent of human history, may be influenced by a cultural mindset centred on control and fear rather than in favour of the infant's and mother's well-being. They may be dominated by fears and anxiety about intimacy and truthfulness and can be supported during pregnancy, since the relationship with the infant begins in the womb and the perinatal practices are simply an extension of it. Prof James McKenna provides robust evidence of the benefits of safe co-sleeping practices to the infant's physiological and psychological well-being and development (McKenna et al., 1994, 2008). Our society may generate fear and excessive control, leading mothers to disconnect from their bodily sensations, which are vital for maintaining a minimum alertness level while sleeping next to the baby and being able to pick up the baby's body cues. Nature has created a wise system of co-regulation between mother and infant that, in normal conditions, is active even at night. This system is altered in mothers with a severe mental condition, although all mothers may disconnect from their bodies and inner wisdom as a consequence of stress, anxiety and depression. Therefore, they need to be supported to allow the mammalian practices to unfold.

A new common-self view implies a shift of consciousness that wisdom traditions unveil: recognising our universal mammalian caring nature and realising that everything around us is part of a whole and affects us – the neighbour, the healthcare practitioner, the music, the trees, the birds, the sunset. The unborn child is a vital element of this whole, and therefore needs to be particularly nurtured, protected and honoured. Thus, he will be able to care for himself, his social and natural environment and the Earth. This expanded view enables us to relate to others, engage with others and have a "communal imagination ethic" (Narvaez, 2014). Competition is against our human nature, our health and well-being. With our imagination and bodily engagement, through attention and wisdom practices, we can transform our suffering, being, personality and culture and have an impact on children's crucial early experiences. Adults can change cultures by developing institutions, services, charities, campaigns and other activities that support pregnancy, birth and parenting, therefore promoting socio-emotional and moral development in children and preventing immorality, violence and selfishness. As adults – parents, healthcare providers and policy makers – we can use our imagination, awareness, heart, engagement and courage to build a society and world in which we all thrive.

Because children depend on adults to support them during early life, adults influence their children's personality predispositions and human traits by the way they treat them from intra-uterine life. Indigenous people clearly teach us that when humans are raised with compassionate care, in healthy nurturing environments, they are more likely to become adults with a humane and moral heritage. Every member of the community considers basic needs a priority, so that every member of the family and community feels loved, safe and supported, thus receive what they need and give it back. Indigenous societies teach us that communal mindfulness and morality, not immorality and violence, develop by default. When communities invest in pregnancy and child-rearing, each child can develop his or her own unique inclinations and thrive as an individual-in-community.

Our human nature is about engaging in meaningful relational interactions, from prenatal life, living cooperatively with other human beings and entities of Mother Nature, and treating them as members of the family. The very first human connection derives from our mother's imagination and embodiment. Although we have moved a long way away from this attitude and these practices, we have the power to re-establish them. But as I have repeatedly observed throughout this book, it is not enough to know intellectually what needs to be done. We must know it from lived personal experience, from continuous practice, which leads to virtuous habits of the mind (e.g. awareness), the heart (e.g. compassion) and the body (e.g. engagement). We must *feel* connected to our child, our mammalian nurturing nature and our companions in the natural world. Children who grow up with the natural and social world as a companion develop a deep sense of how the natural world and community care for them and a sense of gratitude for both. From a sensitive and responsive relationship with caregivers as early as during pregnancy, children learn to believe that the world is a good place and this reduces the risk of them facing disruptive issues in later life. As adults in a compassionate supportive society, they will avoid damaging the sacred relationship with the unborn child, during birth and beyond, with others, and with Nature, letting their bodies, minds and spirits flourish. We then understand that Nature, including our mammalian caregiving resources, has wisdom, sustains and cherishes us and gives us profound lessons.

My final message:

> Live your pregnancy, your babies' and children's lives fully, with curiosity, a sense of joy and wonder, presence and attention. Don't neglect their life in the womb. Take the time to listen to them, talk to them, watch them grow and flourish. Those early moments, days, months and years have life-long effects; yet they slip through your hands like grains of sand, never to return.

> Those early moments, days, months and years have life-long effects; yet they "slip through your hands like grains of sand, never to return".
>
> (Robin Sharma, 2003)

Afterword

The child who is not embraced by the village
will burn it down to feel its warmth.

African proverb

In the last days of finishing this book, coronavirus disease (COVID-19) spread worldwide, requiring people in most countries to go into lockdown, causing a global crisis. Is there a lesson here somewhere? An atonement for all the issues and illnesses man has caused, damaging himself and the only place, the Earth, he can call Home? A massive wake-up call, an opportunity to stop and reflect, relearn to value what has been taken for granted and what really matters?

Humans have believed they could dominate Mother Nature, cross all the boundaries with their intellect and technological inventions. But Nature has its own design and is making it crystal clear: humans were abusing wildlife and their habitats, mothers neglecting their mammalian caregiving primal wisdom resources which have nourished infants for 99.9 per cent of human history and secured stability and well-being. A submicroscopic infectious agent that replicates only inside the living cells of an organism has brought the most arrogant species on the planet to its knees. How can we use this opportunity to reflect and do better?

Issues associated with threats to survival represent one of the most influential sources of stress. The economic stress combined with the fact that a large portion of the population cannot afford healthcare is enough stress to inhibit the immune system and significantly exacerbate the spreading disease. We know stress hormones shut down the immune system when the body is in an adrenal-driven state of fight and flight. Psychoneuroimmunology research clearly reveals that consciousness controls the function of the immune system. Positive consciousness is responsible for the *Placebo Effect*, in which the mind can heal most diseases, while stress and negative thinking create the *Nocebo Effect*, which can contribute to almost any disease. The fear of COVID-19, like any pandemic, coupled with the threats to survival, profoundly inhibits the population's immune system and further exacerbates the epidemic.

This is a critical time for pregnant mothers, couples and their developing babies, as we have learnt throughout this book how high levels of stress, anxiety and depression affect developmental outcomes and have epigenetic effects that can be passed on to the next generations. Now more than ever, those becoming parents need to maintain a healthy lifestyle which enhances their immune system, overcomes fear and keeps them healthy. They need emotional support, human and community connection, mindfulness meditation, compassion and self-compassion, Nature walks, play, dancing and listening to music together and eating nutritious, natural, organic food coming directly from the Earth. They need support from the governments and healthcare systems, as well as from the community to feel united. These practices will all synchronically promote parents' self-psychophysiological regulation so fundamental to the regulation of the foetus/infant's neurological systems underpinning emotional, social and cognitive development.

Our world is in crisis, overwhelmed by political, environmental and mental health issues and endless conflicts. The Earth was begging us to look at the pollution for a very long time and stop all the transport. All these problems are symptoms of the deeper issues of the human condition, so to heal the world, we have to heal the human condition. Much of human life that has characterised the indigenous ways of knowing and living and sustained well-being has to be brought back to life. The human condition is the most important frontier of the natural sciences. It originates from life before birth, before conception. The human condition solves all the problems at the source. It is the responsibility of every human now to understand it, starting from children's basic needs as early as during life in the womb. A solution can be found in the training of the mind, heart and wisdom. This can create an enormous force and change through cooperation but also individual action.

The multisensory awareness fostered by mindfulness practice operates as though:

- The universe is a living expression of divine intelligence, and we are all part of something much greater than our own ego/survival.
- Our intentions and receptive attention are powerful determinants of our reality and have a profound effect on others, and they are both fostered by the practice of mindfulness.
- Our world is designed for us to learn and serve our soul's true purpose.
- With each of our individual self-developments and advancements, the group soul of humanity – what we call our collective unconscious – evolves.
- By becoming open to multisensory awareness, intuition and inspiration, we savour every moment of existence – qualities that we can learn to incorporate into our own lives from before the conception of our children; parents become prophets of the divine potential inside their

children, thus inside every being and the whole community. Mindfulness practice and its fostered primal wisdom virtues can point all of us
towards the path to our higher selves, wholeness, health and well-being.

May all mothers rely on their mammalian caregiving resources, intuitions
and the inner primal wisdom that has passed on to generations through
real human interactions and community-shared childcare and that has
guided them for millennia in their motherhood. May they practice mammalian caregiving such as extended breastfeeding, co-sleeping, singing to
the soul of the child before conception throughout pregnancy and beyond
and group dancing – taking care of the unborn baby and infant in the same
ways Mother Nature takes care of mothers and all of us.

May your body, emotions, mind and spirit be integrated so that you
experience boundless energy and vibrant health benefitting your baby
development before and after birth, and if you are a prenatal or perinatal
professional or any member of the community, enhancing prospective parents' health and well-being, the very generators of humanity welfare.

May your life be filled with beauty, joy, goodness, gratitude, compassion
and love.

Lao-tzu noted, "Conclusions are ignorance arrested on the path to less
ignorance". So, rather than a conclusion, may you find a new beginning
and blessing in the lifelong journey of mindfulness as you receive this book.

References

Abboud, G. (2014). The third Khamtrul Rinpoche. In *The royal seal of Mahamudra*. Shambhala.

Adler, H. M. (2002). The sociophysiology of caring in the doctor-patient relationship. *Journal of General Internal Medicine, 17*(11), 883–890.

Alegria-Torres, J. A., Baccarelli, A., & Bollati, V. (2011). Epigenetics and lifestyle. *Epigenomics, 3*(3), 267–277.

Alessandri, S. M., & Lewis, M. (1996). Differences in pride and shame in maltreated and non-maltreated preschoolers. *Child Development, 67*(4), 1857–1869.

Alhusen, J. L. (2008). A literature update on maternal-foetal attachment. *Journal of Obstetric Gynecologic & Neonatal Nursing, 37*(3), 315–328.

Alhusen, J. L., Hayat, M. J., & Gross, D. (2013). A longitudinal study of maternal attachment and infant developmental outcomes. *Archives of Women's Mental Health, 16*(6), 521–529.

Allman, J. M., Watson, K. K., Tetreault, N. A., & Hakeem, A. Y. (2005). Intuition and autism: A possible role for Von Economo neurons. *Trends in Cognitive Sciences, 9*, 367–373.

Altman, N. (2007). *The oxygen prescription: The miracle of oxidative therapies.* Healing Art Press.

Ammaniti, M., & Gallese, V. (2014). *The birth of intersubjectivity: Psychodynamics, neurobiology, and the self.* W. W. Norton & Company.

Anacker, C., O'Donnell, K. J., & Meaney, M. J. (2014). Early life adversity and the epigenetic programming of hypothalamic-pituitary-adrenal function. *Dialogues in Clinical Neuroscience, 16*(3), 321–333.

Anda, R. F., Felitti, V. J., Bremner, J. D., Walker, J. D., Whitfield, C. H., Perry, B. D., Dube, S. R., & Giles, W. H. (2006). The enduring effects of abuse and related adverse experiences in childhood: A convergence of evidence from neurobiology and epidemiology. *European Archives of Psychiatry and Clinical Neuroscience, 256*(3), 174–186.

Ansermet, F., & Magistretti, P. (2007/2004). *Biology of freedom: Neural plasticity, experience, and the unconscious* (S. Fairfield, trans.). New York: Other Press.

Astin, J. A. (1997). Stress reduction through mindfulness meditation: Effects on psychological symptomatology, sense of control, and spiritual experiences. *Psychotherapy and Psychosomatics, 66*(2), 97–106.

Atkins-Burnett, S., & Allen-Meares, P. (2000). Infants and toddlers with disabilities: Relationship-based approaches. *Social Work, 45*(4), 371–379.

Austin, M. P., Hadzi-Pavlovic, D., Leader, L., Saint, K., & Parker, G. (2005). Maternal trait anxiety, depression and life event stress in pregnancy: Relationships with infant temperament. *Early Human Development, 81*(2), 183–190.

Austin, M. P., Tully, L., & Parker, G. (2007). Examining the relationship between antenatal anxiety and postnatal depression. *Journal of Affective Disorders, 101*(1–3), 169–174.

Bachrach, V. R. G., Schwarz, E., & Bachrach, L. R. (2003). Breastfeeding and the risk of hospitalization for respiratory disease in infancy: A meta-analysis. *Archives of Paediatrics & Adolescent Medicine, 157*(3), 237–243.

Baikie, K. A., & Wilhelm, K. (2005). Emotional and physical health benefits of expressive writing. *Advances in Psychiatric Treatment, 11*(5), 338–346.

Baldoni, F. (2010). Attachment, danger and the role of the father in family life span. *Transilvanian Journal of Psychology (Erdélyi Pszichológiai Szemle, EPSZ), 4*, 375–402.

Baldoni, F., Baldaro, B., & Benassi, M. (2009). Affective disorders and illness behaviour in perinatal period: Correlations between fathers and mothers. *Child Development and Disabilities, 36*(3), 25–44.

Baldoni, F., Matthey, S., Agostini, F., Schimmenti, A., & Caretti, V. (2018). Perinatal assessment of parental affectivity (PAPA): First validation in Italian samples, 16th world association for infant mental health (WAIMH) congress (Rome, May 26–28, 2018). *Infant Mental Health Journal, 39*(Suppl. 77.2), 311.

Baldwin, J. M. (1895). *Mental development in the child and the race.* New York: The Macmillan Company.

Barfoot, J., Meredith, P., Ziviani, J., & Whittingham, K. (2017). Parent-child interactions and children with cerebral palsy: An exploratory study investigating emotional availability, functional ability, and parent distress. *Child Care Health and Development, 43*(6), 812–822.

Barker, D. J. (2004). The developmental origins of well-being. *Philosophical Transactions of the Royal Society of London: Series B, Biological Sciences, 359*(1449), 1359–1366.

Barret, J., Wonch, K. E., Gonzalez, A., Ali, N., Steiner, M., Hall, G. B., & Fleming, A. S. (2012). Maternal affect and quality of parenting experiences are related to amygdala response to infant faces. *Social Neuroscience, 7*(3), 252–268.

Bateson, G. (1972). *Steps to an ecology of mind.* University of Chicago Press.

Bauer, A., Parsonage, M., Knapp, M., Lemmi, V., & Adelaja, B. (2014). *The costs of perinatal mental health problems: Report summary.* London School of Economics and Political Science, School of Mental Health.

Bear, M. F. (2003). Bidirectional synaptic plasticity: From theory to reality. *Philosophical Transactions of the Royal Society of London B, 358*, 649–655.

Berens, A. E., Jensen, S. K. G., & Nelson, C. A. (2017). Biological embedding of childhood adversity: From physiological mechanisms to clinical implications. *Biomed Central (BMC) Medicine, 15*(1), 135.

Bergner, S., Monk, C., & Werner, E. A. (2008). Dyadic intervention during pregnancy? Treating pregnant women and possibly reaching the future baby. *Infant Mental Health Journal, 29*(5), 399–419.

Berkes, F. (1999). *Sacred ecology.* Routledge.

Berlin, L. J., Zeanah, C. H., & Lieberman, A. F. (2008). Prevention and intervention programs for supporting early attachment security. In J. Cassidy & P. R. Shaver (Eds.), *Handbook of attachment: Theory, research, and clinical applications* (pp. 745–761). The Guilford Press.

Bion, W. R. (1962). Container and contained. In W. R. Bion (Ed.), *Elements of psychoanalysis*. Heinemann (Reprinted in 1984 by Karnac Books).

Biringer, Z. (2000). Emotional availability: Conceptualisation and research findings. *American Journal of Orthopsychiatry, 70*(1), 104–114.

Bourgeault, C. (2003). *The wisdom way of knowing: Reclaiming an ancient tradition to awaken the heart.* Jossey-Bass.

Bowlby, J. (1951). *Maternal care and mental health.* Schocken.

Bowlby, J. (1959). Separation anxiety. *International Journal of Psychoanalysts, XLI*, 1–25.

Bowlby, J. (1973). *Attachment and loss: Separation anxiety and anger.* Basic Books.

Boyd, J. E., Lanius, R. A., & McKinnon, M. C. (2018). Mindfulness-based treatments for post- traumatic stress disorder: A review of the treatment literature and neurobiological evidence. *Journal of Psychiatry & Neuroscience, 43*(1), 7–25.

Bradley, R. T., McCraty, R., Atkinson, M., Tomasino, D., Daugherty, A., & Arguelles, L. (2010). Emotion self-regulation, psychophysiological coherence, and test anxiety: Results from an experiment using electrophysiological measures. *Applied Psychophysiology and Biofeedback, 35*(4), 261–283.

Brancato, R. M., Church, S., & Stone, P. W. (2008). A meta-analysis of passive descent versus immediate pushing in nulliparous women with epidural analgesia in the second stage of labour. *Journal of Obstetric, Gynaecologic & Neonatal Nursing, 37*(1), 4–12.

Branjerdporn, G., Meredith, P. J., Strong, J., & Garcia, J. (2016). Associations between maternal- foetal attachment and infant development outcomes: A systematic review. *Maternal and Child Health Journal, 21*(3), 540–553.

Brazelton, T. B. (1995). Foetal observations: Could they relate to another modality, such as touch? In E. Field (Ed.), *Touch in early development* (pp. 11–18). Lawrence Erlbaum Associates.

Bronte-Tinkew, J., Horowitz, A., Kennedy, E., & Perper, K. (2007). *Men's pregnancy Intentions and prenatal behaviours: What they mean for fathers' involvement with their children.* Publication #2007-18. Child Trends.

Bryant, F. B., & Veroff, J. (2007). *Savouring: A new model of positive experience.* Erlbaum.

Buchanan, M. (2009). Behavioural science: Secret signals. *Nature News, 457*(7229), 528–530.

Bujatti, M., & Riederer, P. J. (1976). Serotonin, noradrenaline, dopamine metabolites in transcendental meditation-technique. *Neural Transmission, 39*(3), 257–267.

Cajete, G. (2000). *Native science: Natural laws of interdependence.* Clear Light.

Capra, F. (1976). *The Tao of physics.* Fontana.

Carlsson, M. L. (1998). Hypothesis: Is infantile autism a hypoglutamatergic disorder? Relevance of glutamate – serotonin interactions for pharmacotherapy. *Journal of Neural Transmission, 105*, 525–535.

Carter, C. S., Altemus, M., & Chrousos, G. P. (2001). Neuroendocrine and emotional changes in the post-partum period. *Progress in Brain Research, 133*, 241–249.

Castiello, U., Becchio, C., Zoia, S., Nelini, C., Sartori, L., & Blason, L. (2010). Wired to be social: The ontogeny of human interaction. *PLoS One, 5*, e13199. https://doi.org/10.1371/journal.pone.0013199.

Castonguay, L. G., & Beutler, L. E. (2006). Principles of therapeutic change: A task force on participants, relationships, and techniques factors. *Journal of Clinical Psychology, 62*(6), 631–638.

Centre of the Developing Child at Harvard University. (2009). *Maternal depression can undermine the development of young children.* Working Paper No. 8. https://cascw.umn.edu/wp-content/uploads/2011/06/CDF-MaternalDepression Report.pdf

Chamberlain, D. B. (1994/2011). The sentient prenate: What every parent should know. *Journal of Prenatal and Perinatal Psychology and Health, 26*(1), 37–59.

Chamberlain, D. B. (2003). Communicating with the mind of a prenate: Guidelines for parents and birth professionals. *Journal of Prenatal and Perinatal Psychology and Health, 18*(2), 95–108.

Chamberlain, D. B. (2013). *Windows to the womb: Revealing the conscious baby from conception to birth.* North Atlantic Books.

Champagne, F. A. (2008). Epigenetic mechanisms and the transgenerational effects of maternal care. *Frontiers in Neuroendocrinology, 29*(3), 386–397.

Childre, D., Martin, H., Rozman, D., & McCraty, R. (2016). *Heart intelligence: Connecting with the intuitive guidance of the heart.* Waterfront Press.

Chrousos, G. P., & Gold, P. W. (1992). The concepts of stress and stress system disorders: Overview of physical and behavioural homeostasis. *Journal of the American Medical Association, 267*(9), 1244–1252.

Church, D. (2009). *The genie in your genes: Epigenetic medicine and the new biology of intention.* Energy Psychology Press.

Clark, R. C. (2008). *Building expertise: Cognitive methods for training and performance improvement* (3rd ed.). Pfeiffer.

Cohen, S., & Pressman, S. D. (2006). Positive affect and health. *Current Directions in Psychological Science, 15*(3), 122–125.

Cohn, J. F., Matias, R., Tronick, E. Z., Connell, D., & Lyons-Ruth, K. (1986). Face-to-face interactions, spontaneous and structured, of depressed mothers and their infants. In E. Z. Tronick & T. Field (Eds.), *Maternal depression and infant disturbance: Vol. 34. New directions for child development* (pp. 31–46). Jossey-Bass.

Cohn, J. F., & Tronick, E. (1989). Specificity of infant's response to mother's affective behaviour. *Journal of the American Academy of Child and Adolescent Psychiatry, 28*(2), 242–248.

Condon, J. T. (1993). The assessment of antenatal emotional attachment: Development of a questionnaire instrument. *British Journal of Medical Psychology and Health, 66*(2), 167–183.

Condon, W. S., & Sander, L. W. (1974). Neonate movement is synchronised with adult speech: Interactional participation and language acquisition. *Science, 183*(4120), 99–101.

Coontz, S. (1992). *The way we never were: American families and the nostalgia trap.* Basic Books.

Cooper, M. (2015). *Existential psychotherapy and counselling: Contributions to a pluralistic practice.* Sage.

Cox, D. T., & Gaston, K. (2015). Likeability of garden birds: Importance of species knowledge and richness in connecting people to nature. *PLoS One, 10*(11), 1–14, e0141505.

Cox, D. T., Shanahan, D. F., Hudson, H. L., Plummer, K. E., Siriwardena, G. M., Fuller, R. A., Anderson, K., Hancock, S., & Gaston, K. J. (2017). Doses of neighbourhood nature: The benefits for mental health of living in nature. *Bioscience, 67*(2), 147–155.

Coxhead, N. (1985). *The relevance of bliss.* Wildwood House.

Cozolino, L. J. (2002). *The neuroscience of psychotherapy: Building and rebuilding the human brain*. W. W. Norton & Company.

Cranley, M. S. (1981). Development of a tool for measurement of maternal attachment during pregnancy. *Nursing Research, 30*, 281–284.

Crawford, M. A., & Sinclar, A. J. (1971). Nutritional influences in the evolution of mammalian brain. In K. Elliot & J. A. Knight (Eds.), *Lipids, malnutrition and the developing brain* (pp. 267–292). A Ciba Foundation Symposium, Elsevier.

Creswell, J. D., Taren, A. A., Lindsay, E. K., Greco, C. M., Gianaros, P. J., Fairgrieve, A., Marsland, A. L., Brown, K. W., Way, B. M., Rosen, R. K., & Ferris, J. L. (2012). Alterations in resting-state functional connectivity link mindfulness meditation with reduced interleukin-6: A randomized controlled trial. *Biological Psychiatry, 80*(1), 53–61.

Crocker, J., Canevello, A., Breines, J. G., & Flynn, H. (2010). Interpersonal goals and change in anxiety and dysphoria in first-semester college students. *Journal of Personality and Social Psychology, 98*(6), 1009–1024.

Dahl, C. J. (2016). *Contemplative and scientific perspectives on human flourishing: Psychological dynamics in different families of meditation and a curriculum for the cultivation of well-being* [Doctoral dissertation, University of Wisconsin]. ProQuest Dissertation Publishing.

Dalai Lama. (2006). *His Holiness The Dalai Lama visits Vana Retreat Centre Dehradun, India*, April 6.

Davidson, J. M. (1976). The physiology of meditation and mystical states of consciousness. *Perspectives in Biology and Medicine, 19*(3), 345–380.

Davidson, R. J. (2004). Wellbeing and affective style: Neural substrates and biobehavioural correlates. *Philosophical Transactions Royal Society London, B, 359*, 1395–1411.

Davidson, R. J., & Begley, S. (2012). *The emotional life of your brain*. Plume.

Davidson, R. J., Dunne, J., Eccles, J. S., Engle, A., Geenberg, M., Jennings, P., Jha, A., Jinpa, T., Lantieri, L., Meyer, D., Roeser, R. W., & Vago, D. (2012). Contemplative practices and mental training: Prospects for American education. *Child Development Perspectives, 6*(2), 146–153.

Davidson, R. J., & McEwen, B. S. (2012). Social influences on neuroplasticity: Stress and interventions to promote wellbeing. *Nature Neuroscience, 15*(5), 689–695.

Davies, P. (1993). *The mind of God: The scientific basis for a rational world*. Simon & Schuster Ltd.

Dayan, J., Creveuil, C., Marks, M. N., Conroy, S., Herlicoviez, M., Dreyfus, M., & Tordjman, S. (2006). Prenatal depression, prenatal anxiety, and spontaneous preterm birth: A prospective cohort study among women with early and regular care. *Psychosomatic Medicine, 68*(6), 938–946.

De Bellis, M. D., Woolley, D. P., & Hooper, S. R. (2013). Neuropsychological findings in paediatric maltreatment: Relationship of PTSD, dissociative symptoms, and abuse/neglect indices to neurocognitive outcomes. *Child Development, 18*(3), 171–183.

DeCasper, A. J., Lecanuet, J., Busnel, M., Granier-Deferre, C., & Maugeais, R. (1994). Foetal reaction to recurrent maternal speech. *Infant Behaviour and Development, 17*(2), 159–164.

Decety, J., & Chaminade, T. (2003). Neural correlates of feeling sympathy. *Neuropsychologia, 41*, 127–138.

Decety, J., & Meyer, M. (2008). From emotion resonance to empathic understanding: A social developmental neuroscience account. *Development and Psychopathology, 20*(4), 1053–1080.

Dehaene-Lambertz, G., Montavont, A., Jobert, A., Allirol, L., Dubois, J., Hertz-Pannier, L., & Dehaene, S. (2010). Language or music, mother or Mozart? Structural and environmental influences on infants' language networks. *Brain and Language, 114*(2), 53–65.

Delafield-Butt, J. T., & Gangopadhyay, N. (2013). Sensorimotor intentionality: The origins of intentionality in prospective agent action. *Developmental Review, 33*, 399–425.

D'Elia Riviello, L. (2019). *Involontariamente*. Il Seme Bianco.

Dennis, C. L., & McQueen, K. (2009). The relationship between infant-feeding outcomes and postpartum depression: A quantitative systematic review. *Paediatrics, 123*(4), 736–751.

Dewey, J. (1960/1933). *How we think*. Heath.

Dhillon, A., Sparkes, E., & Rui, V. D. (2017). Mindfulness-based interventions during Pregnancy: A systematic review and meta-analysis. *Mindfulness, 8*(6), 1421–1437.

DiPietro, J. A. (2010). Psychological and psychophysiological considerations regarding the maternal-foetal relationship. *Infant and Child Development, 19*(1), 27–38.

DiPietro, J. A., Costigan, K. A., & Gurewitsch, E. D. (2003). Foetal response to induced maternal stress. *Early Human Development, 74*(2), 125–138.

DiPietro, J. A., Costigan, K. A., Nelson, P., Gurewitsch, E. D., & Laudenslager, M. L. (2008). Foetal responses to induced maternal relaxation during pregnancy. *Biological Psychology, 77*(1), 11–19.

DiPietro, J. A., Novak, M., Costigan, K. A., Atella, L. D., & Reusing, S. P. (2006). Maternal psychological distress during pregnancy in relation to child development at age two. *Child Development, 77*(3), 573–587.

Dozier, M. K., Stovall, K. C., & Albus, K. E. (1999). Attachment and psychopathology in adulthood. In J. Cassidy & P. Shaver (Eds.), *Handbook of attachment* (pp. 497–519). Guilford Press.

Dozier, M. K., Stovall, C., Albus, K. E., & Bates, B. (2001). Attachment for infants in foster care: The role of caregiver state of mind. *Child Development, 72*, 263–304.

Duncan, L. G., & Bardacke, N. (2010). Mindfulness-based childbirth and parenting education: Promoting mindfulness during the perinatal period. *Journal of Child and Family Studies, 19*(2), 190–202.

Dusek, J. A., Otu, H. H., Wohlhueter, A. L., Bhasin, M., Zerbini, L. F., Joseph, M. G., Benson, H., & Libermann, T. A. (2008). Genomic counter-stress changes induced by the relaxation response. *PloS One, 3*(7), e2576.

Edelstein, R. S., Alexander, K. W., Shaver, P. R., Schaaf, J. M., Quas, J. A., Lovas, G. S., & Goodman, G. S. (2004). Adult attachment style and parental responsiveness during a stressful event. *Attachment & Human Development, 6*(1), 31–52.

Edhborg, M., Lundh, W., Seimyr, L., & Widstrom, A. M. (2003). The parent-child relationship in the context of maternal depressive mood. *Archives of Women Mental Health, 6*(3), 211–216.

Eisenberg, L. (1995). The social construction of the human brain. *American Journal of Psychiatry, 152*(11), 1563–1575.

Ekman, P. (2007). The directed facial action task: Emotional responses without appraisal. In J. A. Coan & J. J. Allen (Eds.), *Series in affective science: Handbook of emotion elicitation and assessment* (pp. 47–53). Oxford University Press.

Ekman, P., Freisen, W. V., & Ancoli, S. (1980). Facial signs of emotional experience. *Journal of Personality and Social Psychology, 39*(6), 1125–1134.

Emerson, W. (1996). The vulnerable prenate. *Pre- and Perinatal Psychology Journal, 10*(3), 125–142.

Everett, D. (2009). *Don't sleep, there are snakes: Life and language in the Amazonian Jungle.* Vintage.

Fang, X., Brown, D. S., Florence, C. S., & Mercy, J. A. (2012). The economic burden of child maltreatment in the United States and implications for prevention. *Child Abuse & Neglect, 36*(2), 156–165.

Feldman, R. (2007). Parent-infant synchrony: Biological foundations and developmental outcomes. *Current Directions in Psychological Science, 16*(6), 340–345.

Felitti, V. J., Anda, R. F., Nordenberg, D., Williamson, D. F., Spitz, A. M., Edwards, V., Koss, M. P., & Marks, J. S. (1998). The relationship of adult health status to childhood abuse and household dysfunction. *American Journal of Preventive Medicine, 14*, 245–258.

Ferrari, G. A., Nicolini, Y., Demuru, E., Tosato, C., Hussain, M., Scesa, E., Romeil, L., Boerci, M., Iappinil, E., Rosa Pratil, G. D., Palagi, E., & Ferrari, P. F. (2016). Ultrasonographic investigation of human foetus responses to maternal communicative and non-communicative stimuli. *Frontiers in Psychology.* http://journal.frontiersin.org/journal/36/section/46#archive.

Field, T. M. (1984). Early interactions between infants and their postpartum depressed mothers. *Infant Behaviour and Development, 7*(4), 517–522.

Field, T. M. (1994). The effects of mother's physical and emotional unavailability on emotion regulation. *Monographs of the Society for Research in Child Development, 59*(2–3), 208–227.

Field, T. M. (2011). Prenatal depression effects on early development: A review. *Infant Behaviour and Development, 34*(1), 1–14.

Field, T. M., Diego, M., & Hernandez-Reif, M. (2006). Prenatal depression effects on the foetus and newborn: A review. *Infant Behaviour & Development, 29*(3), 445–455.

Field, T. M., Healy, B., Goldstein, S., Perry, S., Bendell, D., Schanberg, S., Zimmerman, E. A., & Kuhn, C. (1988). Infants of depressed mothers show "depressed" behaviour even with nondepressed adults. *Child Development, 59*(6), 1569–1579.

Firth-Cozens, J. (2016). Interventions to improve physicians' well-being and patient care. *Social Science & Medicine, 52*(2), 215–222.

Fleming, A. S., O'Day, D. H., & Kraemer, G. W. (1999). Neurobiology of mother-infant interaction: Experience and central nervous system plasticity across development and generation. *Neuroscience and Biobehavioural Review, 3*(5), 673–685.

Fletcher, R. (2020). Celebrating dads: New dads to be screened for depression. *Australian Men's Health Forum (AMHF).* www.amhf.org.au.

Flook, L., Goldberg, S. B., Pinger, L., & Davidson, R. J. (2015). Promoting prosocial behaviour and self-regulation skills in preschool children through a mindfulness-based kindness curriculum. *Developmental Psychology, 51*(1), 44–51.

Foley, S., & Hughes, C. (2018). Great expectations? Do mothers' and fathers' prenatal thoughts and feelings about the infant predict parent-infant interaction quality? A meta-analytic review. *Developmental Review, 48*, 40–54.

Fonagy, P., Gergely, G., Jurist, E., & Target, M. (2002). *Affect regulation, mentalisation, and the development of self.* Other Press.

Four Arrows, Cajete, G., & Lee, J. (2010). *Critical neurophilosophy and indigenous wisdom.* Sense.

Frazzetto, G. (2013). *How we feel: What neuroscience can and can't tell us about our emotions.* Random House.

Fredrickson, B. L. (2013). *Love 2.0: How our supreme emotion affects everything we feel, think, do, and become.* Hudson Street Press.

Freud, S. (1911/1953–74). *Formulations on the two principles of mental functioning: Vol. 12 of Thestandard edition of the complete psychological works* (J. Strachey, ed. & trans., pp. 213–226). Hogarth.

Fry, D. P. (2006). *The human potential for peace: An anthropological challenge to assumptions about war and violence*. New York: Oxford University Press.

Fry, D. P. (2014). The environment of evolutionary adaptedness, rough-and-tumble play, and the selection of restraint in human aggression. In D. Narvaez, K. Valentino, Fuentes, J. McKenna, & P. Gray (Eds.), *Ancestral landscapes in human evolution: Culture, childrearing, and social wellbeing* (pp. 167–186). Oxford University Press.

Galea, S., Uddin, M., & Koenen, K. (2011). The urban environment and mental disorders: Epigenetic links. *Epigenetics, 6*(4), 400–404.

Gallese, V. (2003). The roots of empathy: The shared manifold hypothesis and the neural basis of intersubjectivity. *Psychopathology, 36*(4), 171–180.

Gallese, V. (2005). Embodied simulation: From neurons to phenomenal experience. *Phenomenology and the Cognitive Sciences, 4*(1), 23–48.

Gallese, V. (2008). Mirror neurons and the social nature of language: The neural exploitation hypothesis. *Social Neuroscience, 3*(3–4), 317–333.

Gerhardt, S. (2014). *Why love matters: How affection shapes a baby's brain* (new ed.). Taylor & Francis Ltd.

Gilbert, P. (2005). Compassion and cruelty: A biopsychosocial approach. In P. Gilbert (Ed.), *Compassion: Conceptualisations, research and use in psychotherapy* (pp. 9–74). Routledge.

Gilbert, P. (2010). *Compassion-focused therapy*. Routledge.

Gilbert, P., & Choden. (2013). *Mindful compassion*. Constable & Robinson.

Gillath, O., Shaver, P. R., & Mikulincer, M. (2005). An attachment-theoretical approach to compassion and altruism. In P. Gilbert (Ed.), *Compassion: Conceptualisation, research and use in psychotherapy* (pp. 121–147). Routledge.

Gitau, R., Menson, E., Pickles, V., Fisk, N. M., Glover, V., & MacLachlan, N. (2001). Umbilical cortisol levels as an indicator of the foetal stress response to assisted vaginal delivery. *European Journal of Obstetrics & Gynaecology and Reproductive Biology, 98*(1), 14–17.

Glover, V. (2014). Maternal depression, anxiety and stress during pregnancy and child outcome; what needs to be done. *Best Practice & Research Clinical Obstetrics & Gynaecology, 28*(1), 25–35.

Glover, V., & O'Connor, T. G. (2006). Maternal anxiety: Its effect on the foetus and the child. *British Journal of Midwifery, 14*(11), 663–667.

Glover, V., O'Connor, T. G., & O'Donnell, K. (2010). Prenatal stress and the programming of the HPA axis. *Neuroscience & Biobehavioural Reviews, 35*(1), 17–22.

Goldberg, E. (2005). *The wisdom paradox*. Gotham Books.

Goldstein, E. D. (2007). Sacred moments: Implications on wellbeing and stress. *Journal of Clinical Psychology, 63*(10), 1001–1019.

Goleman, D. (1995). *Social intelligence: The new science of human relationships*. Arrow.

Goleman, D., & Davidson, R. (2017). *The science of meditation: How to change your brain, mind and body*. Penguin Books.

Goodman, J. H. (2004). Paternal postpartum depression, its relationship to maternal postpartum depression, and implications for family health. *Journal of Advanced Nursing, 45*(1), 26–35.

Goodridge, J. (1999). *Rhythm and timing of movement in performance: Drama, dance and ceremony*. Jessica Kingsley Publishers.

Gow, R. (2021). *Smart foods for ADHD and brain health: How nutrition influences cognitive function, behavior and mood.* Hachette.

Gray, P. (2013). *Free to learn.* Basic Books.

Greenspan, S. I., & Shanker, S. I. (2004). *The first idea.* Da Capo Press.

Groër, M. W. (2005). Differences between exclusive breastfeeding, formula-feeders, and controls: A study of stress, mood, and endocrine variables. *Biological Research for Nursing, 7*(2), 106–107.

Grossman, P., Niemann, L., Schmidt, S., & Walach, H. (2004). Mindfulness-based stress reduction and health benefits: A meta-analysis. *Journal of Psychosomatic Research, 57*(1), 35–43.

Hagen, E. H., & Barret, H. C. (2007). Perinatal sadness among Shuar women: Support for an evolutionary theory of psychic pain. *Medical Anthropological Quarterly, 21*(1), 22–40.

Hall, H., Beattie, J., Lau, R., East, C., & Biro, M. (2015). The effectiveness of mindfulness training on perinatal mental health; a systematic review. *Women and Birth, 29*(1), 62–71.

Halligan, S. L., Murray, L., Martins, C., & Cooper, P. J. (2007). Maternal depression and psychiatric outcomes in adolescent offspring: A 13-year longitudinal study. *Journal of Affective Disorders, 97*(1–3), 145–154.

Hanington, L., Heron, J., Stein, A., & Ramchandani, P. (2011). Parental depression and child outcomes – is marital conflict the missing link? *Child Care and Health Development, 37*(4), 549–609.

Hardin, J. S., Jones, N. A., Mize, K. D., & Platt, M. (2002). Parent-training with kangaroo care impacts infant neurophysiological development and mother-infant neuroendocrine activity. *Infant Behaviour and Development, 58.* https://doi.org/10.1016/j.infbeh.2019.101416

Harries, V., & Brown, A. (2017). The association between use of infant parenting books that promote strict routines, and maternal depression, self-efficacy, and parenting confidence. *Early Child Development and Care, 189*(8), 1339–1350.

Heidegger, M. (1972). *Being and time.* Harper & Row.

Henderson, J. J., Evans, S. F., Straton, J. A., Priest, S. R., & Hagan, R. (2003). Impact of postnatal depression on breastfeeding duration. *Birth, 30*(3), 175–180.

Hepper, P. G. (1991). An examination of foetal learning before and after birth. *The Irish Journal of Psychology, 12*(2), 95–107.

Hepper, P. G., & Shahidullah, B. S. (1994). The development of foetal hearing. *Foetal and Maternal Medicine Review, 6*(3), 167–179.

Hibbeln, J. R., Davis, J. M., & Steer, C. (2007). Maternal seafood consumption in pregnancy and neurodevelopmental outcomes in childhood (ALSPAC study): An observational cohort study. *Lancet, 369,* 578–585.

Hoekzema, E., Barba-Muller, E., Pozzobon, C., Picado, M., Florencio, L., Garcia-Garcia, D., Soliva, J. C., Tobeña, A., Desco, M., Crone, E. A., Ballesteros, A., Carmona, S., & Vilarroya, O. (2017). Pregnancy leads to long-lasting changes in human brain structure. *Nature Neuroscience, 20*(2), 287–296.

Hofmann, S. G., Grossman, P., & Hinton, D. (2011). Loving-kindness and compassion meditation: Potential for psychological interventions. *Clinical Psychology Review, 31*(7), 1126–1132.

Hoge, E. A., Chen, M. M., Orr, E., Metcalf, C. A., Fischer, L. E., Pollack, M. H., De Vivo, I., & Simon, N. M. (2013). Loving-kindness meditation practice associated with longer telomeres in women. *Brain, Behaviour, and Immunity, 32,* 159–163.

Houston, S. (1989). National aboriginal health strategy working party. *Aboriginal and Islander Health Worker Journal, 13*(4), 7–8.

Hrdy, S. B. (2011). *Mothers and others: The evolutionary origins of mutual understanding.* Belknap Press.

Husserl, E. (1989). *Ideas pertaining to a pure phenomenology and to a phenomenological philosophy: Second book* (R. Rojcewicz & A. Schuwer, trans.). Kluwer Academic.

Ingold, T. (1999). On the social relations of the hunter-gatherer band. In R. B. Lee & R. Daly (Eds.), *The Cambridge encyclopaedia of hunters and gatherers* (pp. 399–410). Cambridge University Press.

Ingold, T. (2011). *The perception of the environment: Essay on livelihood, dwelling and skill.* Routledge.

Irons, C., Gilbert, P., Baldwin, M. W., Baccus, J. R., & Palmer, M. (2006). Parental recall, attachment relating and self-attacking/self-reassurance: Their relationship with depression. *British Journal of Clinical Psychology, 45*(3), 297–308.

Jacobs, T. L., Epel, E. S., Lin, J., Blackburn, E. H., Wolkowitz, O. M., Bridwell, D. A., Zanesco, A. P., Aichele, S. R., Sahdra, B. K. MacLean, K. A., King, B. G., Shaver, P. R., Rosenberg, E. L., Ferrer, E., Wallace, B. A., & Saron, C. D. (2011). Intensive meditation training, immune cell telomerase activity, and psychological mediators. *Psychoneuroendocrinology, 36*(5), 664–681.

Janus, L. (2001). *The enduring effects of prenatal experience: Echoes from the womb.* Heidelberg Mattes.

Jensen, S. K. G., & Nelson, C. A. (2017). Biological embedding of childhood adversity: From physiological mechanisms to clinical implications. *Biomed Central (BMC) Medicine, 15*(1), 135.

Jevning, R., Wilson, A. F., & VanderLaan, E. F. (1978). Plasma prolactin and growth hormone during meditation. *Psychosomatic Medicine, 40*(4), 329–333.

Jung, C. G. (1967). *The I Ching or book of changes* (C. F. Baynes, trans.) Princeton University Press.

Kabat-Zinn, J. (1990). *Full catastrophe living: Using the wisdom of your body and mind to face stress, pain, and illness.* Delta.

Kabat-Zinn, J. (2003a). Mindfulness-based interventions in context: Past, present, and future. *Clinical Psychology: Science and Practice, 10*(2), 144–156.

Kabat-Zinn, J. (2003b). *Coming to our senses: Healing ourselves and the world through mindfulness.* Hyperion Press.

Kabat-Zinn, J., & Kabat-Zinn, M. (1990). *Everyday blessings: The inner work of mindful parenting.* Hyperion Press.

Kaplan, R., & Kaplan, S. (1989). *The experience of nature: A psychological perspective.* Cambridge University Press.

Kashdan, T. B., & Rottenberg, J. (2010). Psychological flexibility as a fundamental aspect of health. *Clinical Psychology Review, 30*(7), 865–878.

Kaufman, J., Plotsky, P. M., Nemeroff, C. B., & Charney, D. S. (2000). Effects of early adverse experiences on brain structure and function: Clinical implications. *Biological Psychiatry, 48*, 778–790.

Keag, O. E., Norman, J. E., & Stock, S. J. (2018). Long-term risks and benefits associated with caesarean delivery for mother, baby, and subsequent pregnancies: Systematic review and meta-analysis. *PLoS Medicine, 15*(1). https://doi.org/10.1371/journal.pmed.1002494.

Kearns, A., Beaty, M., & Barnett, G. (2007). A social-ecological perspective on health in urban environments. *NSW Public Health Bulletin, 18*(3–4), 48–50.

Keltner, D., Kogan, A., Piff, P. K., & Saturn, S. R. (2014). The sociocultural apprais-als, values, and emotions (SAVE) framework of prosociality: Core processes from gene to meme. *Annual Review of Psychology, 65*, 425–460.

Kennel, J., Klaus, M., McGrath, S., Robertson, S., & Hinkley, C. (1991). Continuous emotional support during labour in a US hospital: A randomized controlled trial. *JAMA, 17*, 2197–2201.

Kenny, M. A., & Williams, J. M. G. (2007). Treatment-resistant depressed patients show a good response to mindfulness-based cognitive therapy. *Behaviour Research and Therapy, 45*(3), 617–625.

Khashan, A. S., McNamee, R., Abel, K. M., Mortensen, P. B., Kenny, L. C., Pedersen, M. G., Webb, R. T., & Baker, P. N. (2009). Rates of preterm birth following ante-natal maternal exposure to severe life events: A population-based cohort study. *Human Reproduction, 24*(2), 429–437.

Kimmerer, R. W. (2013). The fortress, the river and the garden: A new metaphor for cultivating mutualistic relationship between scientific and traditional ecological knowledge. In A. Kulnieks, D. Rononhiakewen Longboat, & K. Young (Eds.), *Contemporary studies in environmental and indigenous pedagogies: A curriculum of stories and place*. Sense Publishers.

Kinney, D. K., Munir, K. M., Crowley, D. J., & Miller, A. M. (2008). Prenatal stress and the risk of autism. *Neuroscience & Biobehavioural Reviewers, 32*(8), 1519–1532.

Kisilevsky, B. S., Hains, S. M., Lee, K., Xie, X., Huang, H., Ye, H. H., Zhang, K., & Wang, Z. (2003). Effects of experience on foetal voice recognition. *Psychological Science, 13*(3), 220–224.

Klimecki, O. M., Leiberg, S., Lamm, C., & Singer, T. (2013). Functional neural plas-ticity and associated changes in positive affect after compassion training. *Cerebral Cortex, 23*(7), 1552–1561.

Klimecki, O. M., Leiberg, S., Ricard, M., & Singer, T. (2014). Differential pattern of functional brain plasticity after compassion and empathy training. *Social Cognitive and Affective Neuroscience, 9*(6), 873–879.

Kochanska, G. (2002). Mutually responsive orientation between mothers and their young children: A context for the early development of conscience. *Current Directions in Psychological Science, 11*(6), 191–195.

Kohn, E. (2013). *How forests think: Toward and anthropology beyond the human*. University of California Press.

Kok, B. E., Coffey, K. A., Cohn, M. A., Catalino, L. I., Vacharkulksemsuk, T., Algoe, S. B., Brantly, M., & Fredickson, B. L. (2013). How positive emotions build physical health: Perceived positive social connections account for the upward spiral between positive emotions and vagal tone. *Psychological Science, 24*(7), 1123–1132.

Kok, B. E., & Fredrickson, B. L. (2010). Upward spirals of the heart: Autonomic flexibility, as indexed by vagal tone, reciprocally and prospectively predicts positive emotions and social connectedness. *Biological Psychology, 85*(3), 432–436.

Konner, M. (2005). Hunter-gatherer infancy and childhood: The !Kung and others. In B. Hewlett & M. Lamb (Eds.), *Hunter-gatherer childhood: Evolutionary, developmental and cultural perspectives* (pp. 19–64) Aldine, Transaction.

Konner, M. (2010). *The evolution of childhood: Relationships, emotions, mind*. Harvard University Press.

Kumar, S. (2002). *You are therefore I am: A declaration of dependence*. Green Books.

Kupperman, J. (2005). Morality, ethics, and wisdom. In R. J. Stemberg & J. Jordan (Eds.), *A handbook of wisdom: Psychological perspectives* (pp. 245–271). Cambridge University Press.

Kupperman, J. J. (2010). *Theories of human nature.* Hackett.

Ladd, C. O., Owens, M. J., & Nemeroff, C. B. (1996). Persistent changes in corticotropin-releasing factor neuronal systems induced by maternal deprivation. *Endocrinology, 137*(4), 1212–1218.

Laing, R. D. (1976). *The facts of life.* Pantheon.

Lake, F. (1979). *Studies in constricted confusion: Exploration of a pre- and postnatal paradigm.* Clinical Theology Association.

Latour, B. (2013). *Modes of existence.* Harvard University Press.

Lavretsky, H., Epel, E. S., Siddarth, P., Nazarian, N., St. Cyr, N., Khalsa, D. S., Lin, J., Blackburn, E., & Irwin, M. R. (2013). A pilot study of yogic meditation for family dementia caregivers with depressive symptoms: Effects on mental health, cognition, and telomerase activity. *International Journal of Geriatric Psychiatry, 28*(1), 57–65.

Laxton-Kane, M., & Slade, P. (2002). The role of maternal prenatal attachment in a woman's experience of pregnancy and implications for the process of care. *Journal of Reproductive and Infant Psychology, 20*(4), 253–266.

Lazar, S. W. (2006). *Mind-body connection: Neural correlates of respiration during meditation.* Presented at Mind and Life Summer Research Institute, Garrison.

Lazar, S. W., Bush, G., Golb, R. L., Fricchione, G. L., Khalsa, G., & Benson, H. (2000). Functional brain mapping of the relaxation response and meditation. *Neuroreport, 11*, 1581–1585.

Lecanuet, J. P., Granier-Deferre, C., Jacquet, A. Y., & DeCasper, A. J. (2000). Foetal discrimination of low-pitched musical notes. *Developmental Psychobiology, 36*(1), 29–39.

LeDoux, J. E. (1993). Emotional networks in the brain. In M. Lewis & J. M. Haviland (Eds.), *Handbook of emotions* (pp. 109–118). The Guilford Press.

Lewis, M. D. (2005). Bridging emotions theory and neurobiology through dynamic systems modelling. *Behaviour and Brain Sciences, 28*, 169–194.

Lewis, M. W. (2008). The interactional model of maternal-foetal attachment: An empirical Analysis. *The Journal of Prenatal and Perinatal Psychology and Health, 23*(1), 49–65.

Lewis, T., Amini, F., & Lannon, R. (2000). *A general theory of love.* Vintage.

Lieberman, M. D. (2013). *Social: Why our brains are wired to connect.* Oxford University Press.

Liedloff, J. (1986). *The continuum concept.* Penguin Books.

Lipton, B. H. (2015). *The biology of belief: Unleashing the power of consciousness, matter and miracle.* Hay House.

Longe, O., Maratos, F. A., Gilbert, P., Evans, G., Volker, F., Rockliff, H., & Rippon, G. (2010). Having a word with yourself: Neural correlates of self-criticism and self-reassurance *NeuroImage, 49*(2), 1849–1856.

Luby, J. L., Barch, D. M., Belden, A., Gaffrey, M. S., Tillman, R., Babb, C., Nishino, T., Suzuki, H., & Botteron, K. N. (2012). Maternal support in early childhood predicts larger hippocampal volumes at school age. *Proceedings of the National Academy of Sciences, 109*(8), 2854–2859.

Luders, E., Thompson, P. M., Kurth, F., Hong, J., Phillips, O. R., Wang, Y., Gutman, B. A., Chou, Y. Y., Narr, K. L., & Toga, A. W. (2013). Global and regional alterations of hippocampal anatomy in long-term meditation practitioners. *Human Brain Mapping, 34*(12), 3369–3375.

Luke 1: 41. *Mary visits Elisabeth.* Bible. Biblica.

Luke 17:21. (1973, 1978, 1984, 2011). *Holy Bible* (new international version). Biblica.

Lumey, L. H., Stein, A. D., Kahn, H. S., van der Pal-de Bruin, K. M., Blauw, G. J., Zybert, P. A., & Susser, E. S. (2007). Cohort profile: The Dutch hunger Winter families study. *International Journal of Epidemiology, 36*(6), 1196–1204.

Lupien, S. J., McEwen, B. S., Gunnar, M. R., & Heim, C. (2009). Effects of stress throughout the lifespan on the brain, behaviour and cognition. *Nature Reviews Neuroscience, 10*(6), 434–445.

Lutz, A., Brefczynski-Lewis, J., Johnstone, T., & Davidson, R. J. (2008). Regulation of the Neural circuitry of emotion by compassion meditation: Effects of meditative expertise. *PloS One, 3*(3).

MacLean, P. D. (1990). *The triune brain in evolution: Role in paleocerebral functions.* Plenum.

MacMurray, J. (1992/1962). *Reason and emotion.* Humanity Books.

Magnavita, J. J. (2006). Emotion in short-term psychotherapy: An introduction. *Journal of Clinical Psychology, 62*(5), 517–522.

Maidan, A., & Farwell, E. (1997). *The Tibetan art of parenting: From before conception through early childhood.* Wisdom.

Maina, G., Saracco, P., Giolito, MR, Danelon, D., Bogetto, F., & Todros, T. (2008). Impact of maternal psychological distress on foetal weight, prematurity and intra-uterine growth retardation. *Journal of Affective Disorders, 111*(2–3), 214–220.

Malinowski, P. (2013). Neural mechanisms of attentional control in mindfulness meditation. *Frontiers of Neuroscience,* 7–8. https://doi.org/10.3389/fnins.2013.00008

Marion, W. G. (2000). *Productive men, reproductive women: The agrarian household and the emergence of separate spheres during the German enlightenment.* Berghahn Books.

Martin, C. L. (1999). *The way of human beings.* Yale University Press.

Mason, Z. S., Briggs, R. D., & Silver, E. J. (2011). Maternal attachment feelings mediate between maternal reports of depression, infant social-emotional development, and parenting stress. *Journal of Reproductive and Infant Psychology, 29*(4), 382–394.

Mate, G. (2003). *When the body says no: The cost of hidden stress.* Vintage.

Matousek, R. H., Dobkin, P. L., & Pruessner, J. (2010). Cortisol as a marker for improvement in mindfulness-based stress reduction. *Complementary Therapies in Clinical Practice, 16*(1), 13–19.

McCann, W. J., Marion, G. S., Davis, S. W., Crandall, S. J., & Hildebrandt, C. A. (2013). Applied relaxation and applied mindfulness (ARAM): A practical and engaging approach for mind-body regulation training in medical education. *Annals of Behavioural Science and Medical Education, 19*(2), 10–15.

McCraty, R. (2004). The energetic heart: Bioelectromagnetic communication within and between people. In P. J. Rosch & M. S. Markov (Eds.), *Bioelectromagnetic medicine* (pp. 541–562). Marcel Dekker.

McCraty, R. (2015). *The energetic heart: Biomagnetic communication within and between people, in bioelectromagnetic and subtle energy medicine* (P. J. Rosch, ed., 2nd ed.). Institute of HeartMath.

McCraty, R., Atkinson, M., Tiller, W. A., Rein, G., & Watkins, A. D. (1995). The effects of emotions on short–term power spectrum analysis of heart rate variability. *The American Journal of Cardiology, 76*(14), 1089–1093.

McCraty, R., Atkinson, M., Tomasino, D., & Bradley, R. T. (2009). The coherent heart: Heart-brain interactions, psychophysiological coherence, and the emergence of system-wide order. *Integral Review, 5*(2), 10–115.

McCraty, R., & Childre, D. (2010). Coherence: Bridging personal, social and global health. *Alternative Therapies in Health and Medicine, 16*(4), 10–24.

McCrea, S. M. (2010). Intuition, insight, and the right hemisphere: Emergence of higher sociocognitive functions. *Psychological Research and Behaviour Management, 3*, 1–39.

McDonnell, C. G., & Valentino, K. (2016). Intergenerational effects of childhood trauma: Evaluating pathways among maternal ACEs, perinatal depressive symptoms, and infant outcomes. *Child Maltreatment, 21*(4), 317–326.

McEwen, B. S. (1999). Stress and hippocampal plasticity. *Annual Review of Neuroscience, 22*(1), 105–122.

McFarland, J., Salisbury, A. L., Battle, C. L., Hawes, K., Halloran, K., & Lester, B. M. (2011). Major depressive disorder during pregnancy and emotional attachment to the foetus. *Archives of Women's Mental Health, 14*(5), 425–434.

McGilchrist, I. (2009). *The master and his emissary: The divided brain and the making of the Western world.* Yale University Press.

McGowan, P. O., Sasaki, A., Huang, T. C. T., Unterberger, A., Suderman, M., Emst, C., & Szyf, M. (2008). Promoter-wide hypermethylation of the riboxomal RNA gene promoter in the suicide brain. *PLoS One, 3*(5), 2085.

McKenna, J. J. (2008). Cosleeping and biological imperatives: Why human babies do not and should not sleep alone. *Neuroanthropology.* https://neuroanthropology.net/2008/12/21/cosleeping-and-biological-imperatives-why-human-babies-do-not-and-should-not-sleep-alone/

McKenna, J. J., & Bernshaw, N. J. (2017). Breastfeeding and infant-parent co-sleeping as adaptive strategies: Are they protective against SIDS? *Breastfeeding*, 265–304.

McKenna, J. J., Mosko, S., Richard, C., Drummond, L. H., Cetel, M. B., & Arpaia, J. (1994). Experimental studies of infant-parent co-sleeping: Mutual physiological and behavioural influences and their relevance to SIDS (sudden infant death syndrome). *Early Human Development, 38*(3), 187–201.

Meaney, M. J. (2010). Epigenetics and the biological definition of gene X environment interactions. *Child Development, 81*(1), 41–79.

Mehling, W. E., Acree, M., Steward, A., Silas, J., & Jones, A. (2018). *The multidimensional assessment of interoceptive awareness, version 2 (MAIA-2).* www.osher.ucsf.edu/maia

Meins, E., Fernyhough, C., Wainwright, R., Gupta, M. D., Fradley, E., & Tuckey, M. (2002). Maternal mind-mindeness and attachment security as predictors of theory of mind understanding. *Child Development, 73*(6), 1715–1726.

Melzack, R. (1965). Pain mechanisms: A new theory. *Science, 150*, 971–979.

Mental Health Taskforce. (2016). *NHS report: Implementing the five year forward view for mental health.* Mental Health Taskforce.

Meschino, D., Philipp, D., Israel, A., & Vigod, S. (2016). Maternal-infant mental health: Postpartum group intervention. *Archives of Women Mental Health, 19*(2), 243–251.

Mezzacappa, E. S., Kelsey, R. M., & Katkin, E. S. (2005). Breastfeeding, bottle feeding, and maternal autonomic responses to stress. *Journal of Psychosomatic Research, 58*(4), 351–365.

Mikulincer, M., & Shaver, P. R. (2007). *Attachment in adulthood. Structure, dynamics, and change.* The Guilford Press.

Milgrom, J., Ericksen, J., McCarthy, R., & Gemmill, A. W. (2006). Stressful impact of depression on early mother-infant relations. *Stress and Health: Journal of the International Society for the Investigation of Stress, 22*(4), 229–238.

Miller, L. J. (2002). Postpartum depression. *JAMA, 287*(6), 762–765.

Misri, S., Eng, A. B., Abizadeh, J., Blackwell, E., Spidel, A., & Oberlander, T. F. (2013). Factor impacting decisions to decline or adhere to antidepressant medication in perinatal women with mood and anxiety disorders. *Depression and Anxiety, 30*(11), 1129–1136.

Mohllajee, A. P., Curtis, K. M., Morrow, B., & Marchbanks, P. A. (2007). Pregnancy intention and its relationship to birth and maternal outcomes. *Obstetric Gynaecology, 109*(3), 678–686.

Monk, C., Spicer, J., & Champagne, F. A. (2012). Linking prenatal maternal adversity to developmental outcomes in infants: The role of epigenetic pathways. *Development and Psychopathology, 24*(4), 1361–1376.

Montagu, A. (1986). *Touching: The human significance of the skin.* Harper & Row.

Moore, S. R., McEwen, L. M., Quirt, J., Morin, A., Mah, S. M., Barr, R. G., Boyce, T., & Kobor, M. S. (2017). Epigenetic correlates of neonatal contact in humans. *Development and Psychopathology, 29*(5), 1517–1538.

Morin, E. (1992). From the concept of system to the paradigm of complexity. *Journal of Social and Evolutionary Systems, 15*(4), 371–385.

Murray, L., Arteche, A., Fearon, P., Halligan, S., Croudace, T., & Cooper, P. (2010). The effects of maternal postnatal depression and child sex on academic performance at age 16 years: A developmental approach. *Journal of Child Psychology and Psychiatry, 51*(10), 1150–1159.

Murray, L., Fiori-Cowley, A., & Cooper, P. (1996). The impact of postnatal depression and associated adversity on early mother-infant interactions and later infant outcomes. *Child Development, 67*(5), 2512–2526.

Murray, L., Kempton, C., Woolgar, M., & Hooper, R. (1993). Depressed mothers' speech to their infants and its relation to infant gender and cognitive development. *Journal of Child Psychology and Psychiatry and Allied Disciplines, 34*(7), 1083–1101.

Murray, L., Sinclair, D., Cooper, P., Ducournau, P., Turner, P., & Stein, A. (1999). The socioemotional development of 5-year-old children of postnatally depressed mothers. *The Journal of Child Psychology and Psychiatry and Allied Disciplines, 40*(8), 1259–1271.

Musser, A. K., Ahmed, A. H., Foli, K. J., & Coddington, J. A. (2013). Paternal postpartum depression: What healthcare providers should know. *Journal of Paediatric Care, 27*(6), 479–485.

Narvaez, D. (2012). Moral neuroeducation from early life through the lifespan. *Neuroethics, 5*(2), 145–157.

Narvaez, D. (2013). Development and socialization within an evolutionary context: Growing up to become "a good and useful human being". In D. Fry (Ed.), *War, peace and human human nature: The convergence of evolutionary and cultural views* (pp. 341–358). Oxford University Press.

Narvaez, D. (2014). *Neurobiology and the development of human morality: Evolution, culture, and wisdom.* W. W. Norton & Company.

Narvaez, D., & Gleason, T. (2013). Developmental optimization. In D. Narvaez, J. Panksepp, Schore, & T. Gleason (Eds.), *Evolution, early experience and human development: From research to practice and policy* (pp. 307–325). Oxford University Press.

Narvaez, D., Gleason, T., Wang, L., Brooks, J., Lefever, J., Cheng, A., & Centres for the Prevention of Child Neglect. (2013). The evolved developmental Niche: Longitudinal effects of caregiving practices on early childhood psychosocial development. *Early Childhood Research Quarterly, 28*(4), 759–773.

Nath, S., Ryan, E. G., Trevillion, K., Bick, D., Demilew, J., Milgrom, J., Pickles, A., & Howard, L. M. (2018). Prevalence and identification of anxiety disorders in pregnancy: The diagnostic accuracy of the two-item generalised anxiety disorder scale (GAD-2). *BMJ Open, 8*(9), e023766

National Institute of Child Health and Human Development, Early Child Care Research Network. (2004). Affect dysregulation in the mother-child relationship in the toddler years: Antecedents and consequences. *Developmental Psychopathology, 16*(1), 43–68.

Neff, K. D. (2015). The self-compassion scale is a valid and theoretically coherent measure of self-compassion. *Mindfulness.* Advanced online publication. https://doi.org/10.1007/s12671-015-0479-3

Neff, K. D., & Germer, C. K. (2013). A pilot study and randomised controlled trial of the Mindful self-compassion program. *Journal of Clinical Psychology, 69*(1), 28–44.

Neff, K. D., & McGehee, P. (2010). Self-compassion and psychological resilience among adolescents andyoung adults. *Self and Identity, 9*(3), 225–240.

Neff, K. D., & Seppälä, E. (2016). Compassion, well-being, and the hypo-egoic self. *Oxford Handbook of Hypo-Egoic Phenomena,* 189–202.

Neff, K. D., & Tirch, D. (2013). Self-compassion and ACT. In T. B. Kashdan & J. Ciarrochi (Eds.), *Mindfulness, acceptance, and positive psychology: The seven foundations of well- being* (pp. 78–106). Context Press, New Harbinger.

Negayama, K., Delafield-Butt, J., Momose, K., & Ishijima, K., Kawahara, Lux, E. J., Murphy, A., & Kaliarntas, K. (2015). Embodied intersubjective engagement in mother-infant tactile communication: A cross- cultural study of Japanese and Scottish mother-infant behaviours during infant pick-up. *Frontiers in Psychology, 6,* 1–13.

Nickel, C., Lahmann, C., Muehlbacher, M., Pedrosa, G. F., Kaplan, P., Buschmann, W., Tritt, K., Kettler, C., Bachler, E., Egger, C., Anvar, J., Fartacek, R., Loew, T., Rother, W., & Nickel, M. (2006). Muscle relaxation: A randomized, prospective, controlled trial. *Psychotherapy and Psychosomatics, 75,* 237–243.

Novak, M. (2004). Foetal-maternal interactions: Prenatal psychobiological precursors to adaptive infant development. *Current Topics in Developmental Biology, 59,* 37–60.

Oates, M. (2003). Perinatal psychiatric disorders: A leading cause of maternal morbidity and mortality. *British Medical Bulletin, 67*(1), 219–229.

O'Campo, P., Faden, R. R., Gielen, A. C., & Wang, M. C. (1992). Prenatal factors associated with breastfeeding duration: Recommendations for prenatal interventions. *Birth, 19*(4), 195–201.

O'Connor, T. G., Heron, J., Glover, V., & Alspac Study Team. (2002). Antenatal anxiety predicts child behavioral/emotional problems independently of postnatal depression. *Journal of the American Academy of Child & Adolescent Psychiatry, 41*(12), 1470–1477.

Odent, M. (2015). *Do we need midwives?* Pinter & Martin.

O'Donnell, K., O'Connor, T. G., & Glover, V. (2009). Prenatal stress and neurodevelopment of the child: Focus on the HPA axis and the role of the placenta. *Developmental Neuroscience, 31*(4), 285–292.

O'Donohue, J. (2005). *Beauty, the invisible embrace: Rediscovering the true sources of compassion, serenity, and hope*. Perennial.

O'Donohue, J., & Siegel, D. J. (2006, October). *Awakening the mind*. MindsightInstitute.com, Mindsight Institute Audio Recordings.

O'Hara, M. W., & Swain, A. M. (1996). Rate and risk of postpartum depression: A meta-analysis. *International Review of Psychiatry, 8*, 37–54.

Olds, D. L. (2002). Prenatal and infancy home visiting by nurses: From randomised trials to community replication. *Prevention Science, 3*(3), 153–172.

Olds, D. L. (2007). Preventing crime with prenatal and infancy support of parents: The nurse-family partnership. *Victims and Offenders, 2*(2), 205–225.

Olds, D. L., Henderson, C. R., Tatelbaum, R., & Chamberlin, R. (1986). Improving the delivery of prenatal care and outcomes of pregnancy: A randomized trial of nurse home visitation. *Paediatrics, 77*(1), 16–28.

Olds, D. L., Sadler, L., & Kitzman, H. (2007). Programs for parents of infants and toddlers: Recent evidence from randomized trials. *Journal of Child Psychology and Psychiatry, 48*, 355–391.

Oliver, M. (2005, December 29). George Gerbner, 86: Educator researched the influence of TV viewing on perceptions. *Los Angeles Times*.

Ordway, M. R., Webb, D., & Slade, A. (2015). Parental reflective functioning: An approach to enhancing parent-child relationship in paediatric primary care. *Journal of Paediatric Health Care: Official Publication of National Association of Paediatric Nurse Associations & Practitioners, 29*(4), 325–334.

Orlinsky, D. E., & Howard, K. I. (1986). Process and outcome in psychotherapy. In S. L. Garfield & A. E. Bergin (Eds.), *Handbook of psychotherapy and behaviour change* (pp. 311–381). Wiley.

Panksepp, J. (1991). Affective neuroscience: A conceptual framework for the neurobiological study of emotions. In K. Strongman (Ed.), *International reviews of studies in emotions* (vol. 1, pp. 59–99). Wiley.

Panksepp, J. (1998). *Affective neuroscience: The foundations of human and animal emotions*. Oxford University Press.

Panksepp, J., & Northoff, G. (2009). The trans-species core SELF: The emergence of active cultural and neuro-ecological agents through self-related processing within subcortical-cortical midline networks. *Consciousness and Cognition, 18*, 193–215.

Papousek, H., & Papousek, M. (1992). Beyond emotional bonding: The role of pre-verbal communication in mental growth and health. *Infant Mental Health Journal, 13*(1), 43–53.

Parer, J. T., & King, T. (2000). Foetal heart rate monitoring: Is it salvageable? *American Journal of Obstetrics and Gynaecology, 182*(4), 982–987.

Paris, R., Spielman, E., & Bolton, R. E. (2009). Mother-infant psychotherapy: Examining the therapeutic process of change. *Infant Mental Health Journal, 30*(3), 301–319.

Partanen, E., Kujala, T., Tervaniemi, M., & Huotilainen, M. (2013). Prenatal music exposure induces long-term neural effects. *PloS One, 8*(10), e78946.

Persico, G. (2002). *La ninna nanna: Dall'abbraccio materno alla psicofisiologia della relazione umana*. Gli Incontri.

Persico, G., Antolini, L., Vergani, P., Costantini, W., Nardi, M. T., & Bellotti, L. (2017). Maternal singing of lullabies during pregnancy and after birth: Effects on mother-infant bonding and on newborns' behaviour. Concurrent cohort study. *Women and Birth, 30*(4), e214–e220.

Pert, C. B. (1997). *Molecules of emotion: Why you feel the way you feel.* Simon and Schuster.

Phillips, A. (1998). *The beast in the nursery.* Vintage Books.

Piaget, J. (1954). *The construction of reality in the child.* Basic Books.

Pinto-Gouveia, J., Duarte, C., Marcela, M., & Fráguas, S. (2014). The protective role of self-compassion in relation to psychopathology symptoms and quality of life in chronic and in cancer patients. *Clinical Psychology & Psychotherapy, 21*(4), 311–323.

Piontelli, A. (1992). *From foetus to child.* Routledge.

Piontelli, A. (2002). *Twins: From foetus to child.* Routledge.

Piontelli, A. (2010). *Development of normal foetal movements: The first 25 weeks of gestation.* Springer-Verlag.

Porges, S. W. (1998). Love: An emergent property of the mammalian autonomic nervous system. *Psychoneuroendocrinology, 23*(8), 837–861.

Porges, S. W. (2011). *The polyvagal theory: Neurophysiological foundations of emotions, attachment, communication, self-regulation.* W. W. Norton & Company.

Previc, F. (2009). *The dopaminergic mind in human evolution and history.* Cambridge University Press.

Priel, B., & Besser, A. (2002). Perceptions of early relationships during the transition to motherhood: The mediating role of social support. *Infant Mental Health Journal, 23*(4), 343–360.

Provine, R. R. (2001). *Laughter: A scientific investigation.* Penguin Press.

Pulley, L. V., Klerman, L. V., Tang, H., & Baker, B. A. (2002). The extent of pregnancy mistiming and its association with maternal characteristics and behaviours and pregnancy outcomes. *Perspective on Sexual and Reproductive Health, 34*(4), 206–211.

Queensland Health. (2014). *Queensland centre for perinatal and infant mental health.* Retrieved November 10, 2015, from https://www.health.qld.gov.au/qcpimh/pimh.asp

Raffai, J. (1998). Mother-child bonding-analysis in the prenatal realm: The strange events of a queer world. *International Journal of Prenatal and Perinatal Psychology and Medicine, 10*(2), 163–173.

Ramchandani, P. G., O'Connor, T. G., Evans, J., Heron, J., Murray, L., & Stein, A. (2008a). The effects of pre- and postnatal depression in fathers: A natural experiment comparing the effects of exposure to depression on offspring. *Journal of Child Psychology and Psychiatry, 49*(10), 1069–1078.

Ramchandani, P. G., Stein, A., O'Connor, T., Heron, J., Murray, L., & Evans, J. (2008b). Depression in men in the postnatal period and later child psychopathology: A population cohort study. *Journal of American Academy of Child Adolescent Psychiatry, 47*(4), 390–398.

Reid, V. M., Dunn, K., Young, R. J., Amu, J., Donovan, T., & Reissland, N. (2017). The human foetus preferentially engages with face-like visual stimuli. *Current Biology, 27*(12), 1825–1828.

Reissland, N., Francis, B., Kumarendran, K., & Mason, J. (2015). Ultrasound observations of subtle movements: A pilot study comparing foetuses of smoking and non-smoking mothers. *Acta Paediatrica, 104*(6), 596–603.

Ricard, M. (2015). *Altruism: The power of compassion to change itself and the world.* Atlantic Books.

Rich-Edwards, J. W., Kleinman, K., Abrams, A., Harlow, B. L., McLaughlin, T. J., Joffe, H., & Gillman, M. W. (2006). Sociodemographic predictors of antenatal and postpartum depressive symptoms among women in a medical group practice. *Journal of Epidemiological Community Health, 60*(3), 221–227.

Richens, Y., Hindley, C., & Lavender, T. (2015). A national online survey of UK maternity unit service provision for women with fear of birth. *British Journal of Midwifery, 23*(8), 574–579.

Righetti, P. L. (1996). The emotional experience of the foetus: A preliminary report. *Pre- and Perinatal Psychology Journal, 11*(1), 55–65.

Rizzolatti, G., & Craighero, L. (2004). The mirron-neuron system. *Annual Review of Neuroscience, 27*, 169–192.

Rohr, R. (2011). *Falling upward: A spirituality for the two halves of life.* Jossey-Bass.

Roozendaal, B., McEwen, B. S., & Chattarji, S. (2009). Stress, memory and the amygdala. *Nature Reviews Neuroscience, 10*(6), 423–433.

Røsand, G, B., Slinning, K., Eberhard-Gran, M., Røysamb, E., & Tambs, K. (2012). The buffering effect of relationship satisfaction on emotional distress in couples. *BMC Public Health, 12*(1), 66.

Rubin, R. (1976). Maternal tasks in pregnancy. *Journal of Advanced Nursing, 1*(5), 367–376.

Ruggieri, V. (1991). On the hypothesized physiological correspondence between perceptual and imaginary processes. *Perceptual and Motor Skills, 73*(3), 827–830.

Ruggieri, V. (2001). *L' identita' in psicologia e teatro. Analisi psicofisiologica della struttura dell' io.* Magi Edizioni.

Ryle, G. (1949). *The concept of mind.* University of Chicago Press.

Sabel, V. (2012). *The blossom method: The revolutionary way to communicate with your baby from birth.* Vermilion.

Sable, M. R. (1999). Pregnancy intentions may not be a useful measure for research on maternal and child health outcomes. *Perspectives on Sexual and Reproductive Health, 31*(5), 249–250.

Saeed, G., Fakhar, S., Imran, T., & Abbas, L. K. (2011). The effect of modes of delivery on infants' feeding practices. *Iranian Journal of Medical Sciences, 36*(2), 128–132.

Sandman, C. A., & Davis, E. P. (2012). Neurobehavioral risk is associated with gestational exposure to stress hormones. *Expert Review of Endocrinology & Metabolism, 7*(4), 445–459.

Sandman, C. A., Davis, E. P., Buss, C., & Glynn, L. M. (2012). Exposure to prenatal psychobiological stress exerts programming influences on the mother and her foetus. *Neuroendocrinology, 95*(1), 8–21.

Sansone, A. (2004). *Mothers, babies, and their body language.* Routledge.

Sansone, A. (2007). *Working with parents and infants: A mind-body integration approach.* Routledge.

Sansone, A. (2014). Caesarian birth: Disrupting the human adaptive system. *International Journal of Prenatal and Perinatal Psychology and Medicine, 26*(1–2), 15–31.

Sansone, A. (2018a). When the breast says no. The missing link: A case study. *Journal of Prenatal & Perinatal Psychology & Health, 32*(4), 318–338.

Sansone, A. (2018b). Gems of primal wisdom: From before conception through pregnancy, birth and beyond. A visit to the Himba. *Wissenschaft and Erfahrungseisheit in der ISPPM*, 72–80.

Santarnecchi, E., D'Arista, S., Egiziano, E., Gardi, C., Petrosino, R., Vatti, G., Reda, A., & Rossi, A. (2014). Interaction between neuroanatomical and psychological changes after mindfulness- based training. *PloS One, 9*(10).

Sapolsky, R. M. (1998). *Why zebras don't get ulcers* (2nd ed.). W. H. Freeman & Co Ltd.

Schore, A. N. (1994). *Affect regulation and the origin of the self.* Erlbaum.

Schore, A. N. (2001a). Effects of a secure attachment relationship on right brain development, affect regulation, and infant mental health. *Infant Mental Health Journal, 22,* 7–66.

Schore, A. N. (2001b). The effects of relational trauma on right brain development, affect regulation, and infant mental health. *Infant Mental Health Journal, 22,* 201–269.

Schore, A. N. (2003a). *Affect dysregulation and disorders of the self.* W. W. Norton & Company.

Schore, A. N. (2003b). *Affect regulation and disorders of the self.* W. W. Norton & Company.

Schore, A. N. (2005). A neuropsychoanalytic viewpoint: Commentary on paper by Steven H. Knoblauch. *The International Journal of Relational Perspectives, 15*(6), 829–854.

Schore, A. N. (2011). In conversation with Allan Schore. *Australasian Psychiatry, 19*(1), 30–36.

Schore, A. N. (2012). *The science of the art of psychotherapy.* W. W. Norton & Company.

Schroth, G. (2010). Prenatal bonding (BA): A method for encountering the unborn: Introduction and case study. *Journal of Prenatal & Perinatal Psychology & Health, 25*(1), 3.

Schumacher, M., Zubaran, C., & White, G. L. (2008). Bringing birth-related paternal depression to the fore. *Women & Birth, 21*(2), 65–70.

Schutte, N. S., & Malouff, J. M. (2014). A meta-analytic review of the effects of mindfulness meditation on telomerase activity. *Psychoneuroendocrinology, 42,* 45–48.

Segal, Z. V., Williams, J. M. G., & Teasdale, J. D. (2001). *Mindfulness-based cognitive therapy for depression: A new approach to preventing relapse.* The Guilford Press.

Serpeloni, F., Radtke, K. M., Hecker, T., & Elbert, T. (2016). Epigenetic biomarkers of prenatal maternal stress. *Epigenetics and Neuroendocrinology,* 177–196.

Shapiro, S. L., Schwartz, G. E., & Bonner, G. (1998). Effects of mindfulness-based stress reduction on medical and premedical students. *Journal of Behavioral Medicine, 21,* 581–599.

Shaver, P. R., & Mikulincer, M. (2002). Attachment-related psychodynamics. *Attachment and Human Development, 4*(2), 133–161.

Shaw, R. (2004). The embodied psychotherapist: An exploration of the therapists' somatic phenomena within the therapeutic encounter. *Psychotherapy Research, 14*(3), 271–288.

Shotter, J. (1993). *Conversational realities.* Sage.

Siddiqui, A., & Hagglof, B. (2000). Does maternal prenatal attachment predict postnatal mother-infant interaction? *Early Human Development, 59,* 13–25.

Siegel, D. J. (1999). *The developing mind: How relationships and the brain interact to shape who we are.* The Guilford Press.

Siegel, D. J. (2001). Toward an interpersonal neurobiology of the developing mind: Attachment, "mindsight", and neural integration. *Infant Mental Health Journal, 22*(1–2), 67–94.

Siegel, D. J. (2004). Attachment and self-understanding: Parenting with the brain in mind. *Journal of Prenatal and Perinatal Psychology and Health, 18*(4), 273–285.

Siegel, D. J. (2007). *The mindful brain: Reflection and attunement in the cultivation of well-being.* W. W. Norton & Company.

Siegel, D. J. (2009). Mindful awareness, mindsight, and neural integration: *The Humanistic Psychologist, 37*(2), 137–158.

Siegel, D. J., & Hartzell, M. (2003). *Parenting from the inside out: How a deeper self-understanding can help you raise children who thrive.* Penguin Books.

Siegel, R. D. (2010). *The mindfulness solution: Everyday practices for everyday problems.* The Guilford Press.

Sills, F. (2009). *Being and becoming: Psychodynamics, Buddhism, and the origins of self-hood.* North Atlantic Books.

Sloan Wilson, D. (2019). *This view of life: Completing the Darwinian revolution.* Vintage.

Smith, H. (1991). *The world's religions: Our great wisdom traditions.* Harper & Row.

Solms, M., & Turnbull, O. (2002). *The brain and the inner world: An introduction to the neuroscience of subjective experience.* Karnac Books.

Spitz, R. A. (1945). Hospitalism: An inquiry into the genesis of psychiatric conditions in early childhood. *The Psychoanalytic Study of the Child, 1*(1), 53–74.

Spitz, R. A., & Wolf, K. M. (1946). Anaclitic depression: An enquiry into the genesis of psychiatric conditions in early childhood. *The Psychoanalytic Study of the Child, 2*(1), 313–342.

Sroufe, L. A., Egeland, B., Carlson, E. A., & Collins, W. A. (2005). *The development of the person: The Minnesota study of risk and adaptation from birth to adulthood.* The Guilford Press.

Standley, J. M. (1998). The effect of music and multimodal stimulation on responses of premature infants in neonatal intensive care. *Paediatric Nursing, 24*(6), 532–538.

Stanley, C., Murray, L., & Stein, A. (2004). The effect of postnatal depression on mother-infant interaction: Infant response to the still-face perturbation, and performance on an instrumental learning task. *Developmental Psychopathology, 16*(1), 1–18.

Stein, A., Pearson, R. M., Goodman, S. H., Rapa, E., Rahman, A., McCallum, M., Howard, L. M., & Pariante, C. (2014). Effects of perinatal mental disorders on the foetus and child. *The Lancet, 384*(9956), 1819.

Stenberg, R. J., & Jordan, J. (Eds.). (2005). *A handbook of wisdom: Psychological perspectives.* Cambridge University Press.

Stephens, G. J., Silbert, L. J., & Hasson, U. (2010). Speaker-listener neural coupling underlies successful communication. *Proceedings of the National Academy of Sciences of the United States of America, 107*(32), 14425–14430.

Stern, D. N. (1985). *The interpersonal world of the infant.* Basic Books.

Stern, D. N. (2005a). The present moment in psychotherapy and everyday life. *American Journal of Clinical Hypnosis, 47*(3), 211–214.

Stern, D. N. (2005b). Intersubjectivity. In E. S. Person, A. M. Cooper, & G. O. Gabbard (Eds.), *Textbook of psychoanalysis* (pp. 77–92). American Psychiatric Publishing.

Stern, D. N. (2010). *Forms of vitality: Exploring dynamic experience in psychology, the arts, psychotherapy, and development.* Oxford University Press.

Stevens, L. C., & Woodruff, C. C. (2018). *The neuroscience of empathy, compassion, and self-compassion.* Academic Press.

Swales, D. A., Stout-Oswald, S. A., Glynn, L. M., Sandman, C., Wing, D. A., & Davis, E. P. (2018). Exposure to traumatic events in childhood predicts cortisol production among high risk pregnant women. *Biological Psychology, 139,* 186–192.

Szyf, M., Weaver, I., & Meaney, M. (2007). Maternal care, the epigenome and phenotypic differences in behaviour. *Reproductive Toxicology, 24*(1), 9–19.

Tacey, D. (2003). *The spiritual revolution.* Harper & Row.

Talge, N. M., Neal, C., & Glover, V. (2007). Antenatal maternal stress and long-term effects on child neurodevelopment: How and why? *Journal of Child Psychology and Psychiatry, 48*(3–4), 245–261.

Tashaev, S. S. (2007). Study of the unconscious, pre and postnatal individual perception by means of the age regression model. *International Journal of Prenatal and Perinatal Psychology and Medicine, 19*(1–2), 34–48.

Taylor, J. B. (2008). *My stroke of insight.* Viking.

Taylor, N., Fraser, H., Signal, T., & Prentice, K. (2014). Social work, animal-assisted therapies and ethical considerations: A program example from Central Queensland, Australia. *The British Journal of Social Work, 46*(1), 135–152.

Teixeira, J. M. A., Fisk, N. M., & Glover, V. (1999). Association between maternal anxiety in pregnancy and increased uterine artery resistance index: Cohort based study. *British Medical Journal, 318*(7177), 153–157.

Thich Nhat Hanh. (1991). *Peace is every step: The path of mindfulness in everyday life.* Bantam.

Thich Nhat Hanh. (2012, August 6). The fulness of emptiness. *Lion's Roar.*

Thoman, E. B., & Graham, S. E. (1986). Self-regulation of stimulation by premature infants. *Paediatrics, 78*(5), 855–860.

Thompson, B. L., & Waltz, J. (2008). Self-compassion and PTSD symptom severity. *Journal of Traumatic Stress, 21*(6), 556–558.

Tolle, E. (1999). *The power of now: A guide to spiritual enlightenment.* New World Library.

Tomasello, M., & Carpenter, M. (2007). Shared intentionality. *Developmental Science, 10*(1), 121–125.

Tomatis, A. A. (1981). *La nuit uterine [The uterine night].* Verlag Editions Stock.

Tomatis, A. A. (1987/2004). *The ear and the voice* (P. Prada, P. Sollier, & F. Keeping, trans.). United Nations.

Tomatis, A. A. (1991). *The conscious ear: My life of transformation through listening.* Station Hill Press.

Totton, N. (2011). An extraordinary ordinariness. *European Journal of Psychotherapy and Counselling, 13*(1), 69–75.

Trevarthen, C. (1999). Musicality and the intrinsic motive pulse: Evidence from human psychobiology and infant communication. *Musicae Scientiae, Special Issue,* 157–213.

Trevarthen, C. (2001). Intrinsic motives for companionship in understanding: Their origin, development and significance for infant mental health. *Infant Mental Health Journal, 22*(1–2), 95–131.

Trevarthen, C. (2005). Action and emotion in development of the human self, its sociability and cultural intelligence: Why infants have feelings like ours. In J. Nadel & D. Muir (Eds.), *Emotional development* (pp. 61–91). Oxford University Press.

Trevarthen, C. (2006). First things first: Infants make good use of the sympathetic rhythm of imitation, without reason or language. *Journal of Child Psychotherapy, 31*(1), 91–113.

Trevarthen, C. (2009). Human biochronology: On the source and functions of "musicality". In R. Haas & V. Brandes (Eds.), *Music that works: Contributions of biology, neurophysiology, psychology, sociology, medicine and musicology* (pp. 221–265). Springer-Verlag.

Trevarthen, C., & Aitken, K. J. (2003). Regulation of brain development and age-related changes in infants' motives: The developmental function of "regressive" periods. In M. Heimann (Ed.), *Regression periods in human infancy* (pp. 107–184). Erlbaum.

Trevarthen, C., & Delafield-Butt, J. (2013). Biology of shared experience and language development: Regulation for the intersubjective life of narratives. In M. Legerstee, D. Haley, & M. Bornstein (Eds.), *The developing infant mind: Integrating biology and experience* (pp. 167–199). The Guilford Press.

Trevarthen, W. (2003). Neuroscience and intrinsic psychodynamics: Current knowledge and potential for therapy. In J. Corrigall & H. Wilkinson (Eds.), *Revolutionary connections: Psychotherapy and neuroscience* (pp. 53–78). Routledge.

Tucker, D. M., Luu, P., & Derryberry, D. (2005). Love hurts: The evolution of empathic concern through the encephalisation of nociceptive capacity. *Development and Psychopathology, 17*(3), 699–713.

Turnbull, C. M. (1983). *The human cycle.* Simon & Schuster.

UNICEF. (2007). *An overview of child well-being in rich countries: A comprehensive assessment of the lives and well-being of children and adolescents in the economically advanced nations.* Innocenti Report Card. UNICEF.

Valdesolo, P., & DeSteno, D. (2006). Manipulations of emotional context shape moral judgement. *Psychological Science, 17*(6), 476–477.

Valentine, L., & Gabbard, G. O. (2014). Can the use of humor in psychotherapy be taught? *Academic Psychiatry, 38*(1), 75–81.

Vandekerckhove, M., & Panksepp, J. (2011). A neurocognitive theory of higher mental emergence: From anoetic affective experiences to noetic knowledge and autonoetic awareness. *Neuroscience & Biobehavioural Reviews, 35*(9), 2017–2025.

Van den Bergh, B. R. H., Mulder, E. J. H., Mennes, M., & Glover, V. (2005). Antenatal maternal anxiety and stress and the neurobehavioural development of the foetus and child: Links and possible mechanisms. A review. *Neuroscience & Behavioural Reviews, 29*(2), 237–258.

Van der Bergh, A., & Simons, A. (2009). A review of scales to measure the mother-foetus relationship. *Journal of Reproductive and Infant Psychology, 27*(2), 114–126.

Van der Kolk, B. A. (1987). *Psychological trauma.* American Psychiatric Press.

Van der Kolk, B. A. (2014). *The body keeps the score: Mind, brain and body in the transformation of trauma.* Penguin Books.

Van IJzendoorn, M. H., Sagi, A., & Lambermon, M. W. (1992). The multiple caretaker paradox: Data from Holland and Israel. In R. C. Pianta (Ed.), *Beyond the parents: The role of other adults in children's lives* (pp. 5–24). New Directions for Child Development 57. Jossey-Bass.

Van Zeijl, J., Mesman, J., Van IJzendoom, M. H., Bakermans-Kranenburg, M. J., Juffer, K., Stolk, M. N., Koot, H. M., & Alink, L. R. A. (2006). Attachment-based intervention for enhancing sensitive discipline in mothers of 1-to-3-year-old children at risk for externalizing behaviour problems: A randomized controlled trial. *Journal of Consulting and Clinical Psychology, 74,* 994–1005.

Vastag, B. (2003). Scientists find connection in the brain between physical and emotional pain. *Journal of the American Medical Association, 290*(18), 2389–2390.

Verny, T. R. (1981). *The secret life of the unborn baby: A remarkable and controversial look at life before birth.* Summit Books.

Verny, T. R., & Weintraub, P. (2003). *Pre-parenting: Nurturing your child from conception.* Touchstone.

Vieten, C., & Austin, J. (2008). Effects of a mindfulness-based intervention during pregnancy on prenatal stress and mood: Results of a pilot study. *Archives of Women's Mental Health, 11*(1), 67–74.

Vliegen, N., Luyten, P., & Biringen, Z. (2009). A multimethod perspective on emotional availability in the postpartum period. *Parenting: Science and Practice, 9,* 228–243.

Volz, K. G., Rübsamen, R., & von Cramon, D. Y. (2008). Cortical regions activated by the subjective sense of perceptual coherence of environmental sounds: A proposal for a neuroscience of intuition. *Cognitive, Affective, & Behavioural Neuroscience, 8*(3), 318–328.

Wade, J. (1998). Two voices from the womb: Evidence for physically transcendent and a cellular source of foetal consciousness. *Journal of Prenatal and Perinatal Psychology and Health, 13*(2), 123–147.

Wadhwa, P. D., Culhane, J. F., Rauh, V., & Barva, S. S. (2001). Stress and preterm birth: Neuroendocrine, immune/inflammatory, and vascular mechanisms. *Maternal and Child Health Journal, 5*(2), 119–125.

Wahl, K., & Metzner, C. (2012). Parental influences on the prevalence and development of child aggressiveness. *Journal of Child and Family Studies, 21,* 344–355.

Waite, F., Knight, M. T. D., & Lee, D. (2015). Self-compassion and self-criticism in recovery in psychosis: An interpretative phenomenological analysis study. *Journal of Clinical Psychology, 71*(12), 1201–1217.

Walsh, D. (2007). *Evidence-based care for normal labour and birth: A guide for midwives.* Routledge.

Watson, G. (2008). *Beyond happiness: Deepening the dialogue between Buddhism, psychotherapy and the mind science.* Routledge.

Weaver, I. C., Champagne, F. A., Brown, S. E., Dymov, S., Sharma, S., Meaney, M. J., & Szyf, M. (2005). Reversal of maternal programming of stress responses in adult off-spring through methyl supplementation: Altering epigenetic marking later in life. *Journal of Neuroscience, 25*(47), 11045–11054.

Weaver, I. C., Meaney, M. J., & Szyf, M. (2006). Maternal care effects on the hippocampal transcriptome and anxiety-mediated behaviours in the offspring that are reversible in adulthood. *Proceedings of the National Academy of Sciences U.S.A., 103*(9), 3480–3485.

Weaver, I. C., Szyf, M., & Meaney, M. J. (2002). From maternal care to gene expression: DNA methylation and the maternal programming of stress responses. *Endocrine Research, 28*(4), 699.

Weinstein, A. D. (2016). *Prenatal development and parents' lived experiences: How early events shape our psychophysiology and relationships.* W. W. Norton & Company.

Weng, H. Y., Fox, A. S., Shackman, A. J., Stodola, D. E., Caldwell, J. Z. K., Olson, M. C., Rogers, G. M., & Davidson, R. J. (2013). Compassion training alters altruism and neural responses to suffering. *Psychological Science, 24*(7), 1171–1180.

Wermke, K., Teiser, J., Yovsi, E., Kohlenberg, P. J., Wermke, P., Robb, M., Heidi, K., & Lamm, B. (2016). Fundamental frequency variation within neonatal crying: Does ambient language matter? *Speech, Language and Hearing, 19*(4), 211–217.

Whitehead, R. H. (1988). *Stories from the six worlds: Micmac legends.* Nimbus.

Whittingham, K., Sheffield, J., & Boyd, R. N. (2016). Parenting acceptance and commitment therapy: A randomised controlled trial of an innovative online course for families of children with cerebral palsy. *The British Medical Journal, 6*(10), e012807.

Wielgosz, J., Schuyler, B. S., Lutz, A., & Davidson, R. J. (2016). Long-term mindfulness training is associated with reliable differences in resting respiration rate. *Scientific Report, 6*(1), 1–6.

Williams, J. M. G. (2008). Mindfulness, depression, and modes of mind. *Cognitive Therapy and Research, 32*(6), 721.

Winnicott, D. W. (1960). The theory of the parent-infant relationship. In D. W. Winnicott (Ed.), *The maturational processes and the facilitating environment.* International Universities Press.

Winnicott, D. W. (1965). *The maturational processes and the facilitating environment.* International Universities Press.

Winnicott, D. W. (1971). *Playing and reality.* Tavistock, Routledge.

Winnicott, D. W. (1987). *Babies and their mothers.* Free Association Books.

Wittling, W. (1997). The right hemisphere and human stress response. *Acta Physiologica Scandinavica Supplementum, 640,* 55–59.

World Health Organisation. (1948, June 19–July). *Constitution of the World Health Organisation: Definition of health.* New York International Health Conference, Commission on Social Determinants of Health.

World Health Organisation. (2008). *Closing the gap in a generation: Health equity through action on the social determinants of health: Final report of the commission on social determinants of health.* Commission on Social Determinants of Health.

World Health Organisation. (2018). *Nurturing care for early childhood development: A framework for helping children survive and thrive to transform health and human potential.* Commission on Social Determinants of Health.

Yehuda, R., Daskalakis, N. P., Bierer, L. M., Bader, H. N., Klengel, T., Holsboer, F., & Binder, E. B. (2016). Holocaust exposure induced intergenerational effects of FKBP5 methylation. *Biological Psychiatry, 80*(5), 372–380.

Yue, G. H., & Cole, K. J. (1992). Strength increases from the motor program: Comparison of training with maximal voluntary and imagined muscle contractions. *Journal of Neurophysiology, 67*(5), 1114–1123.

Zeanah, C., & Zeanah, P. D. (2009). The scope of infant mental health. In C. H. Zeanah (Ed.), *Handbook of infant mental health* (pp. 5–21). The Guilford Press.

Zeidan, F., Grant, J. A., Brown, C. A., McHaffie, J. G., & Coghill, R. C. (2012). Mindfulness meditation-related pain relief: Evidence for unique brain mechanisms in the regulation of pain. *Neuroscience Newsletters, 520*(2), 165–173.

Zichella, L. (2002). The anthropological aspects of childbirth: The pain. *The International Journal of Prenatal & Perinatal Psychology and Medicine, 14*(3–4), 213–220.

Zichella, L. (2016). *Alla ricerca della madre.* Edizioni Libra.

Zichella, L., & Janus, L. (2012). Anthropologische aspekte im spannungsfeld von natur und kultur: Das paradigma der komplexität. In S. Hildebrandt, J. Schacht, & H. Blazy (Hgs.), *Wurzeln des Lebens* (pp. 25–29). Mattes.

Zimmer, E. Z., Divon, M. Y., Vilensky, A., Sarna, Z., Peretz, B. A., & Paldi, E. (1982). Maternal exposure to music and foetal activity. *European Journal of Obstetrics and Gynaecology and Reproductive Biology, 13*(4), 209–213.

Zoia, S., Blason, L., D'Ottavio, G., Bulgheroni, M., Pezzetta, E., Scabar, A., & Castiello, U. (2007). Evidence of early development of action planning in the human foetus: A kinematic study. *Experimental Brain Research, 176*(2), 217–226.

Zubrick, S. R., Shepherd, C. C. J., Dudgeon, P., Gee, G., Paradies, Y., Scrine, C., & Walker, R. (2014). Social determinants of social and emotional wellbeing. In *Working together: Aboriginal and Torres Strait Islander mental health and wellbeing principles and practice* (pp. 93–112). Australian Government Department of the Prime Minister and Cabinet.

Index

Printed in the United States
By Bookmasters